NOVEL NANOCARRIERS FOR SKIN DISEASES

Advances and Applications

NOVEL NANOCARRIERS FOR SKIN DISEASES

Advances and Applications

Raj K. Keservani, PhD
Júlia Scherer Santos, PhD
Editors

AAP | APPLE ACADEMIC PRESS

First edition published 2025

Apple Academic Press Inc.
1265 Goldenrod Circle, NE,
Palm Bay, FL 32905 USA

760 Laurentian Drive, Unit 19,
Burlington, ON L7N 0A4, CANADA

CRC Press
2385 NW Executive Center Drive,
Suite 320, Boca Raton FL 33431

4 Park Square, Milton Park,
Abingdon, Oxon, OX14 4RN UK

Apple Academic Press exclusively co-publishes with CRC Press, an imprint of Taylor & Francis Group, LLC

Library and Archives Canada Cataloguing in Publication

CIP data on file with Canada Library and Archives

Library of Congress Cataloging-in-Publication Data

CIP data on file with US Library of Congress

ISBN: 978-1-77491-534-9 (hbk)
ISBN: 978-1-77491-535-6 (pbk)
ISBN: 978-1-03272-595-6 (ebk)

About the Editors

Raj K. Keservani, PhD, MPharm
Associate Professor, Faculty of B. Pharmacy, CSM Group of Institutions, Prayagraj, Uttar Pradesh, India

Raj K. Keservani, PhD, MPharm, is working as an Associate Professor in the Faculty of B. Pharmacy at CSM Group of Institutions, Prayagraj, India. He has more than 12 years of academic (teaching) experience from various institutes in India in pharmaceutical education. He has supervised more than 25 UG students for their research work. He has published over 30 peer-reviewed papers in the field of pharmaceutical sciences in national and international journals, six patents, over 70 book chapters, three co-authored books, and over 40 edited books. He is also active as a reviewer for several international scientific journals. Dr. Keservani graduated with a pharmacy degree from the Department of Pharmacy, Kumaun University, Nainital (Uttarakhand), India. He received his Master of Pharmacy (MPharm) (specialization in pharmaceutics) from the School of Pharmaceutical Sciences, Rajiv Gandhi Proudyogiki Vishwavidyalaya, Bhopal, India. He received his PhD degree from IKG Punjab Technical University, Jalandhar, Punjab, India. Dr. Keservani is a life member of the Society of Pharmaceutical Education and Research (SPER). His research interests include nutraceutical and functional foods, novel drug delivery systems (NDDS), transdermal drug delivery/drug delivery, health science, cancer biology, and neurobiology.

Júlia Scherer Santos, PhD
Department of Chemistry, Federal University of Viçosa, Viçosa, Minas Gerais, Brazil.

Júlia Scherer Santos, PhD, is currently a research fellow at Federal University of Viçosa. She is a specialist in Cosmetology and has a doctorate in Pharmaceutical Nanotechnology. She has experience in the public health area and as a professor of pharmacy. She has published articles and book chapters on the following topics: nanotechnology, cosmetology, nutraceutical and plant bioactive compounds.

Contents

Contributors

Marta Marques Gontijo de Aguiar
Department of Pharmaceutical Products, Faculty of Pharmacy, Federal University of Minas Gerais, Belo Horizonte, Brazil

Tanira Alessandra Silveira Aguirre
Biosciences Graduate Program, Federal University of Health Sciences of Porto Alegre (UFCSPA), Brazil

Eknath D. Ahire
Department of Pharmaceutics, MET's Institute of Pharmacy, Bhujbal Knowledge City, Affiliated to Savitribai Phule Pune University, Adgaon, Nashik, Maharashtra, India

Lucas F. Albuquerque
Laboratory of Food, Drugs, and Cosmetics (LTMAC), University of Brasilia, Brasilia, DF, Brazil

Akash J. Amkar
Shri D.D. Vispute College of Pharmacy and Research Center, Devad-Vichumbe, Panvel, Navi Mumbai, Maharashtra, India

Gabriel Silva Marques Borges
Department of Pharmaceutical Products, Faculty of Pharmacy, Federal University of Minas Gerais, Belo Horizonte, Brazil

Camila O. Cardoso
Laboratory of Food, Drugs, and Cosmetics (LTMAC), University of Brasilia, Brasilia, DF, Brazil

Talita Pizza Anunciato Casarini
Pharmaceutical Sciences Graduate Program, Federal University of Rio Grande do Sul, Brazil.

Renata Vidor Contri
Pharmaceutical Sciences Graduate Program, Federal University of Rio Grande do Sul, Brazil

Dórys Angela Cordenunzzi
Graduate Program in Pharmaceutical Sciences, University of Vale do Itajaí, Itajaí, Santa Catarina, Brazil

Letícia Cruz
Pharmaceutical Technology Laboratory, Postgraduate Program in Pharmaceutical Sciences, Health Sciences Center, Federal University of Santa Maria, Santa Maria, Brazil

Marcílio Cunha Filho
Laboratory of Food, Drugs, and Cosmetics (LTMAC), University of Brasilia, Brasilia, DF, Brazil

Punam S. Gadekar
Shri D.D. Vispute College of Pharmacy and Research Center, Devad-Vichumbe, Panvel, Navi Mumbai, Maharashtra, India

Rafaela Gazzi
Pharmaceutical Sciences Graduate Program, Federal University of Rio Grande do Sul, Brazil

Mailine Gehrcke
Pharmaceutical Technology Laboratory, Postgraduate Program in Pharmaceutical Sciences, Health Sciences Center, Federal University of Santa Maria, Santa Maria, Brazil

Guilherme M. Gelfuso
Laboratory of Food, Drugs, and Cosmetics (LTMAC), University of Brasilia, Brasilia, DF, Brazil

Otto Maurício Santos Gerlach
Graduate Program in Pharmaceutical Sciences, University of Vale do Itajaí, Itajaí, Santa Catarina, Brazil

Graziela Scheuer Gomes
Pharmaceutical Sciences Graduate Program, Federal University of Rio Grande do Sul, Brazil

Gisele Assis Castro Goulart
Department of Pharmaceutical Products, Faculty of Pharmacy, Federal University of Minas Gerais, Belo Horizonte, Brazil

Taís Gratieri
Laboratory of Food, Drugs, and Cosmetics (LTMAC), University of Brasilia, Brasilia, DF, Brazil

Gaurav Gupta
School of Pharmacy, Suresh Gyan Vihar University, Jagatpura, Jaipur, Rajasthan, India; Department of Pharmacology, Saveetha Dental College, Saveetha Institute of Medical and Technical Sciences, Saveetha University, Chennai, Tamil Nadu, India; Uttaranchal Institute of Pharmaceutical Sciences, Uttaranchal University, Dehradun, Uttarakhand, India

Manish Gupta
School of Pharmacy, Suresh Gyan Vihar University, Jagatpura, Jaipur, Rajasthan, India

Ngo Thi Hue
VNU University of Medicine and Pharmacy, Vietnam National University, Ha Noi, Vietnam

Ashish S. Jain
Shri D.D. Vispute College of Pharmacy and Research Center, Devad-Vichumbe, Panvel, Navi Mumbai, Maharashtra, India

Nidhi S. Kate
Shri D.D. Vispute College of Pharmacy and Research Center, Devad-Vichumbe, Panvel, Navi Mumbai, Maharashtra, India

Raj K. Keservani
Faculty of B. Pharmacy, CSM Group of Institutions, Prayagraj, Uttar Pradesh, India

Sanjay J. Kshirsagar
Department of Pharmaceutics, MET's Institute of Pharmacy, Bhujbal Knowledge City, Affiliated to Savitribai Phule Pune University, Adgaon, Nashik, Maharashtra, India

Eduardo Burgarelli Lages
PhyMedExp, Université de Montpellier, INSERM, CNRS, Montpellier, France

Tran Viet Linh
VNU University of Medicine and Pharmacy, Vietnam National University, Ha Noi, Vietnam

Nguyen Viet Long
VNU University of Medicine and Pharmacy, Vietnam National University, Ha Noi, Vietnam

Ruth Meri Lucinda-Silva
Graduate Program in Pharmaceutical Sciences, University of Vale do Itajaí, Itajaí, Santa Catarina, Brazil

Angela Malheiros
Graduate Program in Pharmaceutical Sciences, University of Vale do Itajaí, Itajaí, Santa Catarina, Brazil

Shanti Bhushan Mishra
Department of Pharmacognosy, United Institute of Pharmacy, Prayagraj, Uttar Pradesh, India

Afrasim Moin
University of Hail, Saudi Arabia

Nguyen Thuy Ngoc
VNU University of Medicine and Pharmacy, Vietnam National University, Ha Noi, Vietnam

Aline Ferreira Ourique
Laboratory of Nanotechnology, Graduate Program in Nanosciences, Universidade Franciscana, Santa Maria, Brazil

Karina Paese
Pharmaceutical Sciences Graduate Program, Federal University of Rio Grande do Sul, Brazil

Meenakshi Panchal
Department of Pharmaceutics, Corporate Institute of Pharmacy, Bhopal, Madhya Pradesh, India

Shivani S. Pawar
Shri D.D. Vispute College of Pharmacy and Research Center, Devad-Vichumbe, Panvel, Navi Mumbai, Maharashtra, India

R. S. Raghuwanshi
Department of Pharmaceutical Chemistry, Corporate Institute of Pharmacy, Bhopal, Madhya Pradesh, India

Abhay Raizaday
School of Pharmacy, Suresh Gyan Vihar University, Jagatpura, Jaipur, Rajasthan, India

Bhushan R. Rane
Shri D.D. Vispute College of Pharmacy and Research Center, Devad-Vichumbe, Panvel, Navi Mumbai, Maharashtra, India

Samali S. Raut
Shri D.D. Vispute College of Pharmacy and Research Center, Devad-Vichumbe, Panvel, Navi Mumbai, Maharashtra, India

Virginia Cielo Rech
Laboratory of Nanotechnology, Graduate Program in Nanosciences, Universidade Franciscana, Santa Maria, Brazil

Anna Carolina Furaer da Rocha
Graduate Program in Pharmaceutical Sciences, University of Vale do Itajaí, Itajaí, Santa Catarina, Brazil

Thais Tunes Santos
Department of Physiology and Biophysics, Institute of Biological Sciences, Federal University of Minas Gerais, Belo Horizonte, Brazil

Zípora Morgana Quinteiro Dos Santos
Laboratory of Nanotechnology, Graduate Program in Nanosciences, Universidade Franciscana, Santa Maria, Brazil

Priya Sen
School of Pharmacy, Suresh Gyan Vihar University, Jagatpura, Jaipur, Rajasthan, India

Amit K. Singh
Department of Pharmaceutics, United Institute of Pharmacy, Prayagraj, Uttar Pradesh, India

Amit Kumar Singh
Department of Pharmaceutics, United Institute of Pharmacy, Prayagraj, Uttar Pradesh, India

Santosh Kumar Singh
School of Pharmacy, Suresh Gyan Vihar University, Jagatpura, Jaipur, Rajasthan, India

Jenny Sumara Sozo
Graduate Program in Pharmaceutical Sciences, University of Vale do Itajaí, Itajaí, Santa Catarina, Brazil

Nguyen Đuc Thuan
VNU University of Medicine and Pharmacy, Vietnam National University, Ha Noi, Vietnam

Bui Thanh Tung
VNU University of Medicine and Pharmacy, Vietnam National University, Ha Noi, Vietnam

Hemant K. S. Yadav
School of Pharmacy, Suresh Gyan Vihar University, Jagatpura, Jaipur, Rajasthan, India

Fátima Regina Zan
Director of Planning and Institutional Development, Instituto Federal Farroupilha, Santo Ângelo, Brazil

Abbreviations

AA	alopecia areata
ABLC	amphotericin B lipid complex
ACD	allergic contact dermatitis
AD	atopic dermatitis
AgNPs	silver nanoparticles
ALA	aminolevulinic acid
AmB	amphotericin B
APC	antigen-presenting cells
ASO	antisense-oligonucleotide
atRA	acid therapy
AuNPs	gold nanoparticles
Au-NRs	gold nanorods
BCC	basal cell carcinoma
BMDMs	bone marrow-derived macrophages
BME	bicontinuous microemulsions
BNH	berberine nano-hydrogel
BRB	berberine
BSI	British Standards Institution
CAGR	compound annual growth rate
CD	cyclodextrins
CFL	cationic flexible liposomes
CL	cutaneous leishmaniasis
CNTs	carbon nanotubes
CO2	carbon dioxide
COX	cyclooxygenase
COX-2	cyclo-oxygenase type 2
CTAB	cetyltrimethylammonium bromide
CUBs	cubosomes
CuNPs	copper nanoparticles
CVD	chemical vapor deposition
DDS	drug delivery system
DHEAS	dehydroepiandrosterone sulfate
DLQI	dermatology life quality index
DNA	deoxyribonucleic acid
DNBC	2,4-dinitrochlorobenzene
DOPC	1,2-dioleoyl-sn-glycero-3-phosphocholine
DOTAP	1,2-dioleoyl-3-trimethyl ammonium propane

DPPH	1,1-diphenyl-2-picrylhydrazyl
DSPC	diesteroyl phosphatidylcholine
DSPG	diesteroyl phosphatidylglycerol
EASI	eczema area severity index
ELP	elastin-like polypeptide
ERKs	extracellular signal-regulated kinases
ETOs	ethosomes
FDA	federal drug approval
FDA	Food and Drug Administration
FLG	filaggrin
GA–AuNPs	gallic acid-coated gold nanoparticles
GG-MS	gas chromatography-mass spectrometry
GHK-Cu	glycyl-L-histidyl-L-lysine
HAS	human albumin serum
HF	high frequency
HHSE	human heat-separated epidermis
HIV	human immunodeficiency virus
HPV	human papilloma virus
IFN-γ	interferon-γ
IgE	immunoglobulin E
IGF	insulin-like growth factor
IL-6	interleukin-6
IMQ	imiquimod
iNOS	induced nitric oxide synthase
ISO	International Standard Organization
LNCs	lipid nano-capsules
LUVs	large unilamellar vesicles
MASI	melasma area and severity index
MBC	minimum bactericidal concentration
MEO	melaleuca alternifolia essential oil
MIC	minimal inhibitory concentration
MLVs	multilamellar vesicles
MMA	methyl methacrylate
MMP	matrix metalloproteinase
MnO2	manganese dioxide
MPEG-PCL	monomethoxy-poly(ethylene glycol)-polycaprolactone
MPSA	melanin particle size surface area
MRSA	methicillin-resistant *Staphylococcus aureus*
MSN	mesoporous silica nanoparticles
MTF	miltefosine
MWCNTs	multi-walled carbon nanotubes
NCCN	National Comprehensive Cancer Network
NEs	nano-emulsions

NLC	nanostructured lipid carrier
NPs	nanoparticles
NuBACS	nutraceutical bioavailability classification scheme
OTC	over-the-counter
PASI	psoriasis area severity index
PC	pachyonychia congenita
PCL	poly-ε-caprolactone
PD-1	anti-programed cell death protein-1
PDT	photodynamic therapy
PEG	poly(ethylene glycol)
PEO-PPO-PEO	poly(ethylene oxide)-poly(propylene oxide)-poly(ethylene oxide)
P-G3	PAMAM generation-3
Pg-C-EE	Panax ginseng berry calyx
PHT	phenytoin
PHT-Loaded CuNPs	phenytoin-loaded copper nanoparticles
PLA	poly(D,L-lactide)
PLGA	poly(lactic acid-co-glycolic acid)
PLN	PEGylated lipid nanocarriers
PTT	photothermic therapy
PVA	poly(vinyl acetate)
RA	rheumatoid arthritis
RA	rosmarinic acid
ROS	reactive oxygen species
SC	stratum corneum
SCC	squamous cell carcinoma
SCORAD	scoring AD
SECoplex	SECosome-siRNA complex
SECosomes	surfactant-ethanol-cholesterolosomes
SEDDS	self-emulsifying drug delivery systems
SHS	sponge *Haliclona* sp. spicules
siRNA	small interfering RNA
SLN	solid lipid nanoparticles
SMEDDS	self-micro-emulsifying drug delivery system
SNEDDS	self-nano-emulsifying drug delivery systems
SPION	superparamagnetic iron oxide nanoparticles
SUVs	small unilamellar vesicles
SWCNTs	single-walled carbon nanotubes
TCM	traditional Chinese medicine
TEM	transmission electron microscopy
TEWL	transepidermal water loss
TiO2	titanium dioxide
TLR	toll-like receptors

TNF-α	tumor necrosis factor-alpha
TPGS	d-α-tocopheryl polyethylene glycol succinate
TRAs	transfersomes
TS	technical specifications
TSLP	thymic stromal lymphopoietin
USFDA	U.S. Food and Drug Administration
UV	ultraviolet
UVB	ultraviolet B
VCO	virgin coconut oil
VL	visceral leishmaniasis
WHO	World Health Organization
ZnO	zinc oxide
ZnO-AH	zinc oxide nanoparticles–hot extract

Preface

Drug delivery systems (DDS) have come a long way since its initial days of research. As a result, today there are commercially available nanomedicines for the treatment of various pathologies. Although the development of products based on nanotechnology is more expensive than traditional medicines, the treatment cost can be reduced through the use of lower doses. Moreover, loading currently available drugs into nanocarriers represents a less costly approach than the discovery/development of new drugs.

This book presents the most important contributions that have been published addressing nanocarriers to skin disease treatment. Progress in the treatment of acne, dermatitis, psoriasis, and infections provided by nanocarriers are discussed. Furthermore, follicular delivery is also detailed as a promising strategy for these drug delivery systems due to their reduced particle size. A greater drug deposition into the hair follicles promoted by nanomedicines is discussed which would improve skin disease treatment, mainly skin cancers.

This book is divided into two parts with 13 chapters. In Part I, the use of nanocarriers for skin cancer, topical nanotherapeutics for acne, and topical amphotericin B (AmB) are discussed. In Part II, chapters approaching nanocarriers to non-inflammatory skin diseases are presented. In that regard, relevant information on polymeric and lipid nanoparticles (NPs) in the treatment of skin is highlighted. Chapters on natural ingredients for skin disease treatment are also detailed. Lipid and polymeric carriers for psoriasis and dermatitis are shown. The use of natural polymers, plant extracts, and essential oils is reported as well.

- **Part I: Topically Applied Novel Carriers**

  Chapter 1 – "Nanocarriers for Skin Cancer Topical Treatment," shows research involving the association of these nanostructures with physical methods such as iontophoresis and microneedling to increase drug delivery and reduce the topical application time of these nanoformulations, written by Guilherme M. Gelfuso and associates.

Zípora Morgana Quinteiro Dos Santos et al. discuss novel nanocarriers that represent a recent trend toward improving the solubility/bioavailability of active substances, enabling effective application in the treatment of acne vulgaris, in Chapter 2 – "Topical Nanotherapeutics for the Treatment of Acne Vulgaris."

Chapter 3 – "Topical Delivery of Amphotericin B: Focus on Nanocarriers for the Treatment of Cutaneous Leishmaniasis," written by Gabriel Silva Marques Borges and colleagues, summarizes the main obstacles to the development of formulations for topical delivery of AmB and discusses the potential and advantages of nanomedicine in solving these challenges.

- **Part II: Novel Nanocarriers for Skin Delivery and Disease**

Hemant K. S. Yadav et al. wrote Chapter 4 – "Nanocarriers to Skin Inflammatory Diseases," and discusses the advantages and application of nanocarriers in drug delivery systems. In addition, future aspects of nanocarriers in health care are also discussed.

Chapter 5 – "Small Interfering RNA Nanocarriers to Skin Delivery," written by Shanti Bhushan Mishra et al. provides an update on the nanocarriers-based delivery approaches for siRNA delivery for the management of skin disorders.

The risk of developing skin cancer, including both melanoma and nonmelanoma skin cancers, is linked to exposure to the sun. Use of sunscreen appropriately, limiting sun exposure, and avoiding tanning beds are all preventative methods discussed in Chapter 6 – "Improvement of Skin Cancer by Transdermal Drug Delivery System," written by Bhushan R. Rane and his associates.

Bhushan R. Rane and colleagues wrote Chapter 7 – "Follicular Delivery of Nanocarriers to Improve Skin Disease Treatment," discusses Polymeric nanoparticles, lipid nanoparticles, Metallic nanoparticles, Ethosomes, and niosomes. These are the carriers that show proof of the follicular pathway to give a specific therapeutic effect.

Letícia Cruz and Mailine Gehrcke, report nanotechnology-based approaches to treat atopic dermatitis, more confirmatory in vivo studies about their effectiveness and toxicity are encouraged in Chapter 8 – "Nanocarriers for Atopic Dermatitis Treatment."

Renata Vidor Contri et al. discuss the use of polymeric nanoparticles as a strategy to improve the topical treatment of skin diseases such as acne, melasma, atopic dermatitis, psoriasis, rosacea, mycoses, and skin cancer in Chapter 9 – "Polymeric Nanoparticles Applied to Skin Diseases."

Ruth Meri Lucinda-Silva et al. report nanometric platforms for topical administration of promising plant extracts and phytochemicals, along with their therapeutic applications supported by experimental evidence is presented in Chapter 10 – "Herbal Extracts Loaded-Nanocarriers to Skin Disease Treatment."

Bui Thanh Tung and his associates summarize several studies on this method, thereby giving an overview of it. The results show that the application of nanotechnology in the treatment of skin diseases brings good results and opens a new perspective in the further development of nano-compounds from medicinal plants in Chapter 11 – "Medicinal Plant in Skin Topical Treatment Based on Nanotechnology."

Eknath D. Ahire and his associates summarize the modern-day expertise on how polymeric shipping structures interact with healthful and diseased pores and skin, giving a top-level view of the demanding situations that distinct pathological pores and skin situations pose to the improvement of more secure and greater particular dermal therapies in Chapter 12 – "Biodegradable Nanoparticles to Skin Diseases."

Little is known about the toxicology of these nanotechnology-based formulations, therefore, as future tendencies, more studies should be conducted to ensure the consumers' health and environmental safety. This is discussed in Chapter 13 – "Skin Topical Treatment Based on Nanotechnology," written by Meenakshi Panchal and R. S. Raghuwanshi.

PART I
Topically Applied Novel Carriers

CHAPTER 1

Nanocarriers for Skin Cancer Topical Treatment

LUCAS F. ALBUQUERQUE, CAMILA O. CARDOSO, MARCÍLIO CUNHA FILHO, TAÍS GRATIERI, and GUILHERME M. GELFUSO

Laboratory of Food, Drugs, and Cosmetics (LTMAC), University of Brasilia, Brasilia, DF, Brazil

ABSTRACT

Despite the annually increasing number of cases, advances in research to develop new drugs and formulations have improved the treatment of skin cancers. Recent studies have shown promising results, with increased overall survival and improved quality of life for patients. However, despite the progress, systemic therapy still presents severe adverse reactions, which prevents the continuity of treatment. An alternative to circumvent is the use of topical formulations. However, topical therapy has been limited because of the low penetration of drugs into the skin when incorporated into conventional formulations and toxicity issues. In this context, this chapter presents new research involving nanotechnology to develop safer and more efficient topical formulations for the treatment of skin cancers. The chapter also shows research involving the association of these nanostructures with physical methods such as iontophoresis and microneedling to increase drug delivery and reduce the topical application time of these nanoformulations.

Novel Nanocarriers forSkin Diseases: Advances and Applications.
Raj K. Keservani and Júlia Scherer Santos (Eds.)

1.1 INTRODUCTION

Skin cancers are among the most frequent types of malignancy, originating from different skin cell types of the epidermis, dermis, or skin appendages (Davis et al., 2019; Quaresmini & Guida, 2020). They are divided into two groups: (i) melanoma and (ii) non-melanoma skin cancers, and such classification is a result of the wide variety of presentations and differences in prognosis these diseases present (Catalano et al., 2019).

Melanoma, despite representing only 1 to 5% of skin cancers, is responsible for more than 80% of deaths caused by all skin diseases (Bertrand et al., 2020; Bray et al., 2018). It is worrying to note that melanoma skin cancer is one among malignant diseases that have increased the most annually (Bertrand et al., 2020; Schadendorf et al., 2015). In recent years, melanoma incidence has grown by around 3% per year in the American population (Li & Cai, 2019; Li et al., 2020). Between 1975 and 2018, there was an increase of 320% in melanoma diagnoses. In 1975, for each 1,00,000 Americans, 7.9 developed melanoma. In 2018, for every 1,00,000 inhabitants, 25.3 developed melanoma (Carr et al., 2020; Macdonald, 1975). In Australia, the country with the highest global incidence of skin cancer, the number of new cases of melanoma increased from 26.4 to 51.6 per 1,00,000 inhabitants between 1982 and 2011 (Macdonald, 1975; Raimondi et al., 2020).

This wide variety of incidence rates can be explained by risk patterns associated with a particular population, such as different skin phototypes prevailing in that population (Leonardi et al., 2018). This is evidenced by epidemiological studies, which show Caucasian people (phototypes I and II) have up to 25 times more risk of developing melanoma when compared to Afro-American individuals (phototypes IV, V, and VI) in the same region (Bertrand et al., 2020).

The lethality of melanomas is strongly related to the stage at which the disease is diagnosed. When diagnosed in the early stages (stages I and II), melanoma can be treated with surgical resection, promoting a disease-free survival time of over five years in 98% of patients. Still, this percentage drops substantially in patients who received the diagnosis in the advanced stages of the disease, with a drop of five-year disease-free survival time to about 70% for those with lymph node commitment, and about 5% for patients with metastasis in distant tissues (Carr et al., 2020; Macdonald, 1975).

Differently from melanomas, basal cell carcinoma (BCC) and squamous cell carcinoma (SCC) represent approximately 95% of the incidence of skin cancers (Brandt & Moore, 2019; Collins et al., 2019). In the USA, BCC and SCC together represent about 3 million new cases annually (Brandt & Moore,

2019; Collins et al., 2019). However, even with a high incidence, they are usually of low malignancy and low lethality (Voiculescu et al., 2019).

Amidst keratinocyte carcinoma (non-melanoma skin cancers), approximately 75% of the incidence corresponds to BCC and 25% to SCC (Brandt & Moore, 2019). They can be clinically categorized as superficial, nodular, infiltrative, or sclerosing. The nodular type is the most common, with serous presentation and the presence of elevated papules or nodules (Brandt & Moore, 2019; Catalano et al., 2019). The superficial type, the second most common, is characterized by a horizontal growth with thin and erythematous plaques, which may present telangiectasia (Brandt & Moore, 2019).

Melanoma has four well-described clinical classifications: superficial spreading melanoma, nodular melanoma, malignant lentiginous, and acral melanoma. Each of these classifications has different clinical courses, but all have in common the high capacity for deep invasion and metastasis (Ostrowski & Fisher, 2021).

Superficial spreading melanoma, characterized as an asymmetrical macula with irregular borders and color variation, is defined by an initial period of horizontal growth followed by a period of vertical growth and invasion of the dermis (Carr et al., 2020; Ostrowski & Fisher, 2021). Nodular melanoma is characterized by vertical growth without a previous period of radial growth (Carr et al., 2020; Ostrowski & Fisher, 2021). Its high aggressiveness is responsible for more than 40% of deaths caused by melanoma (Ostrowski & Fisher, 2021).

As for stage of development, melanoma can be classified on a scale that goes from stage I to stage IV. The first is the initial form of melanoma, without the involvement of adjacent tissues; in stage II, there is dermal tissue invasion; in stage III, there is regional spread or in sentinel lymph nodes; and in stage IV, there is distant metastasis (Allemani et al., 2018; Davis et al., 2019; Luke et al., 2017).

The origin and development of skin cancer are multifactorial, occurring both by environmental factors, such as exposure to UV light, and genetic susceptibilities, such as family history and the presence of melanocytic nevi throughout the body (Leachman et al., 2017). Like in other types of cancer, several genetic changes are observed in the course of the disease. These changes can accumulate in discrete stages, progressing from a benign tumor, with limited replication, to a malignant tumor, without replication control and with a high infiltrative capacity (Yeh & Bastian, 2021).

This aggregation of mutations occurs, in part, by the incidence of UV light to which these tumors are exposed, favoring DNA damage and the development of new mutations (Bertrand et al., 2020; Darp & Ceol, 2021; Davis et al., 2019). These genes are known as melanoma drivers, with BRAF and NRAS mutations being the most common (Yeh & Bastian, 2021). It is estimated that 50 to 65% of cutaneous melanomas have the BRAF mutation, while the other 20% have the mutation in the NRAS gene, which are typically mutually exclusive (Leonardi et al., 2018; Shain & Bastian, 2016; Shtivelman et al., 2014). However, these mutations alone are not capable of forming a melanoma. In melanocytic nevi (Leonardi et al., 2018; Yeh & Bastian, 2021), more than 80% of benign melanocytic nevi are mutated in the BRAF gene, usually $BRAF^{V600E}$, resulting in melanocytic proliferation (Leonardi et al., 2018; Ostrowski & Fisher, 2021; Yeh & Bastian, 2021). However, this nevus can remain quiescent for years. This provided evidence to believe that BRAF mutation requires additional mutations for melanoma development, such as mutations in TERT and/or in CDKN2A (Leonardi et al., 2018). Therefore, the accumulation of some molecular alterations in melanocytes is necessary to form melanoma (Yeh & Bastian, 2021). These alterations usually are associated with central control pathways of cell proliferation, such as BRAF, NRAS, and NF1 genes; genes related to cell growth and metabolisms, such as the PTEN and KIT genes; apoptosis resistance regulatory genes, such as p53; cell cycle control, such as CDKN2A; and cell lifespan control genes, such as reverse telomerase TERT (Darp & Ceol, 2021; Leonardi et al., 2018; Lo & Fisher, 2014; Shain & Bastian, 2016).

Another essential factor for melanomas' growth is their angiogenic capacity (Davis et al., 2019; Quaresmini & Guida, 2020). When the size and mass of the tumor increase, nutrient diffusion begins to be limited. Thus, it is necessary to develop a neoplastic vasculature. This process begins with the spread of new blood vessels from pre-existing units, followed by the recruitment of progenitor cells from the bone marrow and the adaptation of tumor cells in a mimesis process (Leonardi et al., 2018; Quaresmini & Guida, 2020).

Another striking feature of melanomas is their immunosuppressive capacity within the tumor microenvironment. Due to the high mutation rate of melanomas, some alterations may be beneficial for immune escape in "immune editing." One of the primary forms of escape is a reduction in the expression of MHC-I molecules, thus reducing aberrant proteins' presentation to cells of the immune system. Furthermore, the production and release of anti-inflammatory mediators or manipulation of immunological checkpoints, such as proteins CTLA-4 and PD-1, block cell death induced by the immune system (Cuevas & Daud, 2018; Davis et al., 2019).

1.2 GENERAL THERAPEUTIC OPTIONS

Melanoma treatment has significantly advanced in the last 10 years with the approval of new drugs by the FDA, including targeted therapy drugs, immune therapies, and drugs used in photodynamic therapy (PDT) (Leonardi et al., 2018; Ostrowski & Fisher, 2021; Patton et al., 2021). The treatment of choice should be based on the size and location of the lesion, in addition to the patient's age (Haque et al., 2015).

In the USA, tumor management is determined by the National Comprehensive Cancer Network (NCCN) (Brandt & Moore, 2019). In fact, surgical resection with a safety edge of at least 4 mm is still the primary clinical treatment of skin tumors (Brandt & Moore, 2019; Moser & Grossman, 2018). Yet, even though this therapeutic approach results in a cure for most patients, there is still a risk of relapse in some cases of BCC and SCC. For melanoma, surgical resection is usually curative only for patients diagnosed in the early stages of the disease. In those diagnosed later or with a history of relapses, there may be impairment of sentinel lymph nodes or regions distant from the tumor, requiring systemic therapy. However, approximately one-third of tumors diagnosed in stage IV have visceral or brain metastases. In these cases, the probability of response to drug treatment is low, representing a limitation of currently available treatments (Leonardi et al., 2018). Drugs currently used to treat skin cancers, regardless of the route of administration and therapeutic modality, are summarized in Table 1.1.

Until 2011, the primary treatment of choice for patients with metastatic melanoma was oral or parenteral chemotherapy, once surgical resection alone was not curative. Nevertheless, alkylating chemotherapy was the first line of choice due to the lack of drug alternatives, with an inadequate response and many severe adverse reactions (Cuevas & Daud, 2018; Davis et al., 2019). After 2011, melanoma therapy was revolutionized with the FDA-approved use of BRAF inhibitors and MEK inhibitors for the systemic treatment of melanoma skin cancer (Davis et al., 2019; Leonardi et al., 2018; Ostrowski & Fisher, 2021), with vemurafenib and dabrafenib being the first drugs approved for this purpose (Davis et al., 2019). After these, other drugs were developed and approved, such as cobimetinib, a MEK inhibitor (Gutzmer et al., 2020).

Initially, the use of BRAF inhibitors showed to be a promising treatment, with an excellent initial response rate to treatment. However, over time, this therapeutic approach caused rapid drug resistance. As a result, BRAF inhibitors are now recommended in patients who are favorable for the $BRAF^{V600E}$

TABLE 1.1 Summary of Systemic and Topical Drugs Indicated for Skin Cancer

Skin Cancer Type	Drug	Control	Follow-Up Time	Outcome	Adverse Events	References
Stage III melanoma	Ipilimumab 10 mg/kg every 3 weeks for 3 months, followed by infusions every 3 months for three years.	Placebo	Seven years	60% OS in the ipilimumab group versus 51.3% OS in the placebo group. Recurrence rate of 57.5% and 67.9% in patients in ipilimumab group and placebo group, respectively.	In ipilimumab group, 53.25% had grade ≥3 adverse events.	Eggermont et al. (2019)
Metastasic melanoma	Nivolumab 3 mg/kg every 2 weeks.	Ipilimumab 10 mg/kg every 3 weeks for 12 weeks, followed by infusions every 12 weeks.	Four years	No difference in recurrence rate was observed between the two groups. However, the PFS was higher in the nivolumab group (52.4 months) than in the ipilimumab group (24.1 months).	N/A	Ascierto et al. (2020)
Advanced melanoma with known BRAF^{v600} mutation.	Pembrolizumab 10 mg/kg every 2 or 3 weeks.	Ipilimumab 3 mg/kg every 3 weeks for 12 weeks.	N/A	Median PFS was longer for the pembrolizumab group (32.7 months) than for the ipilimumab group (15.9 months).	14% and 18% of patients had grade ≥3 adverse events in the pembrolizumab and ipilimumab groups, respectively.	Robert et al. (2019)
Stages III or IV melanoma with known BRAF^{v600} mutation.	Nivolumab 1 mg/kg combined with ipilimumab 3 mg/kg every 3 weeks for 12 weeks, followed by nivolumab 3 mg/kg every 2 weeks.	Nivolumab 3 mg/kg every 2 weeks 3 or ipilimumab 3 mg/kg every 3 weeks for 12 weeks.	Five years	52% OS in the combined treatment group versus 44% and 26% in nivolumab and ipilimumab groups, respectively.	59% had grade ≥3 adverse events in the combined treatment group, versus 23% and 28% in nivolumab and ipilimumab groups, respectively.	Larkin et al. (2019)

TABLE 1.1 *(Continued)*

Skin Cancer Type	Drug	Control	Follow-Up Time	Outcome	Adverse Events	References
Metastasic melanoma with brain metastasis.	Nivolumab 1 mg/kg combined with ipilimumab 3 mg/kg every 3 weeks for 12 weeks, followed by nivolumab 3 mg/kg every 2 weeks.	N/A	14 months.	The intracranial clinical benefit rate was 57%.	55% had grade ≥3 adverse events.	Tawbi et al. (2018)
Patients with a history of at least 2 BCC or SCC in the past five years.	5-FU application twice daily for 2 to 4 weeks.	Placebo.	Three years	No difference was observed between the two groups.	In the 5-FU group, up to 90% had erythema in the first week of treatment.	Weinstock et al. (2018)
Superficial BCC	Imiquimod 5%, 5 weekly applications for 6 weeks.	N/A	39 months	Histologically eradicate up to 82% at a 3-month follow-up, and 89% at 39 months follow-up.	Erythema, itching, and crusting.	Voiculescu et al. (2019)
Nodular and superficial BCC	Curettage and 5 weekly applications of imiquimod 5%.	Surgical excision.	12 months	The rate of patients with recurrence after 12 months was 13.7% for curettage and imiquimod and 0% for surgical excision.	In the imiquimod group, 70% had erythema, 75% erosion, 75% crust, 98.3% squamae and 95% itching.	Sinx et al. (2020)
Nodular and superficial BCC.	Imiquimod, 5 weekly applications.	Surgical excision.	Five years	Five-year free recurrence rates for the imiquimod group were 82.5%, compared with 97.7% for the surgery excision group.	N/A	Williams et al. (2017)
Superficial BCC	Ingenol mebutate applications on days 1 and 2.	Ingenol mebutate applications on days 1 and 8.	85 days	There was a trend of histological clearance in the group with applications on days 1 and 2.	Flaking, scaling, dryness, erythema, itching, edema, headache.	Siller et al. (2010)

Abbreviations: 5-FU: 5-fluorouracil; BCC: basal cell carcinoma; OS: overall survival; PFS: progression-free survival; and SCC: squamous cell carcinoma.

mutation and in combination with other drugs, such as MEK inhibitors or with immunological therapies, like immune checkpoint inhibitors (Gutzmer et al., 2020; Leonardi et al., 2018; Patton et al., 2021). These combinations have shown a response rate in approximately 70% of patients, increasing tumor progression-free survival and symptom control in patients with $BRAF^{V600E}$ (Gutzmer et al., 2020; Leonardi et al., 2018). Notwithstanding, despite this progress, targeted therapy has not resulted in a cure for most patients with metastatic melanoma. A recent study shows overall survival of patients with metastatic melanoma treated with BRAF inhibitors is approximately 10% in five years (Patton et al., 2021).

Another class of FDA-approved systemic drugs that have been used to treat metastatic melanoma are immune checkpoint inhibitors. For this type of cancer, the first immune checkpoint inhibitors approved were anti-CTLA4 drugs, followed by the approval of anti-PD1 drugs. Among anti-CTLA4 drugs, main ones are nivolumab, pembrolizumab, and ipilimumab. As for anti-PD1, vemurafenib and dabrafenib stand out. These drugs have a low response rate when administered alone. Nevertheless, when combined with BRAF inhibitors, they can result in lasting responses in patients responsive to treatment (Ascierto et al., 2020; Eggermont et al., 2019; Leonardi et al., 2018; Robert et al., 2019).

In practice, studies have shown that anti-CTLA4 induces clonal expansion of effector TCD4 lymphocytes, resulting in a Th1-type infiltrative antitumor response (Cuevas & Daud, 2018). This leads to increased recognition of MHC-I proteins and tumor antigens by immune effector cells (Gutzmer et al., 2020). The first FDA-approved regimen was the use of ipilimumab, at a dose of 10 mg per kilogram of the patient in individuals who underwent resection and who had sentinel lymph node participation (Ascierto et al., 2020).

Clinical studies which evaluated this therapeutic regimen were promising, with an improvement in the overall survival of patients after long periods of follow-up. This was reported in a phase III study where 951 patients were followed over seven years. These patients were divided into two groups, where the first received ipilimumab intravenously and the second received a placebo. After seven years of follow-up, overall survival of 60% was observed in the ipilimumab-treated group, compared with 51.3% survival in the placebo group. However, adverse reactions were limiting factors for the study, as 53.25% of patients discontinued treatment because of severe drug reactions (Eggermont et al., 2019).

Regarding the time of disease progression-free survival, it is noted in clinical studies that nivolumab is more advantageous than ipilimumab. Also, in phase III clinical trial, 453 patients received checkpoint inhibitors as adjunctive therapy, with the first group being treated with nivolumab and the second with ipilimumab. At the end of four years of follow-up, the melanoma recurrence rate was similar between the two groups. However, disease-free survival time was higher in the nivolumab-treated group at 52.4 months than at 24.1 months in the ipilimumab-treated group (Ascierto et al., 2020).

Pembrolizumab appears to be more promising in melanoma treatment when compared to ipilimumab. This comparison was described in a different phase III study, in which 834 patients were divided into three groups, the first two receiving different therapeutic regimens of pembrolizumab and the third receiving ipilimumab, all as adjuvant therapy. It was observed median overall survival of patients treated with both pembrolizumab regimens extended survival time to 32.7 months, while those treated with ipilimumab had a lower median survival of 15.9 months (Robert et al., 2019).

To improve immune recognition and prolong overall survival time and disease-free survival time, combinations of checkpoint inhibitors have shown to be promising. However, in these cases, the frequency of adverse reactions is higher, the main limiting factor for treatment. One combination adjuvant therapy that has been studied is treatment with both nivolumab and ipilimumab. However, studies report that despite prolonging disease-free survival time, this combination causes severe adverse reactions in almost 60% of patients, with severe diarrhea being the primary reported reaction (Larkin et al., 2019; Tawbi et al., 2018).

The use of immune checkpoint inhibitors has also been explored in patients with brain involvement due to metastatic melanoma. This was explored in 94 patients with brain metastasis who received a combination of nivolumab and ipilimumab. This study reported that over a 14-month follow-up period of patients, 57% showed tumor stabilization. However, 55% of patients had severe adverse reactions, requiring treatment interruption (Tawbi et al., 2018).

PDT is another treatment modality that has been increasingly used worldwide for superficial tumors (Honors et al., 2018; Wen et al., 2017). Thus, PDT has been used as a complementary and unconventional alternative to superficial skin cancer treatments, having the advantage of being a method with few systemic adverse reactions (Cullen et al., 2020).

PDT consists of applying a photosensitive molecule called photosensitizer at the site to be treated, followed by applying a beam of light with a specific wavelength. This light beam can be emitted by different sources, such as lasers, intense pulsed light, LED, or fluorescent lamps, emitting beams with wavelengths usually varying between 400 and 700 nm (Honors et al., 2018; Mkhobongo et al., 2021). Light beam, in turn, promotes photosensitizer excitation, generating reactive oxygen species (ROS), which cause cellular damage at the treated site, depending on the presence of oxygen in the tissue (Cullen et al., 2020; Honors et al., 2018; Li et al., 2020; Mkhobongo et al., 2021).

Four main classes of photosensitive molecule agents are porphyrins, phthalocyanines, chlorins, and porphycenes, which are non-toxic in their non-irradiating form (Mkhobongo et al., 2021). In tumor treatments, PDT has been shown to destroy both tumor mass and blood vessels associated with tumors (Cullen et al., 2020; Li et al., 2020). In general, studies have observed that photosensitizing agents' influx usually occurs with greater intensity in cells in constant mitotic activity, such as in tumor cells. However, even if the influx is increased in tumor cells, this increase is not specific and can cause damage to cells adjacent to the tumor (Mkhobongo et al., 2021).

PDT has been more used in SCC and superficial BCC treatments, not showing satisfactory action for adjuvant treatment of melanomas since melanin, present in melanomas, acts as a defense against radiation from the light beam and oxidative stress, limiting PDT effectiveness (Cullen et al., 2020; Li et al., 2020; Mkhobongo et al., 2021). In addition, melanin can act as an antioxidant, neutralizing ROS (Li et al., 2020).

Even with all the advances in skin cancer treatment achieved in recent years, the high frequency (HF) of well-known adverse reactions from systemic therapy is limiting. Indeed, there are still many patients who undergo treatment interruption because of such strong adverse reactions. In addition, cancers could acquire drug resistance, again being a limiting factor. In this context, considering that skin cancers are more accessible than those of other organs, allowing a more localized drug intervention, topical formulations for treating melanomas and non-melanoma tumors have been studied, as discussed in the next section.

1.3 TOPICAL ALTERNATIVES FOR SKIN CANCER

Recently, topical therapy has advanced in skin cancer treatments, especially superficial ones. Although surgical intervention is curative for most patients, topical treatment may be considered in specific clinical contexts, such as cases where the tumor is in early stages or developed in exposed areas, like in the face where resection may leave marks (Collins et al., 2019; Haque et al., 2015). However, the choice of topical treatment should consider the size and location of the tumor, as this type of treatment still has a cure rate below surgical intervention (Cullen et al., 2020; Haque et al., 2015), partly limited by the low permeation capacity of some drugs (Collins et al., 2019). Among used drugs in topical therapy, fluorouracil, imiquimod (IMQ), and ingenol mebutate can be highlighted (Haque et al., 2015). From them, fluorouracil and IMQ are FDA-approved for superficial BCC treatment, while ingenol mebutate is commonly used in off-label treatment of superficial BCC (Honors et al., 2018).

Fluorouracil, also known as 5-FU, is a drug belonging to the antimetabolites class. Its mechanism of action involves binding to thymidylate synthase, an enzyme necessary for thymidine synthesis. Thus, 5-FU inhibits cell replication and induces cell death (Collins et al., 2019; Cullen et al., 2020; Haque et al., 2015; Voiculescu et al., 2019). Usually available as a cream containing 5% of the drug, 5-FU can be used to treat superficial BCC without leaving permanent marks on the patient's skin. However, this therapeutic option is limited to patients with small, superficial tumor lesions in low-risk locations (Voiculescu et al., 2019).

The recommended therapeutic regimen of 5-FU is one or two applications a day for up to 11 consecutive weeks (Voiculescu et al., 2019). However, recent studies suggest that the difference in therapeutic regimen adopted can result in a wide variation in the cure rate, ranging between 27% and 90%. This was seen by a study that applied 5-FU twice daily for 11 weeks, showing a cure rate in 90% of patients with superficial BCC, while another study, with the same posology, but for 6 to 8 weeks, showed a cure rate of 54 to 85% (Collins et al., 2019).

Adverse reactions frequency was high, with the onset of pain, erythema, crusting, and pruritus (Collins et al., 2019). Adverse reactions can appear in more than 90% of patients. In clinical practice, adverse reactions are more common in the first week of treatment, reducing the frequency of adverse reactions by up to 65% in the following weeks (Pomerantz et al., 2016). In general, even though 5-FU is widely used in clinical practice, few studies have shown its efficacy. In addition, most studies were without a control group for comparison, which is a limiting factor for evaluating the best therapeutic approach (Cullen et al., 2020).

IMQ, in its turn, is a drug of the immunomodulatory class. Commercially patented as Aldara, IMQ has been approved by the FDA for superficial BCC and actinic keratosis treatment. However, in off-label use, in clinical practice, IMQ has also been used for nodular BCC and superficial melanoma treatments in early stages as adjuvant therapy (Collins et al., 2019; Haque et al., 2015). IMQ's mechanism of action involves binding and activation of toll-like receptors (TLR), mainly TLR-7 and TLR-8, inducing activation of an antitumor immune response (Collins et al., 2019; Cullen et al., 2020; Haque et al., 2015; Voiculescu et al., 2019).

This immune response activation is characterized by stimulation of antigen-presenting cells (APC) and the production of inflammatory cytokines (Voiculescu et al., 2019). The approved therapeutic regimen is one or two applications per day, with five applications per week. However, as with 5-FU use, recent studies have shown that different therapeutic regimens can result in a difference in cure rates, ranging from 43% to 94%. The main adverse reactions reported are similar to those caused by 5-FU, such as erythema, pain, and itching at the application site, with the difference that some patients report hyperchromic appearances at the site (Collins et al., 2019). According to studies, adverse reactions may appear in more than 90% of patients using IMQ, with erythema being the primary reported reaction (Rosenberg et al., 2019).

For superficial BCC treatment, studies suggest IMQ can eradicate tumor cells in more than 80% of patients after three months of treatment. When looking at the long-term effects, almost 90% of patients with superficial BCC were cured, with no cases of tumor recurrence after five years in cured patients. However, tumor clearance is around 80% when it comes to nodular BCC (Voiculescu et al., 2019).

The results of using IMQ are encouraging for superficial BCC treatment. However, as with 5-FU treatment, the cure rate of IMQ still remains below the cure rate of surgical resection. Therefore, some studies have analyzed the association of IMQ with techniques such as curettage. In a 12-month follow-up study, no patients who underwent surgical resection experienced tumor recurrence, while 13.7% of those treated with IMQ and curettage had a recurrence (Sinx et al., 2020). Studies that followed patients for more extended periods observed that patients submitted to surgical intervention, 96.8% remained free of BCC recurrence for three years, while of those treated with IMQ, 85.1% did not have tumor recurrence (Williams et al., 2017).

Another topically applied drug that induces an inflammatory response in tumors is ingenol mebutate, an agent extracted from *Euphorbia peplus*, approved to treat actinic keratosis, but which has also been used off-label for the treatment of superficial BCC (Collins et al., 2019; García-de-la-Fuente et al., 2020; Voiculescu et al., 2019). Ingenol mebutate mechanism of action is not fully understood yet. However, it is known that it induces a rapid cytotoxic response in a mechanism involving neutrophils activation and induces a response mediated by inflammatory cytokines, endothelial adhesion molecules, and the formation of specific antibodies against the tumor

(Collins et al., 2019; García-de-la-Fuente et al., 2020; Haque et al., 2015; Voiculescu et al., 2019).

The immune response induced by ingenol mebutate was evaluated in patients undergoing biopsy on the 3rd and 30th days after treatment. This study observed that the immediate response is mediated by T lymphocytes, while the late response presents an infiltrate of regulatory T cells (García-de-la-Fuente et al., 2020). Regarding its pharmaceutical presentation, ingenol mebutate is available in the gel at 0.0025%, 0.01%, and 0.05%. However, studies suggest the action of ingenol is dose-dependent, as observed in a phase III study, where patients treated with the highest concentration of ingenol had a higher cure rate (Siller et al., 2010).

The adopted therapeutic regimen is one application daily, for two consecutive days, or with an interval of 7 days between two applications. It is still unclear in the literature which is the best therapeutic regimen. However, there are indications that application for two consecutive days increases tumor clearance in patients with superficial BCC (Siller et al., 2010). Regarding adverse reactions, ingenol mebutate usually causes pain, redness, erythema, scaling, and blisters at the site, just like the other topical medications. Still, some systemic reactions were also observed, such as headaches, mainly when applied to large areas (Bucko et al., 2018).

In general, ease of access to skin tumors is a factor that facilitates topical medication use. This offers a great advantage to topical drugs, both in the primary treatment and adjuvant therapy. However, it is evident that topical treatment of skin tumors is still much limited, mainly due to the high toxicity of chemotherapeutic drugs, which often cause adverse effects that compromise the use of dermatological formulations. In addition, the low or incomplete skin penetration of drugs is responsible for compromising the drug's effectiveness or even requiring high amounts of drugs that are often toxic in contact with the skin, which aggravates the situation of toxicity.

In this sense, nanostructured delivery systems emerge as a bet to favor the topical treatment of skin tumors, whether melanoma or non-melanoma. In the next section, the leading research using nanocarriers of different nature will be presented and discussed.

1.4 NANOTECHNOLOGY APPLIED TO TOPICAL TREATMENT OF SKIN CANCERS

New formulations and techniques for treating skin cancer should provide an option to enhance drugs bioavailability, resulting in topical therapies that could reach cancers located in the deeper layers of the skin; also, it makes it possible to decrease dose and circumvent the side effects of systemic administration. Indeed, nanocarriers can be a more stable and less toxic system for the delivery of drugs; they can also increase drug penetration or permeation, enhancing its residence period and controlling its release rate on the skin; thus, it could improve the therapeutic index of the treatment (Goyal et al., 2017). Nanocarriers prepared with different materials, such as polymeric nanoparticles (NPs), silica nanoparticles, lipid nanoparticles, metallic nanoparticles, liposomes, ethosomes (ETOs), nanoemulsions, and nanogels have been researched for topical application in skin cancer treatment, as presented in Figure 1.1. Figure 1.1 is a proposed schematic of the drug delivery mechanism of topical nanocarriers, which can also be associated with other technologies as described in Section 1.5, and Table 1.2 illustrates the potential nanocarriers used in topical therapy to treat skin cancer.

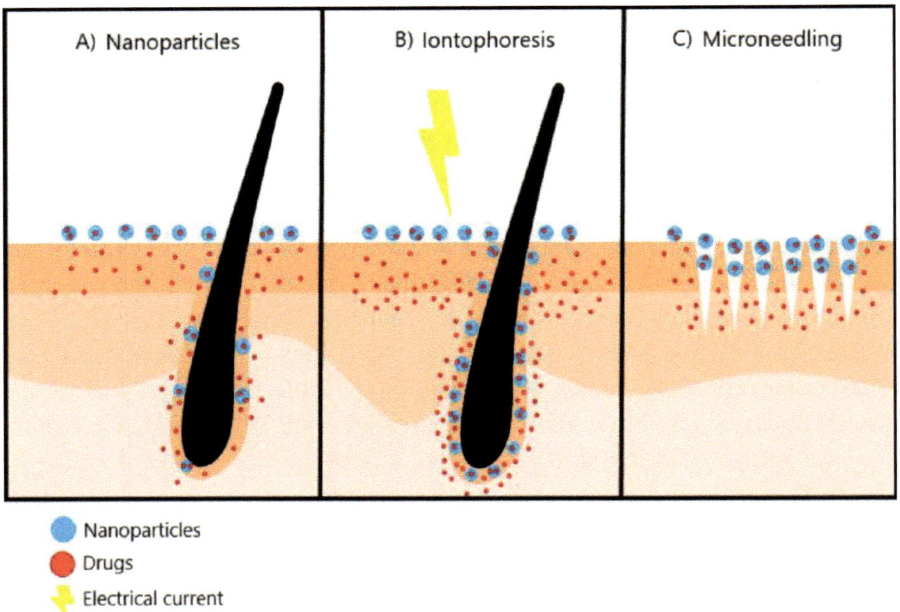

FIGURE 1.1 Scheme of the proposed drug delivery mechanism of topical nanocarriers associated with other technologies. (A) New nanoformulations should increase bioavailability by enhancing drug retention and permeation into deeper skin layers; (B) iontophoresis can increase drug permeation into the skin by electromigration and electroosmosis; and (C) microneedling mechanically generates microchannels in the skin, allowing the drug permeation into deeper skin layers.

TABLE 1.2 Summary of Topically Applied Drugs from Nanocarriers Indicated for Skin Cancer

Type of Nanocarrier	Drug	Size (nm)	Test Model	Outcome	References
Polymeric nanoparticle	5-Fluorouracil	133	Chicken skin (*ex vivo*)	1.7-fold enhanced penetration compared to the control.	Rata et al. (2020)
	Imiquimod	249	Male Swiss mice (*in vivo*)	Provided permeation and retention of the drug in deeper layers of the skin, with higher retention of the drug in the epidermis concerning the dermis.	Dias et al. (2018)
	Imiquimod	180	Newborn pig skin (*ex vivo*)	Penetrated the stratum corneum in 50 min. After 24 h, the drug had already crossed the stratum corneum, and it was found in deeper layers of the skin.	Alvarez-Figueroa et al. (2020)
	Zinc phthalocyanine	189	Female SKH-1 hairless mice (*in vivo*)	Total removal of the tumor after 20 days of treatment, while the control group showed regrowth of the tumor after 10 days of treatment, and it persisted even in the fourth week of the treatment.	Keyal et al. (2018)
	Dacarbazine and zinc phthalocyanine.	259.6	MV3 melanoma cells (*in vitro*).	*In vitro*: enhance the therapeutic efficacy, and it is dose-dependent.	Reis et al. (2021)
			Male Balb/C mice (*in vivo*).	*In vivo* assay: Low accumulation into the stomach, heart, brain, and kidneys suggested that common side effects of dacarbazine could be reduced.	
Silica nanoparticle	5-Fluorouracil	193	Male Wistar rats (*ex vivo*)	4.67-fold enhanced penetration compared to the control. The drug accumulation in skin layers where melanoma cells usually reside was enhanced ~10 times compared to control.	Almomen et al. (2020)
	Methotrexate	~200	Thin slices of the porcine epidermis (*ex vivo*).	Epidermal accumulation of the drug was increased. The glycerolipid lotion and the O/W emulsion increased respectively 2.4- and 2.8-fold compared to the control.	Sapino et al. (2017)

TABLE 1.2 *(Continued)*

Type of Nanocarrier	Drug	Size (nm)	Test Model	Outcome	References
Lipid nanoparticle	5-Fluorouracil and resveratrol.	199–472	*In vitro:* Strat-M™ membrane. *Ex vivo:* Wistar rat skin.	*In vitro* permeation study: 2.4- and 1.7-fold 5-fluorouracil and resveratrol enhanced permeation compared to control. *Ex vivo* study: 5-fluorouracil and resveratrol permeation were increased 2.2- and 1.8-fold compared to control, respectively.	Iqubal et al. (2021)
	Paclitaxel	78–587	Swiss Albino mice (*in vivo*)	A high level of recovery can be observed by a decrease in the size of keratinocyte pearls compared to the poor recovery of control. The growth and volume of tumors formed on the skin were much smaller than control.	Bharadwaj et al. (2016)
	Curcumin	167	Male *Mus musculus* Albino mice (*in vivo*)	2-fold enhanced penetration compared to control.	Abdel Fadeel et al. (2020)
Metallic nanoparticle	5-Fluorouracil	16–150	*Ex vivo*: mice dorsal skin. *In vivo*: A431 tumor-bearing mice.	2-fold higher permeability compared to control. *In vivo* studies: gel and cream formulations achieved 6.8- and 18.4-fold lower tumor volume compared to the control.	Safwat et al. (2018)
	5-Aminolevilinic	17	Female nude mice (*in vivo*).	The tumor grew much slower than the control. Presented a higher percentage of tumor inhibition (64%) compared to control (16%).	Wu et al. (2017)
Liposomes	5-Fluorouracil	156.5	*In vitro:* rat skin. *In vivo:* mice.	*In vitro* permeation: 64.9% of the drug was permeated compared to 36.4% control. *In vivo* experiments: drug deposition was 3-fold higher than drug solution.	Hussain et al. (2016)
	Vismodegib	110	Human skin explants (*ex vivo*).	7-fold enhanced penetration compared to control. The drug was detected along all skin sections.	Calienni et al. (2019)

TABLE 1.2 *(Continued)*

Type of Nanocarrier	Drug	Size (nm)	Test Model	Outcome	References
Ethosomes	Mitoxantrone	78	Ratskin (*in vitro*)	After 6 h, the drug permeated to receptor compartment, and then its penetrating amount gradually increased, while the drug from the control was not detected in the receptor compartment.	Yu et al. (2015)
	Paclitaxel	240	Human stratum corneum and viable epidermis membranes (*in vitro*)	~3.2-fold enhanced penetration compared to control. Increased ~2.2-fold the anti-proliferative activity in a squamous cell carcinoma model compared to control.	Paolino et al. (2012)
	Sulforaphane and curcumin	125	Ratskin (*in vitro*)	~5-fold enhanced penetration compared to control. Deeper penetration in the skin, up to 183 μm, whereas the control penetrated to 44 μm.	Soni et al. (2020)
Nanoemulsions	5-Fluorouracil	66	Cow, goat, and rat skin (*ex vivo*).	Ratskin model: 1.56-enhanced penetration compared to control. Cow and goatskin model: 12.51-fold enhanced penetration compared to control.	Ahmad et al. (2020)
Nanogels	5-Fluorouracil	100–180 nm	*Ex vivo*: porcine skin. *In vivo*: Swiss albino mice.	*Ex vivo* studies: 80–85% of drug release, compared to 40–45% of control. *In vivo* studies: significant reduction in tumor diameter size; significant accumulation of the drug in the dermal region, while the control provides a drug accumulation in tumor nodules and liver, indicating its non-specificity.	Sahu et al. (2019)

1.4.1 POLYMERIC NANOPARTICLES (NPS)

Polymeric nanoparticles are currently the most common among nanocarriers, considering both natural and synthesized polymers, due to some attractive qualities such as high stability and mass production and biocompatibility and nontoxicity of most of the selected polymers. Polymeric nanoparticles can have a vesicular (nanocapsules) where the drug is stored in a polymer cistern, or matrix conformation (nanospheres), in which the drug is scattered on a polymer matrix (Aghebati-Maleki et al., 2020). Eudragit (Dias et al., 2018), chitosan (Alvarez-Figueroa et al., 2020; Keyal et al., 2018; Rata et al., 2020), methoxy polyethylene glycol polylactic acid (CPP) (Keyal et al., 2018), poly(D,L-lactide) (PLA) (Reis et al., 2021) and poly(vinyl acetate) (PVA) (Reis et al., 2021) have been used as matrices to produces nanoparticles encapsulating anticancer drugs.

An innovative approach for skin cancer treatment was developed as a gel formulation to encapsulate 5-FU based on sodium alginate and hyaluronic acid. This study used chitosan and aptamer-functionalized carboxymethyl chitosan as polymers for the nanoformulation. The *ex vivo* experiments showed that the nanocapsules with a diameter of 133 nm could enhance the permeability properties of 5-FU around 1.7-fold compared to the control. In addition, the formulation proved to be non-irritant and manifested a substantial cytotoxic effect on the human basal carcinoma cell line. The results suggested that this formulation is biosafety and has an excellent antitumor effect for skin cancer treatment (Rata et al., 2020).

Another research evaluated the use of nanostructured systems to overcome the high incidence of local and systemic side effects of IMQ and low skin permeation that results in therapeutic ineffectiveness. In this way, polymeric nanoparticles of Eudragit of around 249 nm were obtained. This system provided permeation and retention of the drug in deeper layers of the skin, promoting higher drug retention in the epidermis concerning the dermis. This result is contrary to control, suggesting that this delivery system potentially increased cutaneous permeation (Dias et al., 2018).

The dermal absorption of nanoencapsulated IMQ was also evaluated, in which chitosan nanocapsules were used to load the drug. The experiments showed that the 180 nm-nanocapsules improved the drug penetration to the deeper layers of the skin and that this penetration is dynamic, i.e., the nanocapsules took around 50 min to penetrate the stratum corneum (SC). Furthermore, after 24 h, the bands of IMQ were seen at depths greater than 20 μm, meaning that the drug had already crossed the SC and was found in deeper layers of the skin, where it is available to be absorbed (Alvarez-Figueroa et al., 2020). This outcome was expected once the positively charged nanocapsules were designed to interact with the negative charge of the skin, resulting in more significant transdermal transport of cations (Alvarez-Figueroa et al., 2020), also demonstrates the greater release control of that the encapsulated drug provided by the polymeric nanoparticle.

As mentioned in the sections above, PDT combines the action of photosensitizer, light, and oxygen as a non-invasive treatment modality. The injected photosensitizer can be activated by specific light irradiation to produce ROS that can oxidize subcellular organelles and biomolecules, leading to the destruction of tumor cells (Chi et al., 2020; Wu et al., 2017). Their characteristics of noninvasiveness, fewer side effects, negligible drug resistance, and low systemic toxicity showed that it could be a superior therapy to the traditional forms. Therefore, it has been proposed as an effective modality for skin cancer therapy (Cheng et al., 2017). Several researchers investigated the application of this therapy added to nanotechnology to benefit the effectiveness of antineoplastic treatment, including the production of polymeric nanoparticles.

Nanoparticles of chitosan/CPP were used as a nanosystem to encapsulate zinc phthalocyanine as a photosensitizer for PDT. *In vivo* evaluation of this new system proved that PDT was significantly better with zinc phthalocyanine-CPP when compared to its free form. The nanosystem showed a total removal of the tumor after 20 days of treatment, while the control group showed regrowth of the tumor after 10 days of treatment, and it persisted even in the fourth week of the treatment (Keyal et al., 2018).

A PLA/PVA nanoparticle loading of both dacarbazine and zinc phthalocyanine was produced to improve therapeutic efficacy and reduce the side effects of conventional skin cancer treatments. An *in vitro* PDT test assay using MV3 melanoma cells as a model was performed. Results demonstrated that the combination of dacarbazine and the photodynamic effect of zinc phthalocyanine was essential to enhance the therapeutic efficacy. In addition, *in vivo* assay was performed using radiolabeled PLA/PVA nanoparticles, which results demonstrated that the drug loading affects the biodistribution of the nanoparticle formulations, which nanoparticles with dacarbazine and zinc phthalocyanine were mainly uptake by the liver (90.16%) with a discrete uptake by the stomach (4.03%) and the spleen (3.79%). The nanoparticles that only contained dacarbazine showed a high uptake by the liver (76.12%), stomach (9.55%), and spleen (9.11%). Moreover, the empty nanoparticles showed a high uptake by kidneys (64.78%) and liver (12.43%).

Low accumulation of the nanoparticles into the stomach, heart, brain, and kidneys suggested that common side effects of dacarbazine could be reduced (Reis et al., 2021).

1.4.2 *SILICA NANOPARTICLES*

Silica nanoparticle, a mesostructured type of nanoparticle, is a drug delivery system (DDS) that has a tunable particle size ranging between 50 nm and 300 nm, a high loading capacity due to the large surface (around 1,000 $m^2 g^{-1}$), a uniform hexagonal porous structure, and two functional surfaces, which can selectively be functionalized or conjugated with targeting ligands (Almomen et al., 2020; Sapino et al., 2017).

An amino-functionalized mesoporous silica nanoparticles (MSN-NH_2), in which the amine group was added to further improve the encapsulation of drugs through hydrogen bonding or electrostatic interactions, has already been described (Almomen et al., 2020). A 193 nm-MSN-NH_2 encapsulating 5-FU was formulated in the gel, and the skin permeability study revealed that the enhancement ratio of 5-FU using MSN-NH_2 was 4.67-fold relative to its free drug counterparts. In addition, the accumulation of the drug in skin layers where melanoma cells usually reside was enhanced approximately 10 times with 5-FU when the drug was encapsulated compared to control. These results, therefore, indicated that MSN-NH_2 could be a promising delivery vehicle in the management of melanoma (Almomen et al., 2020).

A methotrexate-based mesoporous silica nanoparticle for topical treatment of skin cancer was also prepared. The obtained nanoparticle presented around 200 nm. *In vitro* permeation experiments were conducted using dermatomed porcine skin, in which several dermal formulations incorporating the nanoparticles were tested. Results showed that the epidermal accumulation of the drug was increased by its inclusion in silica nanoparticles, regardless of the surrounding medium. Two mediums had a pronounced increase in the skin retention of the nanoparticle-loaded drug over the free form, the glycerolipids lotion (70% Butyrospermum Parkii butter, 20% glycine soja oil, 10% glycerin) and the O/W emulsion (Phase A: 3.5% Cetearyl Alcohol and Cetearyl glucoside; 2% potassium cetyl phosphate; 4% dimethicone; 20% paraffin. Phase B: 66.2% aqua; 4% glycerin; 0.3% imidazolidinyl urea), which were respective 2.4- and 2.8-fold. In this way, the MSNs were proven to improve the cutaneous absorption and hence the bioavailability and efficacy of methotrexate (Sapino et al., 2017).

1.4.3 LIPID NANOPARTICLES

The choice for lipid nanoparticles is based on the extreme biocompatibility of the lipids with the skin, which ensures close contact of the drug with the SC and provides its retention on the skin as a thin occlusive film. They also increase skin hydration, leading to an enhancement of drug deposition into the skin and reduce sensibilization of the skin, ensuring less toxicity. In addition, like other nanocarriers, this system, when composed of a mixture of different lipids, provides a capacity for loading more drugs, modulating the drug release profile, and providing stability. For cancer treatment, this lipid-nanosystem has the benefit of being quickly internalized into the cancerous cells due to the greater occlusiveness caused by its lipidic behavior. Further, the presence of lipids that act as an ultraviolet (UV) filter adds UV blocking characteristics to the formulation (Iqubal et al., 2021).

The enhanced skin permeation between epidermis and dermis layers of the skin of 5-FU and resveratrol to obtain a synergistic effect against skin cancer using lipid nanoparticles has already been demonstrated. The nanoparticles exhibited particles ranging from 199–472 nm and were incorporated in a hydrophilic gel to facilitate topical application. An *in vitro* permeation study showed that such nanoparticles could enhance 2.4- and 1.7-fold 5-FU and resveratrol permeation compared to control, respectively. Such result reveals that the dual drug-loaded lipid-nanosystem leads to the production of a formulation capable of significantly improving the permeation of both drugs through the SC towards the deeper skin layers where the tumor is located (Iqubal et al., 2021).

A solid lipid nanoparticle of paclitaxel also showed anticancer efficacy during four weeks of topical treatment. The nanoformulation demonstrated a high level of recovery which can be observed by a decrease in the size of keratinocyte pearls. At the same time, the control showed poor recovery as the size of the keratinocyte pearls was not significantly reduced, and dyskeratosis was observed. Visually, the growth and volume of tumor formed on the skin were much smaller in mice treated with the solid lipid nanoparticle compared to the control. Thus, the formulation proved to be quite efficient in the treatment of skin carcinoma (Bharadwaj et al., 2016).

Another promising study evaluated PEGylated lipid nanocarriers (PLN) loaded with curcumin to target skin cancer by PDT. The 167-PLN encapsulating curcumin was tested *in vivo*. The amount of curcumin extracted from mice's skin was 2-fold higher than the control. Moreover, histopathological analyses showed that the PLN was able to enhance the penetration of curcumin to deeper skin layers, especially after irradiation (Abdel Fadeel et al., 2020).

1.4.4 METALLIC NANOPARTICLES

Several materials can produce metallic nanoparticles, such as iron, gold, silver, titanium dioxide (TiO_2), zinc oxide (ZnO), or iron oxide. These nanoparticles can entrap the drug both into the nucleus or adsorbed on the nanoparticle surface and have shown high stability and biocompatibility (Krishnan & Mitragotri, 2020).

Gold nanoparticles (AuNPs) have the potential to maximize anticancer drug efficacy and minimize off-target side effects, which makes this material an investigational target for drug delivery applications. 5-FU loaded onto AuNPs prepared with different molar ratios of 5-FU/cetyltrimethylammonium bromide (CTAB) was tested using different techniques, where the optimum 5-FU/CTAB-gold nanoparticles (molar ratio 1:1 5-FU/CTAB, pH 11.5) were incorporated into gel and cream bases. The *ex vivo* permeability was evaluated in mice's dorsal skin, and the *in vivo* anticancer efficacy was evaluated in A431 tumor-bearing mice. These nanoparticles presented a spherical shape and a size of ~16–150 nm, sustained the drug release, and provided around 2-fold higher permeability through mice skin compared with free 5-FU incorporated in gel and cream formulations. The *in vivo* studies showed that the gel and cream formulations achieved 6.8- and 18.4-fold lower tumor volume compared with the untreated control, respectively, confirming the potential of topical 5-FU/CTAB-gold nanoparticles to enhance drug efficacy against skin cancer (Safwat et al., 2018).

A study investigated whether the AuNPs encapsulating 5-aminolevulinic acid (5-ALA) and metalloproteinase-2-activatable cell-penetrating peptides could enhance the antitumor efficiency of PDT in skin cancer. The photodynamic therapeutic effect was evaluated *in vivo* using mice as a model. The SCC-7 tumor-bearing nude mice were treated with the AuNPs by tail vein injection after irradiating the tumor tissues with 635 nm light for four hours. The tumor of mice treated with the developed formulation grew much slower than the control. The tumor inhibition rate was also calculated and showed that the mice treated with the nanoparticle had a higher percentage of tumor inhibition (64%) than the control of free ALA (16%), suggesting significantly improved therapeutic efficacy (Wu et al., 2017).

1.4.5 LIPOSOMES AND ETHOSOMES (ETOS)

Liposomes are phospholipids and cholesterol-containing bilayers vesicular systems with highly high biocompatibility (Katharotiya et al., 2021). Ultra-deformable liposomes are highly elastic liposomes capable of penetrating the

SC instead of merging with this layer. Also, the presence of an edge activator that increases the deformability of the bilayer allowed them to pass through pores much smaller than their size. This property makes this vesicle system a versatile and advantageous carrier for topical drug delivery (Calienni et al., 2019; Hussain et al., 2016).

An elastic liposome containing 5-FU was investigated for increased drug permeation through the SC. The formulation was incorporated in a hydrophilic gel and compared with the marketed cream. The results showed that the selected formulation enabled the permeation of 64.9% drug, compared to 36.4% provided by the control (Hussain et al., 2016). *In vivo* experiments were also performed to justify the permeation potential and drug deposition of the 5-FU-loaded formulation into the skin after topical application for 24 h, using confocal laser scanning microscopy. The results showed that drug deposition of optimized elastic liposome was about three-fold higher than drug solution. It was capable of delivering 5-FU into the epidermal area for enhanced topical delivery than drug solution (Hussain et al., 2016).

Another study incorporated vismodegib to ultra-deformable liposomes to obtain a nano-DDS via a topical route. The obtained liposomes presented an average size of 110 nm, and 7-fold significantly enhanced their penetration in human skin compared to the free drug. Moreover, the drug was detected along with all skin layers, which penetrated deeper into the skin (Calienni et al., 2019).

ETOs are multilayer vesicles, much like liposomes, but filled with high ethanol concentrations (20–45%) to also incorporate apolar drugs into the nanostructure core (Bellefroid et al., 2019; Soni et al., 2020; Yu et al., 2015). An ethosome gel was researched to entrap mitoxantrone and provide a new topical therapy for melanomas. Indeed, 78 nm–ETOs gel was significantly more permeable across the rat skin than the free drug incorporated in an aqueous solution. The drug from the nanoformulation was found in the receptor compartment in Franz diffusion six hours after the experiment was initiated. Then its penetrating amount gradually increased, while the drug from the control was not detected in the receptor compartment (Yu et al., 2015).

Paclitaxel-loaded ETOs were also proposed as a topical alternative for skin cancer treatment. The skin application of paclitaxel-loaded ETOs could improve the drug permeation in a SC-epidermis membrane model, ~3.2-fold higher than the control. Moreover, it increased ~2.2-fold the anti-proliferative activity in a squamous cell carcinoma (SCC) model as compared to the free drug (Paolino et al., 2012).

Among the strategies to produce an ethosome for topical delivery in skin cancer, an optimized ethosomal nanogel encapsulating natural compounds with anticancer properties was evaluated. The study obtained a formulation with an average size of 125 nm, incorporating sulforaphane and curcumin. *In vitro* skin permeation and retention studies corroborated the drug delivery from ethosome formulation into the distinguished layer of skin. The results indicated that the permeation capability of the drugs from nanoformulation was significantly higher than the free drugs solution. Moreover, the total co-delivered curcumin and sulforaphane from nanocarrier retained in the epidermis were ~5-fold higher than the control containing free drugs. The ethosome formulation also provided a deeper penetration in the skin, up to 183 μm. In contrast, the control penetrated to 44 μm, which could benefit the therapy as the melanoma is in deeper skin layers (Soni et al., 2020).

1.4.6 NANOEMULSIONS

Nanoemulsions are colloidal dispersions of polar and apolar phases stabilized by some surfactants. This system has a transparent or slightly turbid color due to its small droplet size, improving its stability compared to conventional emulsions. Unlike microemulsions, this system may be obtained with less surfactant, is not thermodynamically stable, and requires significant energy input for formation (Giacone et al., 2020). Indeed, the effects of nanoemulsions for topical application of 5-FU bioavailability have already been evaluated. The formulation was composed of castor oil (oil), transcutol HP (surfactant), and polyethylene glycol (PEG)–400 (cosurfactant), and the optimized formulation contained 40% of oil, 20% of water, and 40% of surfactant: cosurfactant (1:1) was incorporated in carbopol gel. The permeation studies were performed *in vitro* in different skin models (cow, goat, and rat). The permeation of the drug from gel nanoemulsion for the rat skin model was 1.56-fold higher than the nanoemulsion and 12.51-fold higher than the control for the cow and goatskin model (Ahmad et al., 2020).

1.4.7 NANOGELS

Nanogels are a nanosized polymeric three-dimensional network composed of hydrogel nanoparticles in aqueous dispersions. Their structure resembles the extracellular matrix of the epidermal tissue. Their ease of preparation, tunable size, and low toxicity make this vehicle interesting to be explored for topical drug delivery in cancer therapy (Soni et al., 2020).

A novel chitosan-based pH-responsive biodegradable nanogel was developed to encapsulate 5-FU to treat melanoma via a topical route. The *ex vivo* permeation experiments were performed using porcine corneas. The 100 nm nanoformulation revealed a significant permeation compared to the free drug solution. The cationic property of chitosan provided an enhanced penetration efficiency due to better mucoadhesion over skin facilitation sustained release of the drug. After 24 h, the permeation of 5-FU from nanogel showed about 80–85% of drug release, while 40–45% of the drug was released from the drug solution. *In vivo* studies were performed using Swiss albino mice. The tumor growth and diameter profile were measured, and the results showed that the nanogel system exhibits a significant reduction in tumor diameter size.

Moreover, the sustained release of the drug by its formulation allowed only one dose to be applied daily, while conventional gel requires twice or thrice application in a day. To understand the localization potential of nanogels in melanoma nodules, experiments of gamma scintigraphy screening were performed, and it demonstrated that nanogel formulation provides a significant accumulation of the drug in the dermal region. In contrast, the control provides a drug accumulation in tumor nodules and the liver, indicating non-specificity. This work proved that the developed formulation portends to be a promising platform for efficient and sustained delivery of 5-FU for topical chemotherapy (Sahu et al., 2019).

1.5 PHYSICAL METHODS ASSOCIATED WITH NANOCARRIERS

Research proved that the development of nanosystems is an excellent strategy to enhance cancer therapy efficacy both for increasing drug penetration into the target tissue and for promoting significant outcomes in terms of stability, biocompatibility, and safety.

Currently, some approaches investigate how synergistic effects of nanosystems, and physical methods could further improve oncologic treatment. For example, technologies such as iontophoresis, alternating current, and microneedling added to nanotechnology showed to be promising substitutes in skin cancer therapies. In general, the strategic integration of physical methods and nanocarriers exhibited superior advantages in drug delivery, providing the most significant penetration of drugs (Huber et al., 2015b), better recovery of tumors (Suneet, De, Rangarajan et al., 2020), and greatest tumor inhibition (Hao et al., 2020b). Furthermore, the application time of the formulation can also be shortened, considering that physical methods can considerably speed up the time for large amounts of the drug to reach the target tissue.

In this way, the association of these strategies could improve skin cancer treatment and could be used as an alternative treatment modality. Table 1.3 summarizes technological approaches added to nanotechnology in skin cancer therapy.

Iontophoresis is a physical non-invasive technique in which a small electrical current is applied to the skin to stimulate the topical and transdermal delivery of molecules. It can promote the permeation of both charged and uncharged drugs through electromigration and electroosmosis (Byrne et al., 2018; Huber et al., 2015a). A study examined the potential of the anodic iontophoresis of doxorubicin-loaded cationic solid lipid nanoparticles (SLNs) to increase drug penetration. A formulation containing 136 nm-nanoparticle under passive conditions increased the drug penetration in the SC and the viable epidermis by 2.7-fold and 3.4-fold, respectively, compared to the control of the free drug. Under iontophoretic conditions, the lipid nanoparticles' drug penetration was increased by 59.9-fold and 41.2-fold, respectively. When evaluated *in vivo*, the anodic iontophoresis of the lipid nanoparticles effectively inhibited tumor cell survival and tumor growth in nude BALB/c mice affected with SCC, accompanied by an increase in keratinization consequent cell death. Thus, the strong synergistic effect of iontophoresis with nanoencapsulation provides a potential strategy for treating skin cancer (Huber et al., 2015a).

Another promising method to treat cancer is hyperthermia therapy, which promotes heat energy delivery to increase the surrounding temperature (40°C–45°C). This therapy can boost anticancer drug efficacy by modifying responsible gene expression and increasing drug sensitivity (Suneet, De, & Jain, 2020). A doxorubicin hydrochloride was incorporated in a magnetic nanofibrous mat-based bandage was developed to treat skin cancer using an external alternating current to induce hyperthermia. It fabricated Fe_3O_4 nanoparticles incorporating PCL fibers, and its efficacy was observed using the BALB/c mice model in the presence of an external alternating current magnetic field. The *in vivo* experiment confirmed the full recovery of chemically induced skin tumors on BALB/c mice within a month after five hyperthermic doses for 15 minutes, without any sign of inflammation and recurrence of cancer post-therapy. The study showed that the PCL-Fe_3O_4

TABLE 1.3 Summary of Other Technological Approaches Added to Nanotechnology to Improve the Topical Treatment of Skin Cancer

Type of Technology	Type of Nanocarrier/ Drug	Size (nm)	Test Model	Outcome	References
Iontophoresis	Solid lipid nanoparticle/ doxorubicin	136	*In vitro*: pig ears. *In vivo*: nude BALB/c mice	*In vitro*-passive conditions: increased the penetration 2.7-fold in the stratum corneum and 3.4-fold in the viable epidermis. *In vitro*-iontophoretic conditions: increased the penetration 59.9-fold in the stratum corneum and 41.2-fold in the viable epidermis. *In vivo* antitumor potential: effective inhibition of tumor cell survival and tumor growth, increased keratinization, and cell death.	Huber et al. (2015a)
Hyperthermia therapy	PCL-Fe_3O_4 nanofibrous/ Doxorubicin.	100–1,000	BALB/c mice (*in vivo*).	Complete recovery of tumors within a month after five hyperthermic doses for 15 minutes, without any sign of inflammation and recurrence of cancer post-therapy.	Suneet, De, & Jain (2020)
Microneedling	MPEG-PCL nanoparticle/5-Fu and indocyanine green.	217	BALB/cA-nu mice (*in vivo*)	Most outstanding tumor inhibition compared to controls, and the mice were all cured without recurrence.	Hao et al. (2020a)
	Zeolitic imidazolate framework-8 nanoparticle/ camptothecin.	50	C57BL/6 female mice (*in vivo*).	The tumor grew merely to 190 mm^3 on the 12th day, which was smaller than the control groups.	Zhao et al. (2021)
	Lipid nanoparticle/ cisplatin and anti-PD-1.	57.6	Male and female. C_3H/HeJ mice (*in vivo*).	75.95% of infiltration of CD^{8+} T-cells among tumor cells. The tumor volume (18.312 ± 8.286 mm^3) and tumor weight (0.012 ± 0.005 g) were significantly decreased compared to the control (tumor volume of 192.799 ± 79.824 mm^3 and tumor weight of 0.219 ± 0.061 g).	Lan et al. (2020)

nanofibrous-based bandages could effectively treat skin cancer with the help of an external alternating current magnetic field (Suneet, De, & Jain, 2020).

Microneedles are minimally invasive devices fabricated by micro-nano-processing technology. It can penetrate the SC of the skin or the mucosa, allowing a transdermal delivery through mechanical microchannels. This highly efficient system can conveniently transport drugs, proteins, genes, RNA, vaccines, and other biological macromolecules (Hao et al., 2020a; Kennedy et al., 2017; Lan et al., 2020; Zhao et al., 2021).

A near-infrared light-responsive 5-Fu and indocyanine green (as a photothermal agent) loaded monomethoxy-poly(ethylene glycol)-polycaprolactone (MPEG-PCL) nanoparticle was developed and integrated with a hyaluronic acid dissolvable microneedle system. *In vivo* experiments were performed to evaluate the system's antitumor ability. Results showed that the intratumor administration of the developed nanosystem under photothermal and microneedle therapy exhibited the most significant tumor inhibition compared to the controls, and the mice were all cured without recurrence (Hao et al., 2020a).

A multifunctional metal-organic nanoparticle-integrated dissolving microneedle DDS was similarly constructed as a new approach to skin cancer therapy. The nanoparticle was prepared based on the framework incorporating the photothermal agent copper sulfide (CuS) into zeolitic imidazolate framework-8 and functionalized by hyaluronic acid, which also encapsulated the chemotherapeutic drug, camptothecin. The tumor in mice treated with the developed nanoparticle, added to the microneedle delivery and photothermal therapy, had the lowest weight compared to controls. It grew merely to 190 mm^3 on the 12th day, which was almost negligible than the control groups (Zhao et al., 2021).

A lipid nanoparticle was developed encapsulating both chemotherapeutic–cisplatin and immunotherapeutic agents–anti-programed cell death protein-1 (PD-1) – added to this technology was used the microneedle-mediated local delivery device. In such a case, the nanoparticle delivered through microneedles effectively boosted the immune response, exhibiting the highest T-cell infiltration, 75.95% of CD^{8+} T-cells among tumor cells. Thereby, a remarkable effect on tumor regression was realized. The anti-tumor efficiency *in vivo* exhibited that the tumor weight of the developed nanoparticle delivered through microneedles showed the most notable tumor regression effect compared with any other group. The tumor volume (18.312 $\pm$ 8.286 mm^3) and tumor weight (0.012 $\pm$ 0.005 g) of the group treated with the nanoformulation delivered through microneedles were significantly decreased compared to its control, which presented a tumor volume of 192.799 ± 79.824 mm^3 and a tumor weights of 0.219 ± 0.061 g (Lan et al., 2020). Such results have implied that the microneedle system has a broad application prospect for skin cancer treatment. Moreover, when acting synergistically with other therapies, such as chemotherapy and photothermal therapy, this device can improve the anticancer action of drugs, resulting in promising outcomes.

1.6 CONCLUSION

The improved formulations for skin cancer treatment with nanotechnology have shown promising results with several therapeutic advantages, such as increased drug penetration, higher stability, increased safety, and more outstanding biocompatibility. In addition, current studies have shown that the addition of nanotechnology to the use of physical methods capable of promoting permeation could further improve the bioavailability of drugs. In this way, the synergistic action of these two approaches may allow the treatment against skin cancer to achieve results that are even more promising.

KEYWORDS

- **biocompatibility**
- **iontophoresis**
- **microneedling**
- **nanocarriers**
- **nanotechnology**
- **skin cancer**
- **topical delivery**

REFERENCES

Abdel, F. D. A., Kamel, R., & Fadel, M., (2020). PEGylated lipid nanocarrier for enhancing photodynamic therapy of skin carcinoma using curcumin: In-vitro/in-vivo studies and histopathological examination. *Scientific Reports, 10*(1), 1–10. https://doi.org/10.1038/s41598-020-67349-z.

Aghebati-Maleki, A., Dolati, S., Ahmadi, M., Baghbanzhadeh, A., Asadi, M., Fotouhi, A., Yousefi, M., & Aghebati-Maleki, L., (2020). Nanoparticles and cancer therapy: Perspectives for application of nanoparticles in the treatment of cancers. *Journal of Cellular Physiology, 235*(3), 1962–1972. https://doi.org/10.1002/jcp.29126.

Ahmad, N., Ahmad, R., Mohammed, B. T., Al Homoud, S. H., Al-Nasif, H. A., & Sarafroz, M., (2020). A comparative *ex vivo* permeation evaluation of a novel 5-fluorocuracil nanoemulsion-gel by topically applied in the different excised rat, goat, and cow skin. *Saudi Journal of Biological Sciences, 27*(4), 1024–1040. https://doi.org/10.1016/j.sjbs.2020.02.014.

Allemani, C., Matsuda, T., Di Carlo, V., Harewood, R., Matz, M., Nikšić, M., Bonaventure, A., et al., (2018). Global surveillance of trends in cancer survival 2000-14 (CONCORD-3): Analysis of individual records for 37 513 025 patients diagnosed with one of 18 cancers from 322 population-based registries in 71 countries. *The Lancet, 391*(10125), 1023–1075. https://doi.org/10.1016/S0140-6736(17)33326-3.

Almomen, A., El-Toni, A. M., Badran, M., Alhowyan, A., Kalam, M. A., Alshamsan, A., & Alkholief, M., (2020). The design of anionic surfactant-based amino-functionalized mesoporous silica nanoparticles and their application in transdermal drug delivery. *Pharmaceutics, 12*(11), 1–19. https://doi.org/10.3390/pharmaceutics12111035.

Alvarez-Figueroa, M. J., Narváez-Araya, D., Armijo-Escalona, N., Carrasco-Flores, E. A., & González-Aramundiz, J. V., (2020). Design of chitosan nanocapsules with compritol 888 ATO® for imiquimod transdermal administration. Evaluation of their skin absorption by Raman microscopy. *Pharmaceutical Research, 37*(10), 195. https://doi.org/10.1007/s11095-020-02925-6.

Ascierto, P. A., Del Vecchio, M., Mandalá, M., Gogas, H., Arance, A. M., Dalle, S., Cowey, C. L., et al., (2020). Adjuvant nivolumab versus ipilimumab in resected stage IIIB–C and stage IV melanoma (CheckMate 238): 4-year results from a multicenter, double-blind, randomized, controlled, phase 3 trial. *The Lancet Oncology, 21*(11), 1465–1477. https://doi.org/10.1016/S1470-2045(20)30494-0.

Bellefroid, C., Lechanteur, A., Evrard, B., Mottet, D., Debacq-Chainiaux, F., & Piel, G., (2019). *In vitro* skin penetration enhancement techniques: A combined approach of ethosomes and microneedles. *International Journal of Pharmaceutics, 572*, 118793. https://doi.org/10.1016/j.ijpharm.2019.118793.

Bertrand, J. U., Steingrimsson, E., Jouenne, F., Bressac-De, P. B., & Larue, L., (2020). Melanoma risk and melanocyte biology. In: *Acta Dermato-Venereologica* (Vol. 100, Issue 100-year theme Skin malignancies, pp. 272–283). Medical Journals/Acta D-V. https://doi.org/10.2340/00015555-3494.

Bharadwaj, R., Das, P. J., Pal, P., & Mazumder, B., (2016). Topical delivery of paclitaxel for treatment of skin cancer. *Drug Development and Industrial Pharmacy, 42*(9), 1482–1494. https://doi.org/10.3109/03639045.2016.1151028.

Brandt, M. G., & Moore, C. C., (2019). Nonmelanoma skin cancer. In: *Facial Plastic Surgery Clinics of North America* (Vol. 27, No. 1, pp. 1–13). W.B. Saunders. https://doi.org/10.1016/j.fsc.2018.08.001.

Bray, F., Ferlay, J., Soerjomataram, I., Siegel, R. L., Torre, L. A., & Jemal, A., (2018). Global cancer statistics 2018: GLOBOCAN estimates of incidence and mortality worldwide for 36 cancers in 185 countries. *CA: A Cancer Journal for Clinicians, 68*(6), 394–424. https://doi.org/10.3322/caac.21492.

Bucko, A. D., Jarratt, M., Stough, D. B., Kyhl, L., Villumsen, J., & Hall, A., (2018). Pharmacokinetics of ingenol mebutate gel under maximum use conditions in large treatment areas. *Journal of Dermatological Treatment*, *29*(1), 74–79. https://doi.org/10.1080/09546634.2017.1329506.

Byrne, J. D., Yeh, J. J., & DeSimone, J. M., (2018). Use of iontophoresis for the treatment of cancer. *Journal of Controlled Release*, *284*, 144–151. https://doi.org/10.1016/j.jconrel.2018.06.020.

Calienni, M. N., Febres-Molina, C., Llovera, R. E., Zevallos-Delgado, C., Tuttolomondo, M. E., Paolino, D., Fresta, M., et al., (2019). Nanoformulation for potential topical delivery of Vismodegib in skin cancer treatment. *International Journal of Pharmaceutics*, *565*, 108–122. https://doi.org/10.1016/j.ijpharm.2019.05.002.

Carr, S., Smith, C., & Wernberg, J., (2020). Epidemiology and risk factors of melanoma. In: *Surgical Clinics of North America* (Vol. 100, No. 1, pp. 1–12). W.B. Saunders. https://doi.org/10.1016/j.suc.2019.09.005.

Catalano, O., Roldán, F. A., Varelli, C., Bard, R., Corvino, A., & Wortsman, X., (2019). Skin cancer: Findings and role of high-resolution ultrasound. In: *Journal of Ultrasound* (Vol. 22, No. 4, pp. 423–431). Springer Science+Business Media. https://doi.org/10.1007/s40477-019-00379-0.

Cheng, Y., Chang, Y., Feng, Y., Liu, N., Sun, X., Feng, Y., Li, X., & Zhang, H., (2017). Simulated sunlight-mediated photodynamic therapy for melanoma skin cancer by titanium-dioxide-nanoparticle–gold-nanocluster–graphene heterogeneous nanocomposites. *Small*, *13*(20), 1–12. https://doi.org/10.1002/smll.201603935.

Chi, Y. F., Qin, J. J., Li, Z., Ge, Q., & Zeng, W. H., (2020). Enhanced anti-tumor efficacy of 5-aminolevulinic acid-gold nanoparticles-mediated photodynamic therapy in cutaneous squamous cell carcinoma cells. *Brazilian Journal of Medical and Biological Research*, *53*(5), 1–12. https://doi.org/10.1590/1414-431x20208457.

Collins, A., Savas, J., & Doerfler, L., (2019). Nonsurgical treatments for nonmelanoma skin cancer. In: *Dermatologic Clinics* (Vol. 37, No. 4, pp. 435–441). W.B. Saunders. https://doi.org/10.1016/j.det.2019.05.003.

Cuevas, L., & Daud, A., (2018). Immunotherapy for melanoma. *Seminars in Cutaneous Medicine and Surgery*, *37*(2), 127–131. https://doi.org/10.12788/j.sder.2018.028.

Cullen, J. K., Simmons, J. L., Parsons, P. G., & Boyle, G. M., (2020). Topical treatments for skin cancer. In: *Advanced Drug Delivery Reviews* (Vol. 153, pp. 54–64). Elsevier B.V. https://doi.org/10.1016/j.addr.2019.11.002.

Darp, R., & Ceol, C., (2021). Making a melanoma: Molecular and cellular changes underlying melanoma initiation. *Pigment Cell and Melanoma Research*, *34*(2), 280–287. https://doi.org/10.1111/pcmr.12950.

Davis, L. E., Shalin, S. C., & Tackett, A. J., (2019). Current state of melanoma diagnosis and treatment. In: *Cancer Biology and Therapy* (Vol. 20, No. 11, pp. 1366–1379). Taylor and Francis Inc. https://doi.org/10.1080/15384047.2019.1640032.

Dias, M. F., Figueiredo, B. C. P. De., Teixeira-Neto, J., Guerra, M. C. A., Fialho, S. L., & Silva, C. A., (2018). *In vivo* evaluation of antitumoral and antiangiogenic effect of imiquimod-loaded polymeric nanoparticles. *Biomedicine and Pharmacotherapy*, *103*, 1107–1114. https://doi.org/10.1016/j.biopha.2018.04.079.

Eggermont, A. M. M., Chiarion-Sileni, V., Grob, J. J., Dummer, R., Wolchok, J. D., Schmidt, H., Hamid, O., et al., (2019). Adjuvant ipilimumab versus placebo after complete resection of stage III melanoma: Long-term follow-up results of the European organization for research and treatment of cancer 18071 double-blind phase 3 randomized trial. *European Journal of Cancer*, *119*, 1–10. https://doi.org/10.1016/j.ejca.2019.07.001.

García-de-la-Fuente, M. R., Santacana, M., Verdaguer, J., Vilardell, F., Garí, E., & Casanova, J. M., (2020). Characterization of the inflammatory response triggered by topical ingenol mebutate 0.05% gel in basal cell carcinoma. *Australasian Journal of Dermatology*, *61*(2), e200–e207. https://doi.org/10.1111/ajd.13229.

Giacone, D. V., Dartora, V. F. M. C., De Matos, J. K. R., Passos, J. S., Miranda, D. A. G., De Oliveira, E. A., Silveira, E. R., et al., (2020). Effect of nanoemulsion modification with chitosan and sodium alginate on the topical delivery and efficacy of the cytotoxic agent piplartine in 2D and 3D skin cancer models. *International Journal of Biological Macromolecules*, *165*, 1055–1065. https://doi.org/10.1016/j.ijbiomac.2020.09.167.

Goyal, N., Thatai, P., & Sapra, B., (2017). Skin cancer: Symptoms, mechanistic pathways, and treatment rationale for therapeutic delivery. *Therapeutic Delivery*, *8*(5), 265–287. https://doi.org/10.4155/tde-2016-0093.

Gutzmer, R., Stroyakovskiy, D., Gogas, H., Robert, C., Lewis, K., Protsenko, S., Pereira, R. P., et al., (2020). Atezolizumab, vemurafenib, and cobimetinib as first-line treatment for unresectable advanced BRAFV600 mutation-positive melanoma (IMspire150): Primary analysis of the randomized, double-blind, placebo-controlled, phase 3 trial. *The Lancet*, *395*(10240), 1835–1844. https://doi.org/10.1016/S0140-6736(20)30934-X.

Hao, Y., Chen, Y. W., He, X. L., Yang, F., Han, R. X., Yang, C. L., Li, W., & Qian, Z. Y., (2020a). Near-infrared responsive 5-fluorouracil and indocyanine green loaded MPEG-PCL nanoparticle integrated with dissolvable microneedle for skin cancer therapy. *Bioactive Materials*, *5*(3), 542–552. https://doi.org/10.1016/j.bioactmat.2020.04.002.

Hao, Y., Chen, Y. W., He, X. L., Yang, F., Han, R. X., Yang, C. L., Li, W., & Qian, Z. Y., (2020b). Near-infrared responsive 5-fluorouracil and indocyanine green loaded MPEG-PCL nanoparticle integrated with dissolvable microneedle for skin cancer therapy. *Bioactive Materials*, *5*(3), 542–552. https://doi.org/10.1016/j.bioactmat.2020.04.002.

Haque, T., Rahman, K. M., Thurston, D. E., Hadgraft, J., & Lane, M. E., (2015). Topical therapies for skin cancer and actinic keratosis. In: *European Journal of Pharmaceutical Sciences* (Vol. 77, pp. 279–289). Elsevier B.V. https://doi.org/10.1016/j.ejps.2015.06.013.

Honors, C. N., Kruger, C. A., & Abrahamse, H., (2018). Photodynamic therapy for metastatic melanoma treatment: A review. In: *Technology in Cancer Research and Treatment* (Vol. 17). SAGE Publications Inc. https://doi.org/10.1177/1533033818791795.

Huber, L. A., Pereira, T. A., Ramos, D. N., Rezende, L. C. D., Emery, F. S., Sobral, L. M., Leopoldino, A. M., & Lopez, R. F. V., (2015a). Topical skin cancer therapy using doxorubicin-loaded cationic lipid nanoparticles and iontophoresis. *Journal of Biomedical Nanotechnology*, *11*(11), 1975–1988. https://doi.org/10.1166/jbn.2015.2139.

Huber, L. A., Pereira, T. A., Ramos, D. N., Rezende, L. C. D., Emery, F. S., Sobral, L. M., Leopoldino, A. M., & Lopez, R. F. V., (2015b). Topical skin cancer therapy using doxorubicin-loaded cationic lipid nanoparticles and iontophoresis. *Journal of Biomedical Nanotechnology*, *11*(11), 1975–1988. https://doi.org/10.1166/jbn.2015.2139.

Hussain, A., Samad, A., Ramzan, M., Ahsan, M. N., Ur Rehman, Z., & Ahmad, F. J., (2016). Elastic liposome-based gel for topical delivery of 5-fluorouracil: *In vitro* and *in vivo* investigation. *Drug Delivery*, *23*(4), 1115–1129. https://doi.org/10.3109/10717544.2014.976891.

Iqubal, M. K., Iqubal, A., Imtiyaz, K., Rizvi, M. M. A., Gupta, M. M., Ali, J., & Baboota, S., (2021). Combinatorial lipid-nanosystem for dermal delivery of 5-fluorouracil and resveratrol against skin cancer: Delineation of improved dermatokinetics and epidermal drug deposition enhancement analysis. *European Journal of Pharmaceutics and Biopharmaceutics*, *163*, 223–239. https://doi.org/10.1016/j.ejpb.2021.04.007.

Katharotiya, K., Shinde, G., Katharotiya, D., Shelke, S., Patel, R., Kulkarni, D., & Panzade, P., (2021). Development, evaluation and biodistribution of stealth liposomes of 5-fluorouracil for effective treatment of breast cancer. *Journal of Liposome Research*, 1–13. https://doi.org/10.1080/08982104.2021.1905661.

Kennedy, J., Larrañeta, E., McCrudden, M. T. C., McCrudden, C. M., Brady, A. J., Fallows, S. J., McCarthy, H. O., et al., (2017). *In vivo* studies investigating biodistribution of nanoparticle-encapsulated rhodamine B delivered via dissolving microneedles. *Journal of Controlled Release*, *265*, 57–65. https://doi.org/10.1016/j.jconrel.2017.04.022.

Keyal, U., Luo, Q., Bhatta, A. K., Luan, H., Zhang, P., Wu, Q., Zhang, H., et al., (2018). Zinc pthalocyanine-loaded chitosan/mPEG-PLA nanoparticles-mediated photodynamic therapy for the treatment of cutaneous squamous cell carcinoma. *Journal of Biophotonics*, *11*(11). https://doi.org/10.1002/jbio.201800114.

Krishnan, V., & Mitragotri, S., (2020). Nanoparticles for topical drug delivery: Potential for skin cancer treatment. *Advanced Drug Delivery Reviews*, *153*, 87–108. https://doi.org/10.1016/j.addr.2020.05.011.

Lan, X., Zhu, W., Huang, X., Yu, Y., Xiao, H., Jin, L., Pu, J. J., et al., (2020). Microneedles loaded with anti-PD-1-cisplatin nanoparticles for synergistic cancer immuno-chemotherapy. *Nanoscale*, *12*(36), 18885–18898. https://doi.org/10.1039/d0nr04213g.

Larkin, J., Chiarion-Sileni, V., Gonzalez, R., Grob, J. J., Rutkowski, P., Lao, C. D., Cowey, C. L., et al., (2019). Five-year survival with combined nivolumab and ipilimumab in advanced melanoma. *New England Journal of Medicine*, *381*(16), 1535–1546. https://doi.org/10.1056/nejmoa1910836.

Leachman, S. A., Lucero, O. M., Sampson, J. E., Cassidy, P., Bruno, W., Queirolo, P., & Ghiorzo, P., (2017). Identification, genetic testing, and management of hereditary melanoma. *Cancer and Metastasis Reviews*, *36*(1), 77–90. https://doi.org/10.1007/s10555-017-9661-5.

Leonardi, G. C., Falzone, L., Salemi, R., Zanghì, A., Spandidos, D. A., Mccubrey, J. A., Candido, S., & Libra, M., (2018). Cutaneous melanoma: From pathogenesis to therapy (review). In: *International Journal of Oncology* (Vol. 52, No. 4, pp. 1071–1080). Spandidos Publications. https://doi.org/10.3892/ijo.2018.4287.

Li, X. Y., Tan, L. C., Dong, L. W., Zhang, W. Q., Shen, X. X., Lu, X., Zheng, H., & Lu, Y. G., (2020). Susceptibility and resistance mechanisms during photodynamic therapy of melanoma. In: *Frontiers in Oncology* (Vol. 10). Frontiers Media S.A. https://doi.org/10.3389/fonc.2020.00597.

Li, X., & Cai, Y., (2019). Better prognostic determination and feature characterization of cutaneous melanoma through integrative genomic analysis. *Aging*, *11*(14), 5081–5107. https://doi.org/10.18632/aging.102099.

Lo, J. A., & Fisher, D. E., (2014). The melanoma revolution: From UV carcinogenesis to a new era in therapeutics. *Science*, *346*(6212), 945–949. https://doi.org/10.1126/science.1253735.

Luke, J. J., Flaherty, K. T., Ribas, A., & Long, G. V., (2017). Targeted agents and immunotherapies: Optimizing outcomes in melanoma. *Nature Reviews Clinical Oncology*, *14*(8), 463–482. https://doi.org/10.1038/nrclinonc.2017.43.

Macdonald, E. J., (1975). Epidemiology of melanoma. *Progress in Clinical Cancer*, *6*, 139–149. https://doi.org/10.3390/medsci9040063.

Mkhobongo, B., Chandran, R., & Abrahamse, H., (2021). The role of melanoma cell-derived exosomes (Mtex) and photodynamic therapy (pdt) within a tumor microenvironment. In: *International Journal of Molecular Sciences* (Vol. 22, No. 18). MDPI. https://doi.org/10.3390/ijms22189726.

Moser, J., & Grossman, K., (2018). Adjuvant therapy for resected high-risk melanoma. *Seminars in Cutaneous Medicine and Surgery*, *37*(2), 109–111. https://doi.org/10.12788/j.sder.2018.022.

Ostrowski, S. M., & Fisher, D. E., (2021). Biology of melanoma. In: *Hematology/Oncology Clinics of North America* (Vol. 35, No. 1, pp. 29–56). W.B. Saunders. https://doi.org/10.1016/j.hoc.2020.08.010.

Paolino, D., Celia, C., Trapasso, E., Cilurzo, F., & Fresta, M., (2012). Paclitaxel-loaded ethosomes®: Potential treatment of squamous cell carcinoma, a malignant transformation of actinic keratoses. *European Journal of Pharmaceutics and Biopharmaceutics*, *81*(1), 102–112. https://doi.org/10.1016/j.ejpb.2012.02.008.

Patton, E. E., Mueller, K. L., Adams, D. J., Anandasabapathy, N., Aplin, A. E., Bertolotto, C., Bosenberg, M., et al., (2021). Melanoma models for the next generation of therapies. In: *Cancer Cell* (Vol. 39, No. 5, pp. 610–631). Cell Press. https://doi.org/10.1016/j.ccell.2021.01.011.

Pomerantz, H., Korgavkar, K., Lee, K. C., Lew, R., & Weinstock, M. A., (2016). Validation of photograph-based toxicity score for topical 5-fluorouracil cream application. *Journal of Cutaneous Medicine and Surgery*, *20*(5), 458–466. https://doi.org/10.1177/1203475416643952.

Quaresmini, D., & Guida, M., (2020). Neoangiogenesis in melanoma: An issue in biology and systemic treatment. In: *Frontiers in Immunology* (Vol. 11). Frontiers Media S.A. https://doi.org/10.3389/fimmu.2020.584903.

Raimondi, S., Suppa, M., & Gandini, S., (2020). Melanoma epidemiology and sun exposure. *Acta Dermato-Venereologica*, *100*(100-year theme Skin Malignancies), 250–258. https://doi.org/10.2340/00015555-3491.

Rata, D. M., Cadinoiu, A. N., Atanase, L. I., Popa, M., Mihai, C. T., Solcan, C., Ochiuz, L., & Vochita, G., (2020). Topical formulations containing aptamer-functionalized nanocapsules loaded with 5-fluorouracil – an innovative concept for the skin cancer therapy. *Materials Science and Engineering C*, *119*(11), 111591. https://doi.org/10.1016/j.msec.2020.111591.

Reis, S. R. R., Helal-Neto, E., Da Silva De, B. A. O., Pinto, S. R., Portilho, F. L., De Oliveira, S. L. B., Alencar, L. M. R., et al., (2021). Dual encapsulated dacarbazine and zinc phthalocyanine polymeric nanoparticle for photodynamic therapy of melanoma. *Pharmaceutical Research*, *38*(2), 335–346. https://doi.org/10.1007/s11095-021-02999-w.

Robert, C., Ribas, A., Schachter, J., Arance, A., Grob, J. J., Mortier, L., Daud, A., et al., (2019). Pembrolizumab versus ipilimumab in advanced melanoma (KEYNOTE-006): Post-hoc 5-year results from an open-label, multicenter, randomized, controlled, phase 3 study. *The Lancet Oncology*, *20*(9), 1239–1251. https://doi.org/10.1016/S1470-2045(19)30388-2.

Rosenberg, A. R., Tabacchi, M., Ngo, K. H., Wallendorf, M., Rosman, I. S., Cornelius, L. A., & Demehri, S., (2019). Skin cancer precursor immunotherapy for squamous cell carcinoma prevention. *JCI Insight*, *4*(6). https://doi.org/10.1172/jci.insight.125476.

Safwat, M. A., Soliman, G. M., Sayed, D., & Attia, M. A., (2018). Fluorouracil-loaded gold nanoparticles for the treatment of skin cancer: Development, *in vitro* characterization, and *in vivo* evaluation in a mouse skin cancer xenograft model. *Molecular Pharmaceutics*, *15*(6), 2194–2205. https://doi.org/10.1021/acs.molpharmaceut.8b00047.

Sahu, P., Kashaw, S. K., Sau, S., Kushwah, V., Jain, S., Agrawal, R. K., & Iyer, A. K., (2019). pH responsive 5-fluorouracil loaded biocompatible nanogels for topical chemotherapy of aggressive melanoma. *Colloids and Surfaces B: Biointerfaces*, *174*, 232–245. https://doi.org/10.1016/j.colsurfb.2018.11.018.

Sapino, S., Oliaro-Bosso, S., Zonari, D., Zattoni, A., & Ugazio, E., (2017). Mesoporous silica nanoparticles as a promising skin delivery system for methotrexate. *International Journal of Pharmaceutics*, *530*(1, 2), 239–248. https://doi.org/10.1016/j.ijpharm.2017.07.058.

Schadendorf, D., Fisher, D. E., Garbe, C., Gershenwald, J. E., Grob, J. J., Halpern, A., Herlyn, M., et al., (2015). Melanoma. *Nature Reviews Disease Primers*, *1*. https://doi.org/10.1038/nrdp.2015.3.

Shain, A. H., & Bastian, B. C., (2016). From melanocytes to melanomas. *Nature Reviews Cancer*, *16*(6), 345–358. https://doi.org/10.1038/nrc.2016.37.

Shtivelman, E., Davies, M. A., Hwu, P., Yang, J., Lotem, M., Oren, M., Flaherty, K. T., & Fisher, D. E., (2014). Pathways and therapeutic targets in melanoma. *Oncotarget*, *5*(7), 1701–1752. https://doi.org/10.18632/oncotarget.1892.

Siller, G., Rosen, R., Freeman, M., Welburn, P., Katsamas, J., & Ogbourne, S. M., (2010). PEP005 (ingenol mebutate) gel for the topical treatment of superficial basal cell carcinoma: Results of a randomized phase IIa trial. *Australasian Journal of Dermatology*, *51*(2), 99–105. https://doi.org/10.1111/j.1440-0960.2010.00626.x.

Sinx, K. A. E., Nelemans, P. J., Kelleners-Smeets, N. W. J., Winnepenninckx, V. J. L., Arits, A. H. M. M., & Mosterd, K., (2020). Surgery versus combined treatment with curettage and imiquimod for nodular basal cell carcinoma: One-year results of a noninferiority, randomized, controlled trial. *Journal of the American Academy of Dermatology*, *83*(2), 469–476. https://doi.org/10.1016/j.jaad.2020.04.053.

Soni, K., Mujtaba, A., Akhter, M. H., Zafar, A., & Kohli, K., (2020). Optimization of ethosomal nanogel for topical nano-CUR and sulphoraphane delivery in effective skin cancer therapy. *Journal of Microencapsulation*, *37*(2), 91–108. https://doi.org/10.1080/02652048.2019.1701114.

Suneet, K., De, T., & Jain, S., (2020). Magnetic nanofibers-based bandage for skin cancer treatment: A non-invasive hyperthermia therapy. *Cancer Reports*, *3*(6), e1281. https://doi.org/10.1002/cnr2.1281.

Suneet, K., De, T., Rangarajan, A., & Jain, S., (2020). Magnetic nanofibers-based bandage for skin cancer treatment: A non-invasive hyperthermia therapy. *Cancer Reports*, *3*(6). https://doi.org/10.1002/cnr2.1281.

Tawbi, H. A., Forsyth, P. A., Algazi, A., Hamid, O., Hodi, F. S., Moschos, S. J., Khushalani, N. I., et al., (2018). Combined nivolumab and ipilimumab in melanoma metastatic to the brain. *New England Journal of Medicine*, *379*(8), 722–730. https://doi.org/10.1056/nejmoa1805453.

Voiculescu, V. M., Lisievici, C. V., Lupu, M., Vajaitu, C., Draghici, C. C., Popa, A. V., Solomon, I., et al., (2019). Mediators of inflammation in topical therapy of skin cancers. In: *Mediators of Inflammation* (Vol. 2019). Hindawi Limited. https://doi.org/10.1155/2019/8369690.

Weinstock, M. A., Thwin, S. S., Siegel, J. A., Marcolivio, K., Means, A. D., Leader, N. F., Shaw, F. M., et al., (2018). Chemoprevention of basal and squamous cell carcinoma with a single course of fluorouracil, 5%, cream: A randomized clinical trial. *JAMA Dermatology*, *154*(2), 167–174. https://doi.org/10.1001/jamadermatol.2017.3631.

Wen, X., Li, Y., & Hamblin, M. R., (2017). Photodynamic therapy in dermatology beyond non-melanoma cancer: An update. In: *Photodiagnosis and Photodynamic Therapy* (Vol. 19, pp. 140–152). Elsevier B.V. https://doi.org/10.1016/j.pdpdt.2017.06.010.

Williams, H. C., Bath-Hextall, F., Ozolins, M., Armstrong, S. J., Colver, G. B., Perkins, W., & Miller, P. S. J., (2017). Surgery versus 5% imiquimod for nodular and superficial basal cell carcinoma: 5-year results of the SINS randomized controlled trial. *Journal of Investigative Dermatology*, *137*(3), 614–619. https://doi.org/10.1016/j.jid.2016.10.019.

Wu, J., Han, H., Jin, Q., Li, Z., Li, H., & Ji, J., (2017). Design and proof of programmed 5-aminolevulinic acid prodrug nanocarriers for targeted photodynamic cancer therapy. *ACS Applied Materials and Interfaces*, *9*(17), 14596–14605. https://doi.org/10.1021/acsami.6b15853.

Yeh, I., & Bastian, B. C., (2021). Melanoma pathology: New approaches and classification*. *British Journal of Dermatology*, *185*(2), 282–293. https://doi.org/10.1111/bjd.20427.

Yu, X., Du, L., Li, Y., Fu, G., & Jin, Y., (2015). Improved anti-melanoma effect of a transdermal mitoxantrone ethosome gel. *Biomedicine and Pharmacotherapy*, *73*, 6–11. https://doi.org/10.1016/j.biopha.2015.05.002.

Zhao, Y., Zhou, Y., Yang, D., Gao, X., Wen, T., Fu, J., Wen, X., et al., (2021). Intelligent and spatiotemporal drug release based on multifunctional nanoparticle-integrated dissolving microneedle system for synergetic chemo-photothermal therapy to eradicate melanoma. *Acta Biomaterialia*, *135*, 164–178. https://doi.org/10.1016/j.actbio.2021.09.009.

CHAPTER 2

Topical Nanotherapeutics for the Treatment of Acne Vulgaris

ZÍPORA MORGANA QUINTEIRO DOS SANTOS,[1,2] FÁTIMA REGINA ZAN,[3] VIRGINIA CIELO RECH,[1,2] and ALINE FERREIRA OURIQUE[1,2]

[1]*Laboratory of Nanotechnology, Universidade Franciscana, Santa Maria, Brazil*

[2]*Graduate Program in Nanosciences, Universidade Franciscana, Santa Maria, Brazil*

[3]*Director of Planning and Institutional Development, Instituto Federal Farroupilha, Santo Ângelo, Brazil*

ABSTRACT

Acne vulgaris an inflammatory skin disease which attack large portion of the world population, which is subject to multifactorial interpretation and is challenging to classify regarding severity and epidemiology. Global expenses for the treatment of acne vulgaris were estimated to account for more than 10% of general expenses for the treatment of skin disorders. However, the structural characteristics of the skin can be a barrier to the permeation of active ingredients, limiting the effectiveness of conventional topical products. The search for more effective therapeutic systems with fewer associated problems has proportionate to the creation of different nanocarriers, with the ability of vectorization, controlled and sustained release, greater permeation, and better stability of the active ingredients increasing their bioavailability and protecting the active substances from enzymatic degradation or chemical and increasing their bioavailability. This has increased therapeutic efficacy on the skin surface, improved permanence of the active

Novel Nanocarriers forSkin Diseases: Advances and Applications.
Raj K. Keservani and Júlia Scherer Santos (Eds.)

ingredient on the skin, resulted in products capable of adapting to the physiological variations of the skin, enhanced results even in lower percentages, granted to the sensory optimization in the application on the skin. Nanostructures such as liposomes, niosomes, ethosomes (ETOs), transferosomes, phytosomes, nanoemulsions, polymeric nanoparticles, lipid nanoparticles, micelles, fullerenes, dendrimers, and cyclodextrins (CDs) represent a recent trend towards improving the solubility/bioavailability of active substances, enabling effective application in the treatment of acne vulgaris.

2.1 INTRODUCTION

2.1.1 BACKGROUND ON ACNE VULGARIS AND TREATMENT TRENDS

The normal structure of the skin consists essentially of three large layers of tissue: a top layer – the epithelial portion of ectodermal origin, the epidermis; a middle layer – the conjunctival portion of mesodermal origin, the dermis or chorion; and a deep-conjunctival portion of mesodermal origin, the hypodermis or subcutaneous cellular tissue (Moniz et al., 2020).

Sebaceous glands are distributed throughout the skin, except for the palmoplantar regions. They are found in the dermis and its ducts always flow into the pilosebaceous follicle, with or without hair (Abdo et al., 2020). Under normal conditions, the size of the sebaceous glands is inversely proportional to the dimensions of the hair in the corresponding follicle (Roger et al., 2019).

The secretion of the sebaceous glands is of the holocrine type, and the product of its activity is an oily substance called *sebum* that covers not only the hair but also the surface of the skin; for its maintenance and texture, this product is released along with cellular debris. The activity of the sebaceous glands is stimulated by androgens and is independent of nerve stimulation (Vela-Romera et al., 2019).

Acne vulgaris is an inflammatory disease that affects and develops in the pilosebaceous follicle. It is considered the most prevalent skin disease in the world, affecting approximately 650 million people (about 9.4% of the world's population) (Ahmad et al., 2018; Sánchez-Dueñas & Tovar-Garza, 2019). It has multi-factorial origins, involving such factors as age, sex, stress, hereditary factors, hormonal factors, environmental factors, eating habits, hygiene habits, and use of comedogenic products, among others (dos Santos et al., 2020).

These factors are related to increased levels of dehydroepiandrosterone sulfate (DHEAS), hyperkeratinization with consequent obstruction of the follicular opening, and changes in sebum composition in the sebaceous gland, favoring the proliferation of the bacteria causing acne vulgaris, which leads to the release of such cytokines as interleukin-6 (IL-6) and interleukin-8 (IL-8) by infundibular keratinocytes and IL-8 and Interleukin-12 (IL-12) by macrophages, in addition to proinflammatory mediators, resulting in the induction of signaling in the pilosebaceous unit, an essential component in the initial process of acne lesions (Cunha et al., 2020; dos Santos et al., 2020).

In 2015, global expenses for the treatment of acne vulgaris were estimated to account for more than 10% of general expenses for the treatment of skin disorders (Lima, Barros, & Lúcio, 2020). In the United States alone, spending on the treatment of this pathology exceeded US$ 2 billion in 2017 (Augusto, 2017).

Studies have shown that this chronic dermatosis can manifest lesions in up to 99% of the face, 60% of the back and 15% of the chest (Flores-Rojas, Cabello-Carlos, & Paucar-Lescano, 2020), which are characterized by the presence of open comedones, closed comedones, papules, pustules, and in more advanced stages, some lesions with greater inflammation such as nodules, cysts, and abscesses (Lima, Barros, & Lúcio, 2020).

Although acne vulgaris is not accompanied by high morbidity and mortality, level of basic and supplementary conditions of human life is highly affected, and it can leave serious scars with consequent psychological impacts that may alter mood, self-esteem, and interpersonal relationships (Tasoula et al., 2012). This strengthens the need for timely and effective treatment to reduce sequelae (Sánchez-Dueñas & Tovar-Garza, 2019).

Topical treatment of this pathology is done in general with the use of antibiotics, retinoids, bactericides, seboregulators or keratolytics (Montagner & Costa, 2010; Sampaio & Bagatin, 2008). And although these products have significant effects in the treatment of acne vulgaris, their use against the acne-promoting bacteria *Cutibacterium acnes* (*C. acnes*), previous name *Propionibacterium acnes* (*P. acnes*) (Dréno et al., 2018), *Staphylococcus aureus* (*S. aureus*), and *Staphylococcus epidermidis* (*S. epidermidis*) may trigger non-tolerable adverse effects, such as non-acceptance of therapy by the patient, severe dryness of the skin, sensitization, burning sensation, peeling, erythema, dermatitis, allergies, sebocyte toxicity, dyschromias, in addition to bacterial resistance (Gollnick & Schramm, 1998; Purdy & de Berker, 2011; Tripathi et al., 2013).

Due to its multi-factorial nature and the clinical manifestations involved in this dermatosis, topical therapy is a challenge. In recent years, the diagnosis and classification of the severity of acne vulgaris have been studied extensively in order to update and develop new topical therapeutic options (Flores-Rojas, Cabello-Carlos, & Paucar-Lescano, 2020). It is known that people still prefer topical treatment to the use of other routes, obviously in order to minimize side effects (Działo et al., 2016; Kumar et al., 2007).

The history of cosmetics follows human history itself, and it has always been linked to man's scientific and cultural evolution. Archaeological evidence dates their first use to around 4000 BC as personal care products and later, as aids to in topical esthetic therapy (Kumar, 2005).

Although in the past they were considered luxury goods, the development of their formulations over the years changed their status to a skin therapeutic option, protection against solar radiation, preventive, and corrective care against unesthetic changes, and as aids for the improvement of physical appearance (in products popularly known as cosmeceuticals) (Lin, 2010). As such, pharmaceutical ingredients started being a part of cosmetic formulations, requiring greater rigor and investments from the industry (Oliveira et al., 2018).

Over the years, substances of synthetic origin and natural products or their derivatives have been widely employed in the topical treatment of skin dysfunctions and dermatological disorders. Historically, there have been reports of their use especially in the treatment of inflammations, wounds, cuts, and burns (Silva, 2009). However, the structural characteristics of the skin can be a barrier to the permeation of active ingredients, limiting the effectiveness of conventional topical products (Roger et al., 2019).

Nanotechnology innovations applied to the manufacture of new products have opened up great opportunities for development in various segments of the production chain, especially in the manipulation of nanostructured systems for dermal application through the use of natural products, raw materials, personal hygiene products or cosmetics (Prairna et al., 2020).

Positive expectations regarding the application potential of topical nanotherapeutics for the treatment of acne vulgaris are intensifying (Oliveira et al., 2018; dos Santos et al., 2019). However, even with the clear applications in clinical settings, few topical nanotherapeutics or nanocosmeceuticals (cosmetics with considerable pharmacological effects) are known to the population with regard to their active ingredients, effects, the nanostructures that compose them, and where to find them (Dhapte-Pawar et al., 2020).

Although science is continuously developing, there are still considerable gaps in knowledge regarding the applicability of the different topical nanostructures applied to the treatment of acne vulgaris. This justifies and encourages the increasing scientific research and technological interest. Figure 2.1 can serve as a demonstration of the evolution (in years) of the importance of this topic, revealing the growing interest in research involving the terms: "acne vulgaris*, nano* and topic*."

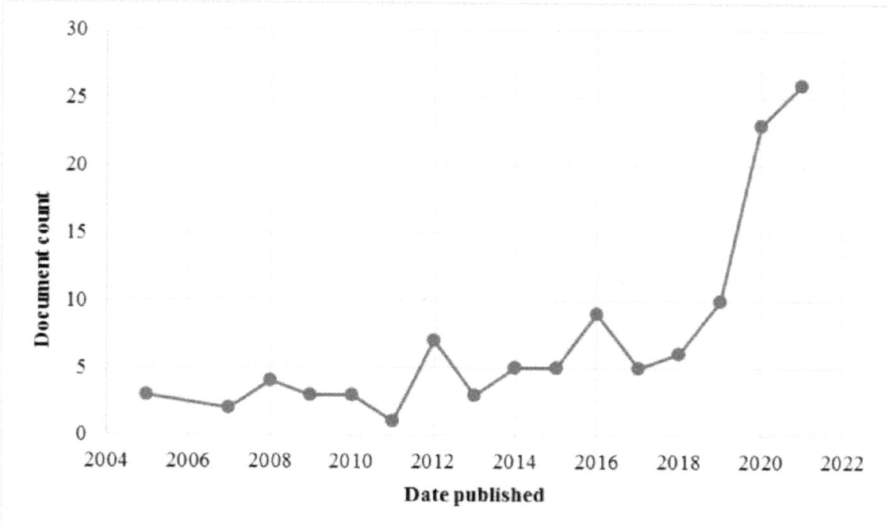

FIGURE 2.1 Scientific articles involving Acne Vulgaris * AND Nano * AND Topic * from 2005 to 2021.

2.2 TREATMENT OF ACNE VULGARIS

The classic treatment for acne vulgaris seeks to correct one or more factors related to its genesis. For a compound to be effective in treating acne vulgaris, it must be able to inhibit *C. acnes*, reduce pro-inflammatory lipids in sebocytes, and reduce the formation of post-acne scars (Ribeiro et al., 2015).

It is therefore desirable that the substances indicated for the control of acne vulgaris have an antioxidant, antibacterial, anti-inflammatory, seboregulatory, keratolytic, and healing activity (Figure 2.2) (Campos et al., 2007).

Substances intended for treatment range from the use of topical products to the use of oral and intravenous drugs (Dessinioti & Dreno, 2020). Although the use of these products may have significant effects in the treatment of acne vulgaris, they can trigger non-tolerable adverse effects (Sandru, 2019; Zasada & Budzisz, 2019). In addition, few of them are concerned about controlling oxidative stress, which can act as the "match" that ignites the cascade of events related to the clinical manifestations of acne vulgaris (dos Santos et al., 2019).

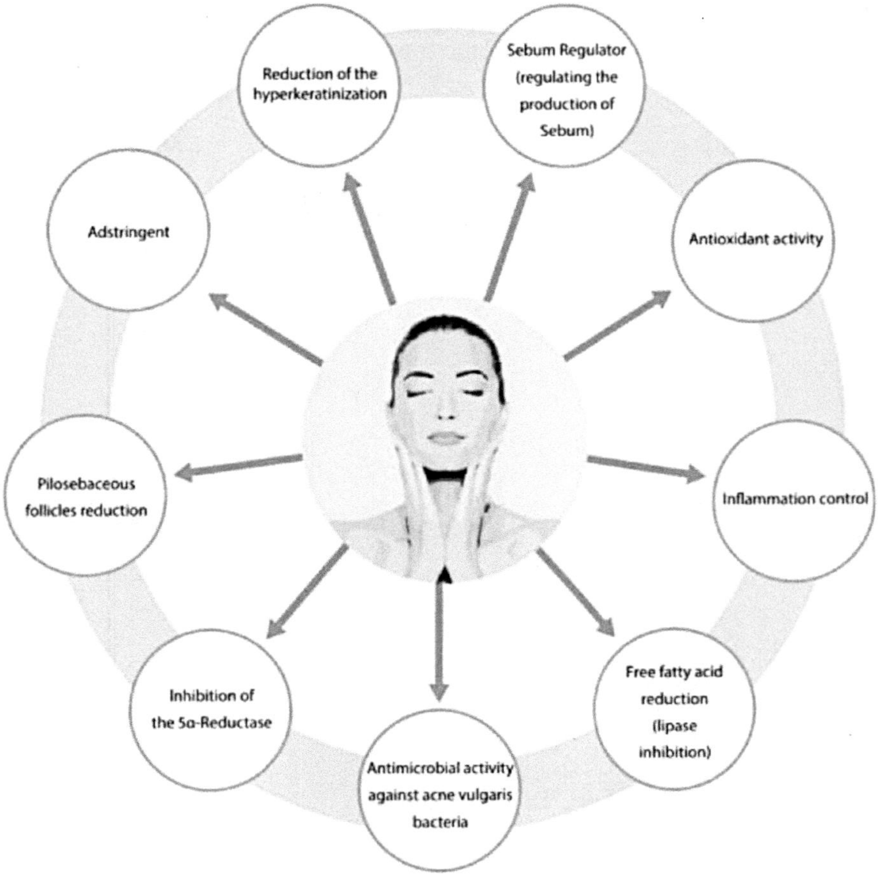

FIGURE 2.2 Flowchart of the expectations for an ideal treatment of acne vulgaris.

Bactericides such as benzoyl peroxide, sebostatic agents such as azelaic acid, topical antibiotics including clindamycin 1% and erythromycin 2%, dapsone 5% or 7.5%, and retinoids such as adapalene, isotretinoin, and tretinoin, are the first choice topical treatment agents for acne vulgaris (Montagner & Costa, 2010; Sampaio & Bagatin, 2008), but they have significant adverse effects (Table 2.1) such as burning sensation, erythema, dryness, peeling, hypersensitivity, photosensitivity, hypopigmentation, bacterial resistance, alteration of the skin's microbiota, and restriction of use for pregnant and lactating women (Gollnick & Schramm, 1998; Purdy & de Berker, 2011; Tripathi et al., 2013). Such adverse effects hinder the maintenance and adherence to treatment (da Silva et al., 2014; Thiboutot et al., 2009).

TABLE 2.1 Side Effects of the Main Compounds Administered in the Topical Therapeutic of Acne Vulgaris

Product	Erythema	Peeling	Burning Sensation	Resistance
Azelaic acid	Occasional	Occasional	Frequent	No
Benzoyl peroxide	Frequent	Frequent	Occasional	No
Adapalene	Occasional	Occasional	Occasional	No
Tretinoin	Very frequent	Very frequent	Frequent	No
Isotretinoin	Frequent	Frequent	Occasional	No
Clindamycin	Frequent	Frequent	Very occasional	Very frequent
Erythromycin	Frequent	Frequent	Very occasional	Very frequent
Dapsone	Occasional	Occasional	Very occasional	No

The therapeutic substances for acne vulgaris have changed little since the last decade, but the recognition that acne vulgaris is an inflammatory and non-transmissible condition has resulted in a reduction in the use of antibiotics, leading to a reassessment of therapeutic options by researchers and companies, and consequently, opening space for new therapeutic products, technologies, and complementary therapies for the treatment of acne vulgaris (Araviiskaia et al., 2019; Dikicier, 2019; Marson & Baldwin, 2019).

2.2.1 NATURAL PRODUCTS FOR THE TREATMENT OF ACNE VULGARIS

The use of natural products with the therapeutic purpose of preventing, treating, and curing diseases has accompanied humanity since the dawn of civilization (Lacerda et al., 2013; Maciel et al., 2002). Written records show that plants were being used as early as the II and III centuries BC. It is therefore believed that the use of plants for health disorders is as old as the human species (Andrade et al., 2007; Campesato, 2005). Such evidence demonstrates that knowledge about medicinal plants is often the only healer wellspring of a population (Megersa & Tamrat, 2022; Pan et al., 2014).

A vast body of popular knowledge has formed as a result of experimentation, trial-and-error, and especially, observation during the performance of treatment. The empirical use of natural products for therapeutic purposes was followed by evaluation, however rough and imperfect, of the signs and symptoms that appeared after their use in order to classify whether the plant species were beneficial or not based on the quality of the response (Maciel et al., 2002). This reinforces that popular knowledge is the basis of scientific development in many situations (Pan et al., 2014).

At the end of the 18th century, the active constituents of the products of natural origin endowed with medicinal properties began being isolated and their chemical structures being determined (Campesato, 2005). Indirectly, this popular knowledge ignited the interest of researchers and much of this empirical knowledge was scientifically proven (Maciel et al., 2002), justifying the use of natural products as raw material for the synthesis of bioactive substances (Viegas et al., 2006).

As such, the need to expand therapeutic options using the resources of biodiversity drove the development of the pharmaceutical industry (Simões & Schenkel, 2002). Sources of natural substances, including plant-derived compounds, have been used as a strategy for obtaining new biologically active compounds because of their vast diversity in terms of structure and physicochemical and biological properties (Maciel et al., 2002). It is estimated that up to 30% of all products evaluated as therapeutic agents are derived from natural products (Calixto, 2005), but the term "natural products" should inspire caution, since it implies these products can be easily accessed, which can lead to adverse reactions and even compromise other therapies (Maciel et al., 2002; Simões & Schenkel, 2002; Viegas et al., 2006).

The therapeutic effect of plants or plant extracts and derivatives is very useful in the treatment of skin disorders because they have a wide distribution in nature, show benefits in the control and progression of acne vulgaris lesions, and have minor side effects, such as sensitization, dryness, peeling, and hyperchromias. Natural products that have currently been applied clinically for this therapy are gallic acid (Iriguchi, 2012), *Melaleuca alternifolia* (Ahmad & Popli, 2019), nicotinamide (Walocko et al., 2017), *Nigella sativa* (Aljabre et al., 2015), propolis (Barbosa et al., 2014), quercetin (Działo et al., 2016), and resveratrol (Taylor et al., 2014). Table 2.2 shows some characteristics of these compounds in the treatment of acne vulgaris.

2.2.2 COMPLEMENTARY TREATMENTS FOR ACNE VULGARIS

Other therapeutic options for acne vulgaris involve modalities such as:

1. **High Frequency (HF):** Equipment that uses HF alternating currents. When the electromagnetic currents come into contact with oxygen they cause ozone to form, exerting an oxidizing, bactericidal, healing, and antiseptic effect on acne lesions (Antonio et al., 2017; Coqueiro & Santos, 2019; Lovato et al., 2018).

TABLE 2.2 Compounds Commonly Administered in the Topical Therapeutic of Acne Vulgaris and Their Limitations on Application

Effect	Application for Acne Vulgaris	Limitations of Use
Gallic acid	Antioxidant (Kim et al., 2002), astringent, anti-inflammatory, anti-aging (Kroes et al., 1992), anti-seborrheic (Iriguchi, 2012).	Low solubility and high light sensitivity (Puton, 2019).
Melaleuca alternifolia	Bactericidal (Low et al., 2013), healing, antiseptic, anti-inflammatory (Hart et al., 2000), antioxidant (Zhang et al., 2018).	Can be easily absorbed into the skin, which points to caution in its application and the possibility of contact dermatitis in a hydroalcoholic vehicle (Andrade et al., 2018; Cross et al., 2008).
Nicotinamide	Anti-inflammatory (Franco Codevilla et al., 2015; Morganti et al., 2011), antimicrobial (Shahtalebi et al., 2014), whitening of residual hyperpigmentation, seboregulatory (Biedroń et al., 2008)	Hyperpigmentation, pruritus, erythema, burning sensation and irritation at the site of application (Mohammed et al., 2013; Morganti et al., 2011).
Nigella sativa	Anti-inflammatory (Amin & Hosseinzadeh, 2016), antioxidant, healing (Yaman et al., 2010), antibacterial (Chaieb et al., 2011; Hariharan et al., 2016; Jrah Harzallah et al., 2011), antimicrobial (Chaieb et al., 2011).	Can cause contact dermatitis, phototoxicity, and burning (Burits & Bucar, 2000; Eid et al., 2017; Hadi & Ashor, 2010).
Propolis	Healing, antioxidant (Barbosa et al., 2014; Bonamigo et al., 2017; Melo et al., 2012), antibacterial (Cao et al., 2017; Zaccaria et al., 2017), anti-inflammatory (Barbosa et al., 2014; Sforcin, 2007; Sforcin & Bankova, 2011; Volpi & Bergonzini, 2006), seboregulator (Mohammad Ali et al., 2015).	Can cause skin irritation and sensitization (Gregory et al., 2002).
Quercetin	Antioxidant, anti-inflammatory (Kwon et al., 2014; Li et al., 2016; Moon et al., 2003; Wang et al., 2013), reduces keloids and hypertrophic scars (Działo et al., 2016; Tsai et al., 2013), antimicrobial (Camargo et al., 2008; Działo et al., 2016).	Has difficult permeability and limited bioavailability, can be photodegraded (Baby et al., 2008; Gomathi et al., 2003; Scalia et al., 2013).
Resveratrol	Antioxidant (Kerem et al., 2006; Lange et al., 2009), anti-inflammatory (Baur & Sinclair, 2006; Chan, 2002), antimicrobial (Docherty et al., 2007; Pettit et al., 2009; Taylor et al., 2014), suppresses the growth of sebocytes (Kim et al., 2015), stimulates healing, reduces the proliferation of keratinocytes (Wu et al., 2014), reduces the formation of comedones (Fabbrocini et al., 2011).	Low bioavailability (Ndiaye et al., 2011), not very stable and can be photodegraded (Park & Boo, 2013).

2. **Microcurrents:** Subsensory electric current equipment. When the current is applied to the skin, it causes an increase in cutaneous microcirculation and consequently improves tissue nutrition and oxygenation, promoting anti-inflammatory, healing, and bactericidal effects and reducing the signs of edema (Gentzkow, 1993; Saniee et al., 2012; Trivedi et al., 2018).

3. **Cryotherapy:** Therapy that uses carbon dioxide (CO_2) or liquid nitrogen to cauterize localized and severe lesions that do not respond to topical and/or systemic treatment (Al-turfy, 2015; Zimmerman & Crawford, 2012).

4. **Laser Therapy and Photo Therapy:** Electromagnetic current equipment that uses a photosensitizer combined with a light and oxygen source to reorganize collagen in order to produce an anti-inflammatory, bactericidal effect and treat inflammatory, non-inflammatory, and moderate to severe acne (Boen et al., 2017; Marson & Baldwin, 2019).

5. **Techniques of Traditional Chinese Medicine (TCM):** Oriental techniques such as acupuncture, auriculotherapy, moxa therapy, cupping therapy and phytotherapy that seek to promote the homeostatic balance of the individual with acne vulgaris. These therapies approach the disorder both from the physical, psychic, emotional, and hormonal point of view and seek to reduce inflammation and the oiliness of the skin (Cao et al., 2013, 2016; Xu et al., 2013).

Although these alternative methods to the use of topical formulations may be indicated for the treatment of acne vulgaris, sufficient efficacy and safety information has not been found in the scientific literature. As such, the methodological limitations and quality of reports in the acne vulgaris studies weaken any evidence.

In addition, the application of these techniques has limitations, such as the high cost of treatment, the displacement of the patient to a center, the need for trained professionals for the handling of electrothermophototherapeutic equipment and the application of acupuncture, auriculotherapy, moxa therapy, or cupping techniques. There is therefore a need for innovative alternatives for the development of new treatments, such as the use of nanotechnology in the development of nanostructures for topical use, reducing the previously mentioned limitations of the compounds and optimizing their delivery at the desired site (Prairna et al., 2020).

2.3 FUNDAMENTALS OF NANOTECHNOLOGY

Nanoscience is a science with a high degree of interdisciplinarity that studies the fundamental principles of molecules and structures with a size between 1 and 100 nanometers (Riehemann et al., 2009; Stopar et al., 2016). To this end, it uses techniques from physics, biology, chemistry, medicine, materials engineering, and other sciences (Baril et al., 2012). Through these techniques, it is possible to discover new properties of materials, enabling the application of innovative products for society (Fernandes & Filgueiras, 2008).

Nanotechnology is an innovative scientific field that includes the design, production, characterization, and application of materials, devices, and systems, controlling the manipulation of atoms at the nanometer scale (1 nm = 10^{-9} m), enabling the creation of new organizational structures that have different behaviors and properties than the currently known materials (Quevedo, 2019).

With the growing use of nanostructured products, the concept of nanotechnology has aroused metrological controversies regarding what is to be considered for nano-scale classifications (Bailo, 2018; Martines et al., 2016).

The International Organization for Standardization (ISO) established criteria for defining nanotechnology through the technical specifications (ISO/TS) 27,687 of 2008 and Technical Committee (ISO/TC) 229 of 2005. These criteria involve the responsibility of preparing, analyzing, and publishing standards relating to nanotechnology (Tanaka, 2019).

Thus, according to ISO/TS 27687: 2008, a nano-object is defined as a material with one, two, or three external dimensions in the size range of approximately 1–100 nm (Lazzaretti, 2018; Nolasco & dos Santos, 2017).

And according to ISO/TC 229 of 2005, nanotechnology comprises the understanding and control of matter and processes at the nanoscale, typically, but not exclusively, below 100 nanometers, in one or more dimensions. At these scales, the emergence of size-dependent phenomena provides new applications and/or properties for nanoscale materials that are different from the properties of the individual atoms, molecules, or macroscopic materials, enabling the creation of better materials, devices, and systems that exploit these new properties (Alencar et al., 2017).

Since 2005, a considerable amount of articles involving nanotechnology (according to the Scopus database from 2005 to 2021, using the descriptor *nanotechnology*) have been published (Figure 2.3). This demonstrates the rising scientific and technological interest and research and development funding being dedicated to nanotechnology. Such investments have led to rapid developments in such fields as chemistry, material science, energy, medicine, biotechnology, agriculture, food, electronic devices, and consumer products (Cheng et al., 2016).

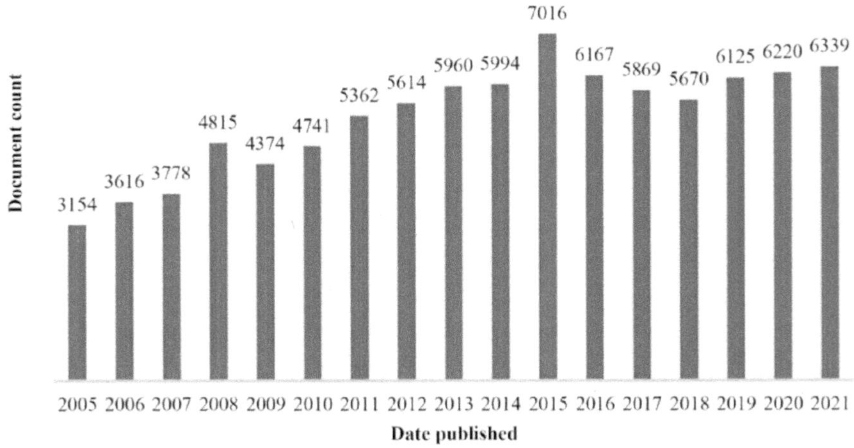

FIGURE 2.3 Scientific papers involving nanotechnology from 2005 to 2021.

The field of nanotechnology includes several sub-fields; in the health care sector, nanomedicine, nanopharmaceuticals, medical physics, nanotheranostics, and nanocosmetics stand out (Alves, 2006; Marques et al., 2009; Silva, 2004; Wong et al., 2020).

The principle of this new technology is based on the fact that materials on the nanometer scale may have chemical, physicochemical, and behavioral properties that differ from those presented on larger scales (Etheridge et al., 2013). With the reduction of their size, nanomaterials applied to the development of topical nanotherapeutics change the properties related to stability, reactivity, surface area, degree of dispersion, and the ability to interact with other molecules and systems (Baril et al., 2012). This may provide characteristics that were previously not presented by a particular product (Alencar et al., 2017; Schulz, 2018).

2.3.1 NANOCOSMETICS: THE REVOLUTION IN COSMETIC PRODUCTS

In recent years, the cosmetic industry has been thriving with a growth rate of about 15%. In 2017, the global cosmetic products market was valued at US$ 532.43 billion, and it is estimated that by 2023 it will reach US$ 805.61

billion, recording a compound annual growth rate (CAGR) of 7.14% in the 2018–2023 period. For the global nanocosmetics market, an average growth rate of 16.6% is estimated each year (Bilal & Iqbal, 2020).

The competitive market, the technological advances, the growing demand for cosmetics and an increasingly demanding public, has focused the attention of the cosmetics industry on the development of increasingly elaborate products. As such, simple cosmetics, which previously only involved cleaning, protective, and disguising characteristics, started being incorporated with pharmacological ingredients, receiving the designation "cosmeceuticals" (Dhapte-Pawar et al., 2020; Kushwaha et al., 2020).

The term "cosmeceutical" was coined by Raymond Reed and researched by Dr. Albert Kligman in the late 1970s (Kligman, 2005). This term suggests a new generation of cosmetic products, incorporated into biologically active ingredients, that possess therapeutic benefits for personal appearance, but that don't qualify as a drug or pharmaceutical product (Lohani et al., 2014). According to Kligman, a cosmeceutical product represents "a topical preparation that is sold as a cosmetic but has performance characteristics that suggest pharmaceutical action."

Currently, therefore, cosmeceuticals are considered a niche between pharmaceutical and cosmetic preparations, where products are enriched with the measurable therapeutic efficacy of bioactive components and formulations are diversified for topical application, expanding the possibilities for medical professionals and therapists to treat patients with disorders of the skin and skin appendages as well as esthetic dysfunctions (Kaul et al., 2018; Lohani et al., 2014).

With the advent of nanotechnology, the cosmetic industry has found an ally in this emerging field to meet the sector's innovation needs and increase the effectiveness of cosmeceuticals. Although there is still no global consensus today regarding the use of the term cosmeceuticals, several countries have written their own guidelines to regulate cosmetic and cosmeceutical products, seeking to consider the application, demand, and effectiveness of cosmeceuticals driven by nanotechnology (Dhapte-Pawar et al., 2020).

In addition to the designated characteristics of the term cosmeceuticals, nanocosmeceuticals present even better prepared cosmetic formulations, with desirable attributes such as efficacy, safety, targeting of the desired site, formulation stability, novelty, and patent protection, metabolism in the skin, and the possibility of industrial scaling (Effiong et al., 2020; Kaul et al., 2018).

Currently, different materials in nanometric scale, with distinct and specific characteristics are being used in cosmetic formulations or recommended for future use as nanosystems or nanocarriers to encapsulate the active ingredients for their efficient delivery through skin layers (Bilal & Iqbal, 2020).

According to statistical data collected by Euromonitor, the European Union is the world's largest producer of cosmetic products, followed by the United States, China, Japan, and Brazil, which are also the countries with the highest numbers of cosmetics consumers in the world (Verde, 2017).

The growth of the sector can be explained by such factors as the increase in life expectancy, an increasingly young population in the labor market, global advertisement investments in social media, the appreciation of male esthetics, and especially the technological advances in innovative cosmetic products and resources, which employ nanotechnology to enable the development of better quality products with different properties and better performance (Dimer et al., 2013; Faria et al., 2013; Rattner, 2005). This exponential growth has increased the interest in investments from major international companies in order to launch nanocosmetics (Baril et al., 2012; Melo et al., 2015; Verde, 2017).

Cosmetics in scale nanometric they are known as a topical formulation that delivers active or other nanostructured ingredients and that has superior properties when compared to conventional products (Baril et al., 2012).

Nanocosmetics are included in the pharmaceutical and cosmetic industry and are classified as a specific sector of personal care, perfumery, and cosmetic products (Ferreira & Rangel, 2009; Fronza, 2006). In the pharmaceutical area, the nanoparticles used in cosmetics have an approximate size of 100 to 600 nm, but in some nanocosmetics it is possible to find sizes inferior to 50 nm (Fronza, 2006).

The search for more effective therapeutic systems with fewer associated problems has led to the development of different nanocarriers, with the ability of vectorization, controlled and sustained release, greater permeation, and better stability of the active substances (Mora-Huertas et al., 2010; Patra et al., 2018; Tiwari et al., 2012), protecting the active ingredients from chemical or enzymatic degradation and increasing their bioavailability. This has increased therapeutic efficacy on the skin surface, improved permanence of the active ingredient on the skin (Fronza, 2006), resulted in products capable of adapting to the physiological variations of the skin, increased effectiveness even in smaller doses (Ereno, 2008), and led to the sensory optimization in the application on the skin (Garvil et al., 2013).

Given the expectations of the application, the route on the skin should be extensively evaluated and well defined. After all, a precise and sustained adjustment in the delivery system may reduce the potential for irritation of the active substance or raw materials used and enable the use of lower concentrations (Chaudhri et al., 2015; Open et al., 2017; Tsujimoto & Hara, 2018).

2.3.2 ADVANTAGES AND DISADVANTAGES OF TOPICAL NANOTHERAPEUTICS

The skin is the body's first protective barrier to the external environment. It plays an important role against mechanical and electrical trauma, invasion of pathogenic microorganisms, excessive ultraviolet (UV) radiation, and the loss of water and electrolytes through the transepidermal route, in addition to being a selective barrier to the permeation of various substances (Roger et al., 2019). However, despite its importance, the structure of the skin, especially the stratum corneum (SC) in the epidermis, can be an obstacle to the action of topical nanotherapeutic products (Kou et al., 2018).

The penetration mechanism consists of three pathways: the intracellular pathway where the active ingredient penetrates the keratinous cells, which is a very difficult passage (Trommer & Neubert, 2006); the intercellular pathway where the active ingredient diffuses through a lipid matrix (Goh et al., 2017); and the follicular pathway where the active ingredients passes through the hair follicles and glands (Lademann et al., 2011). Although the follicular pathway represents only 0.1% of the human skin surface, these appendages have a remarkable importance in the permeability of ions, polar, and apolar molecules, in addition to presenting a reservatory capacity of active substances applied topically (Barbero & Frasch, 2017).

Each nanostructure has particular advantages and disadvantages. The application of a cosmetic product is carried out on the surface of the skin, and its permeation or not is linked to the desired function and result. In the case of cosmetic products for therapeutic (cosmeceutical) purposes, the clinical efficacy of the product is measured by the diffusion capacity of the active substances through the skin appendages and the intact epidermis, passing through the subsequent layers to the dermis and hypodermis (Alves, 2015; Goh et al., 2017). This effectiveness can be limited when large molecules, poorly soluble or active substances are found in the formulation that can be photodegraded, for example. Such limitations can lead to a decrease or loss of effectiveness and even degradation of the product before it exerts the desired effect (Mihranyan et al., 2012).

Permeation through the intact skin is very difficult for molecules larger than 200–350 Daltons (Da) and 400 Da is considered the maximum size. In addition, the molecule must not be hydrophobic, must possess affinity for both lipophilic and hydrophilic phases, possess a short half-life time and not be irritating (Palmer & DeLouise, 2016).

A constraint factor for nanoparticle penetration throughout the pathway is the high intracellular diffusion resistance for particles greater than 5 nm. Theoretically, therefore, the follicular pathway may represent the predominant penetration pathway for nanoparticles greater than 5 nm (Carvalho, 2018).

Regarding the topical application in different areas of the body, Nasir & Friedman (2010) reported that, in general, structures of up to 1,000 nm permeate the intact skin in flexural zones, while in other regions particles of up to 7,000 nm are capable of reaching deeper cutaneous strata provided the skin has disruptions in continuity.

To overcome these obstacles and improve consumer acceptance, new topical administration systems based on nanotechnology have been developed in order to increase efficiency in the skin layers (Hua, 2015).

Topical nanotherapeutics are therefore being developed in order to provide a host of benefits, such as reducing the amount of active ingredients needed to have an equal or greater effect than a conventional topical therapeutic product, protecting the active ingredients by increasing their stability to degradation, improving therapeutic performance, reducing the risks of skin irritation through a gradual release of the active ingredient, thus decreasing the contact time with the skin, ensuring lower toxicity because some particles are made up of biodegradable lipids, increasing therapeutic adherence (Pardeike et al., 2009; Shelke et al., 2015), improving the apparent solubility of active ingredients, enabling the formation of a film, allowing for controlled occlusion, keeping the skin hydrated, and allowing a blend of active substances (Pandey et al., 2016). In addition, nanoparticles in topical products may optimize the chemical stability of compounds sensitive to light, oxidation, and hydrolysis (Montenegro et al., 2016).

2.4 NANOSTRUCTURES EMPLOYED IN THE DEVELOPMENT OF TOPICAL NANOTHERAPEUTICS

Several studies in the field of nanotechnology focused on cosmeceuticals have pointed to better therapies for skin conditions, such as topical nanotherapeutics for the treatment of acne vulgaris (Kaul et al., 2018).

Commonly, skin changes induced by acne vulgaris can easily result in an unesthetic appearance and form scars that often result in emotional and psychological problems related to the self-image and low self-esteem (dos Santos et al., 2019). A treatment capable of bypassing the skin barrier, exerting an anti-acne therapeutic effect, and minimizing the adverse effects of conventional products is therefore essential to meet the treatment objectives (Gupta et al., 2012; Prow et al., 2011).

Although the public consuming cosmeceuticals has increased greatly in recent years, just as the diversity of cosmeceuticals available on the market, the topical application of active compounds is still a challenge with regard to the safety, control, and determination of the exact amount of active ingredients that reach the different skin layers (Dhapte-Pawar et al., 2020; Nanda et al., 2016). The characteristics of the active ingredient and the physicochemical parameters of both the formulation (pH, concentration, molecular weight, and solubility) and transport system are responsible for the different distribution in the skin, and the same nanostructure can be used for various applications (Müller-Goymann, 2004).

As such, significant investments are being made in nanocarrier technologies as a way to increase the variety of nanostructures, improving the local bioavailability of several active compounds for topical administration (Goyal et al., 2016).

Nanostructures such as liposomes (Soni et al., 2016), SLNs (Souto & Müller, 2008), nanocapsules (Lohani et al., 2014), micelles (Yukuyama et al., 2016), niosomes, nanoemulsions (Ahmad et al., 2018), nanospheres (Kushwaha et al., 2020), fullerenes, ethosomes (ETOs) (Hameed et al., 2019), and phytosomes (Surini et al., 2018), among others, represent a recent trend towards improving the solubility/bioavailability of active substances (Bilal & Iqbal, 2020).

In addition, nanotechnology-based dermal formulations are an interesting strategy for the transport of several classes of substances, both hydrophilic and lipophilic, representing an alternative to overcome challenges related to the skin barrier and the kinetic and dynamic characteristics of various formulations when used through other pathways (Effiong et al., 2020).

2.4.1 MAIN NANOSTRUCTURES USED IN THE DEVELOPMENT OF TOPICAL NANOTHERAPEUTICS FOR THE TREATMENT OF ACNE VULGARIS

2.4.1.1 NANOEMULSIONS

Nanoemulsions (Figure 2.4) are systems measuring between 20 and 400 nm (Rai et al., 2018; Sugumar et al., 2014), made from oily materials in a process that mixes water with oil, resulting in stable, clear, and translucent droplets that withstand large temperature variations (Behera et al., 2010; Canavez, 2011).

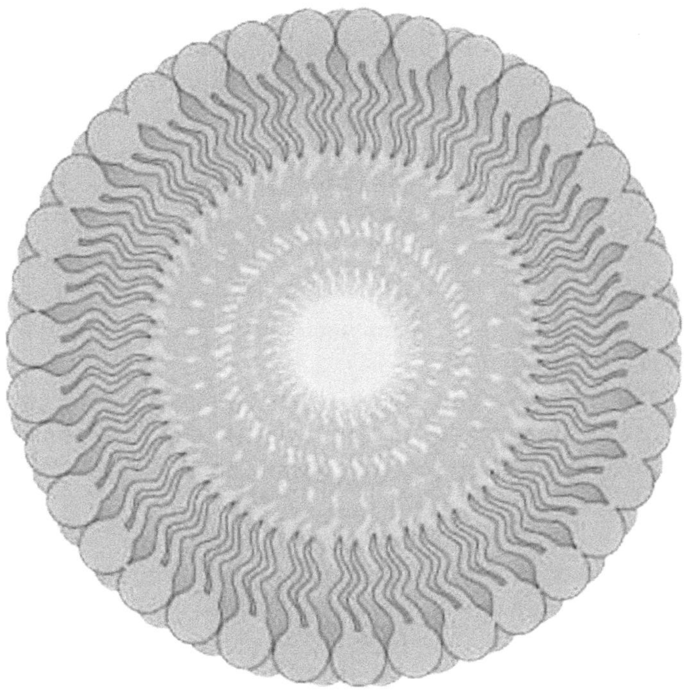

FIGURE 2.4 Schematic representation of nanoemulsion.

The flexible composition of nanoemulsions offers a wide range of applications in the food, pharmaceutical and personal care industries (Faria-Tischer & Tischer, 2012). Because nanoemulsions can increase the permeability of the active ingredients, have easy spreadability and pleasant sensory characteristics, they are commonly used in cosmetic products in formulations of bath oils, moisturizing products for the skin, hair, and mucous membranes, and in anti-wrinkle and anti-aging creams (Daudt et al., 2013).

Some of the advantages of nanoemulsions over other nanostructures include increased absorption rate, favoring of the solubilization of lipophilic substances, increased bioavailability, application through different administration routes, ability to carry lipophilic and hydrophilic substances, and the ability to perform the orderly delivery of active ingredients (Sonneville-Aubrun et al., 2004; Tadros et al., 2004). Regarding the negative effects, the following stand out: limited solubilization for substances with a high melting point, stability influenced by temperature and pH (Daudt et al., 2013; Faria-Tischer & Tischer, 2012).

Regarding the development of nanoemulsions for the topical treatment of acne vulgaris, Zidan et al. positively evaluated the controlled release capacity and antibacterial activity *in vitro* of nanoemulsions containing nicotinamide (Zidan et al., 2016). A study conducted by Taleb et al. (2018), on the other hand, aimed to evaluate the antiacne activity potential *in vitro* and *in vivo* of *Origanum vulgare L.* A nanoemulsion containing oregano oil was tested in an animal model of acne. The formulation showed healing effects as a result. In addition, the researchers suggest that the oregano oil nanoemulsion is a potential natural and effective alternative to treat acne and overcome emerging antibiotic resistance.

Janani et al. (2019) hypothesized that the combination of polyphenol and adapalene in a nanoemulgel could be beneficial for the treatment of acne vulgaris. In addition, a recent *in vitro* study satisfactorily evaluated the encapsulation of retinol palmitate in nanoemulsion and its subsequent incorporation into a hydrogel system to improve topical delivery and stability (Algahtani et al., 2020). According to a clinical pilot study conducted by Sabori et al. (2018), the treatment with tretinoin-containing nanoemulsions was able to reduce the number of acne lesions on the face, reduce the size of papules and pustules, and mitigate the adverse effects and intensity of porphyrin production.

2.4.1.2 POLYMERIC NANOPARTICLES

Polymeric nanoparticles (Figure 2.5) are solid and spherical structures ranging from 10 to 1,000 nm in size. They can be prepared from biodegradable materials such as polymers (natural or synthetic) (Ramos, 2018). They are highly stable systems, capable of releasing the active ingredient only at the desired target, thus increasing effectiveness and reducing side effects and toxicity (Rajesh & Lillard, 2000; Keservani et al., 2017).

They are widely applied in the treatment of skin conditions to optimize the permeation of therapeutic agents in the skin, and in the development of new sunscreen formulations since they are capable of transporting highly lipophilic substances that are poorly soluble in water (Baril et al., 2012; Carvalho, 2018; Raj et al., 2012).

In general, there are two types of polymeric nanoparticles: nanospheres, composed of a polymeric matrix, which carries the drug on the surface or mixed in the matrix; and nanocapsules, characterized by a vesicular system that confines substances in a nucleus or center (oil or water) surrounded by a polymeric shell (Faria-Tischer & Tischer, 2012; Mora-Huertas et al., 2010; Schaffazick et al., 2003; Vrignaud et al., 2011).

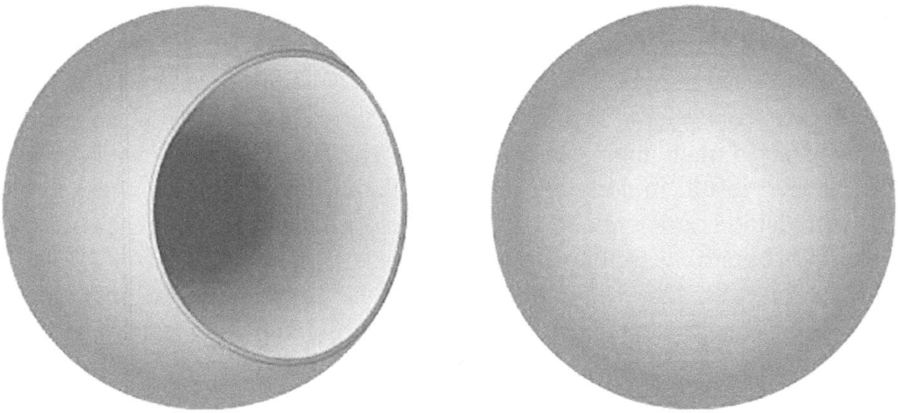

FIGURE 2.5 Schematic representation of polymeric nanoparticles: nanocapsule and nanosphere, respectively.

2.4.1.2.1 Nanospheres

Nanospheres differ from nanocapsules (Keservani et al., 2018) in that they form solid matrix systems where a polymerized material constitutes a three-dimensional network in which the active substance can be adsorbed, incorporated, or covalently bonded on the particle surface, forming dissolution, dispersion, or porous systems (Baril et al., 2012; Delgado, 2013). As such, the active ingredients can be adsorbed on the surface of the sphere or encapsulated inside the particle. Nanospheres in cosmetics are efficiently used to encapsulate such ingredients as vitamins and fragrances (Daudt et al., 2013; Letchford & Burt, 2007; Souto & Müller, 2008).

Adapalene-containing nanospheres have been formulated to increase efficacy and improve skin tolerability in the treatment of acne. Skin irritation was assessed *in vitro* and comedolytic activity *in vivo* in an animal model. According to the results of a skin irritation study, the secretion of proinflammatory cytokines such as interleukin 1 *alpha* (IL-1) and interleukin 8 (IL-8) was significantly reduced, confirming that the formulation is less irritating and has better comedolytic properties, significantly reducing the size of acne lesions when compared to the commercial Differin gel® (Ramezanli & Michniak-Kohn, 2018).

2.4.1.2.2 Nanocapsules

In nanocapsules, the active substance can be found in the nucleus or included in the wall or shell. The release of the active substance is usually conditioned to the dissolution and disintegration of the polymer shell and the diffusion phenomena of the substance in the particle (Schaffazick et al., 2003).

Nanocapsules are widely used as vehicles for sunscreens and can form a protective film on the surface of the skin, regulating the penetration of encapsulated substances. When applied in cosmetic products they can also avoid incompatibilities between the ingredients of the formulation, reduce undesirable odors and protect ingredients that are sensitive to photodegradation (Daudt et al., 2013; Helgason et al., 2009).

Nanocapsules containing retinoic acid were evaluated *in vitro* demonstrating effective results regarding encapsulation and antibacterial activity (Lara, 2008). In the same year, another study evaluated isotretinoin nanocapsules incorporated in a hydrophilic gel regarding their skin penetration capacity through the *tape stripping* technique in healthy volunteers. The results revealed the ability of isotretinoin-containing nanocapsules to permeate the SC faster than its free form. The authors concluded that isotretinoin-containing nanocapsules are a promising system for cutaneous application and capable of improving the protection of the drug against light (Felippi, 2008).

Another study conducted by Ourique et al. (2011) obtained satisfactory results in tretinoin nanoencapsulation, increasing photostability and reducing cutaneous permeation of tretinoin when compared to formulations containing the unencapsulated drug.

Recently, a successful *in vivo* and *in vitro* study used flutamide-loaded zein nanocapsules in a hydrogel formulation to optimize the topical administration of flutamine. The results minimized the permeation of flutamine in the skin with a low-cost, biocompatible, and promising delivery system for the dermal treatment of pilosebaceous unit disorders (Sallam & Elzoghby, 2018).

2.4.1.3 LIPID NANOPARTICLES

Lipid nanoparticles are aqueous dispersions of particles organized through solid lipids (Figure 2.6). They range in size from 50 to 1,000 nm, can be stabilized by one or more surfactants, and have the ability to modify the polarity of the surface, improving the administration of substances at the topical and systemic level (Souto et al., 2012).

Their main characteristics include excellent physicochemical stability, the ability to protect unstable substances from degradation, the ability to control release, excellent tolerability, occlusive ability, modulation of encapsulated substance delivery, and the absence of problems related to large-scale production and sterilization (González et al., 2016; Soni et al., 2016).

As disadvantages, lipid nanoparticles have less capacity to preserve effectively the active substance encapsulation, potentially causing the formation of alternative colloidal structures, such as micelles, liposomes, micelle, and nanocrystal mixtures, in addition to presenting physical instability during storage or administration due to the complexity of the lipid's physical state (Daudt et al., 2013; Guterres et al., 2007).

There are two generations of lipid nanoparticles: the first generation are SLNs, and the second generation are nanostructured lipid carriers (NLC) (Müller et al., 2002; Souto & Müller, 2008).

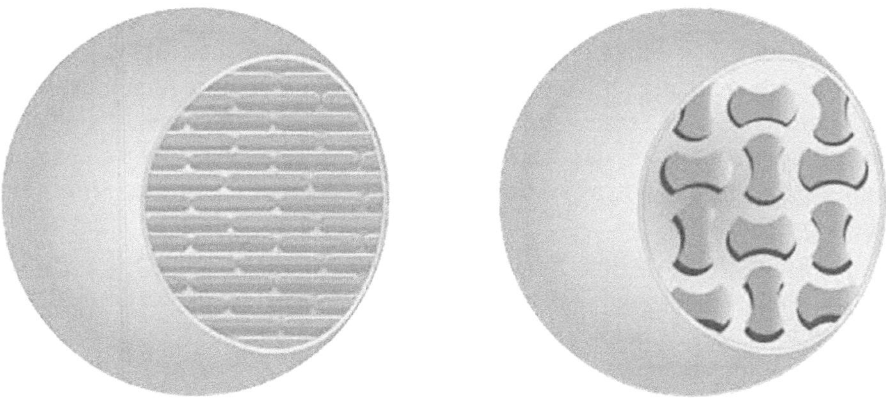

FIGURE 2.6 Schematic representation of lipid nanoparticles: On the left is the solid lipid nanoparticle and on the right, is the nanostructured lipid carrier.

2.4.1.3.1 Solid Lipid Nanoparticles (SLNs)

Solid lipid nanoparticles have a matrix consisting of a solid lipid core and an active substance. They are ideal for transporting lipophilic substances that can be formulated in aqueous systems, with potential effective applications in sunscreen formulations (Marcato, 2009). Their main disadvantage is linked to the high degree of crystallinity, reducing the space available for the active substance, and therefore decreasing the encapsulation effectiveness due to stability problems, including the release of the substance, particle growth and gelation (Müller et al., 2002; Wu & Guy, 2009).

An *in vitro* study developed by Kelidari et al. (2015) evaluated the optimization of the formulation and penetration into the skin of SLNs loaded with spironolactone. Subsequently, the same group conducted a prospective randomized, *in vivo*, double-blind study and effectively evaluated the topical application of SLNs containing spironolactone. The results revealed that the adverse effects of the oral administration for acne treatment were minimized (Kelidari et al., 2016).

SLNs containing nicotinamide also demonstrated satisfactory results in the treatment of skin inflammations in an *in vitro* and *in vivo* study (Pan et al., 2016).

2.4.1.3.2 Nanostructured Lipid Carriers (NLC)

This second generation of lipid nanoparticulate systems has a matrix formed by a mixture of solid and liquid lipids, nonetheless, this matrix remains solid at under normal temperature conditions (Mehnert & Mader, 2001). This characteristic minimizes the low encapsulation efficacy of NLCs. Their composition and structure form a film on the skin that increases the penetration of molecules or increases the amount of water in the upper layers of the epidermis, promoting the desired effect (Chen et al., 2010; Müller et al., 2011).

The incorporation of isotretinoin into NLCs was evaluated *in vitro* and *in vivo*. The results confirmed the potential of the nanostructured lipid form to incorporate drugs that are poorly soluble in water into topical applications, in addition to reducing skin irritation (Patwekar et al., 2018).

Dapsone was incorporated into the lipid matrix of NLCs. The trial evaluated the *in vitro* release and *ex vivo* skin permeation. The formulation had a controlled release with good occlusive effect. In addition, it improved dapsone permeation in the skin, increased the amount of active substance retained in the skin in a controlled manner, and improved anti-rosacea activity (Elmowafy et al., 2019).

In order to develop, optimize, and characterize a gel of NLCs containing clindamycin phosphate for better topical administration in the treatment of acne, Fatima et al. (2019) conducted an *in vitro* and *in vivo* study. The results regarding the skin retention study, tape stripping technique and confocal laser scanning microscopy revealed greater retention and permeation depth, suggesting that clindamycin NLCs are promising agents for the treatment of acne.

The combinatorial effect of Carrot Extract and Marigold Extract on NLCs was evaluated *in vitro* and *in vivo*. The results demonstrated high biocompatibility, a significant ability to capture free radicals, reduced expression of inflammatory cytokines, and better transdermal absorption (Lacatusu et al., 2020).

2.4.1.4 LIPOSOMES

Liposomes (Figure 2.7) have a concentric shape consisting of one or more membranes as phospholipid bilayers involving an aqueous nucleus, resembling a cell membrane (Mihranyan et al., 2012). Due to the amphipathic nature of phospholipids, they are able to incorporate both lipophilic substances and water-soluble substances, modulating the delivery of the substance to the desired target (Torchilin, 1997). Another advantage of liposomes is that they can easily interact deeply with the cells of the body because they are biocompatible and biodegradable (Edwards & Baeumner, 2006; Schaffazick et al., 2003).

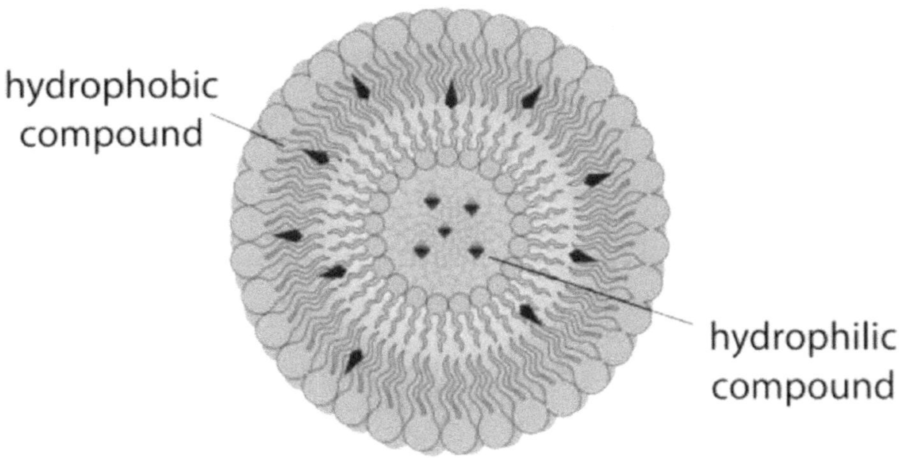

FIGURE 2.7 Schematic representation of liposomes.

The main lipid component of the liposome is phosphatidylcholine. Cholesterol is usually included in the composition to stabilize the structure and thus form more rigid liposomes (Tiwari et al., 2012). Like other vesicular systems, liposomes can reduce toxicity and increase the stability of encapsulated ingredients (Chorilli et al., 2007).

Liposomes can encapsulate a variety of active substances and be incorporated into various types of cosmetic products, being able to replenish or increase the endogenous lipids of the SC, increasing hydration and reducing skin dryness (Coderch et al., 1999). In addition, they are effectively applied in skin moisturizers, anti-cellulite, anti-aging, and eye-care products, after-shaves, sunscreens, and makeup (Ahmadi Ashtiani et al., 2016; Bochicchio et al., 2020).

The main disadvantage of liposomes is related to stability because of the formation of crystals, oxidation, and hydrolysis of the phospholipids, in addition to the instability of the bilayers after emptying the retained material. Liposomes also have a short half-life and high production costs (Apolinário et al., 2017).

According to Sætern et al. (2005), depending on their process conditions, chemical composition and morphology, liposomes can be classified as large multilamellar vesicles (MLVs) with diameters ranging from 400 to 3,500 nm; large unilamellar vesicles (LUVs), with diameters ranging from 100 to 1,000 nm, and small unilamellar vesicles (SUVs), with diameters from 20 to 50 nm (Lee et al., 2006; Sahoo & Labhasetwar, 2003; Santos & Castanho, 2002).

In addition to liposomes, there are studies involving other nanoencapsulation methods using transferosomes, ETOs, and niosomes, which are other vesicles that have a similar structure, and which are being employed in order to increase the penetration of substances through the skin (Marianecci et al., 2014).

The penetration and retention of transcutol-containing liposomes for tretinoin delivery was determined in a trial using mouse skin. According to the results of the study, the authors concluded that the formulation can be successfully used for the dermal delivery of tretinoin (Bavarsad et al., 2016).

A study conducted by Hasanpouri et al. (2018) found good results in the *in vitro* release of liposomal tetracycline hydrochloride and its permeation through the skin in an *ex vivo* model. Liposomes containing retinoic acid was also evaluated in of an *in vitro* study in order for to optimize the release through the skin into treatment acne vulgaris was also evaluated in an *in vitro* study in order to optimize the release through the skin (Lu et al., 2019).

Dermal bioavailability *ex vivo*, dermal distribution, anti-acne efficacy *in vivo* and skin irritation studies were performed using a combination containing benzoyl peroxide and adapalene liposomes compared to the free compounds and the commercial formulation Epiduo. The study results revealed that the association of liposomes with benzoyl peroxide and adapalene significantly increased dermal bioavailability and reduced skin irritation and papule density in an animal model when compared to the same free compounds and Epiduo. The authors concluded, therefore, that the combination of liposomes with benzoyl peroxide and adapalene for topical application can provide an alternative, effective, and safe approach for the co-delivery of anti-acne dermo-cosmetics (Jain et al., 2018).

2.4.1.5 TRANSFEROSOMES

Due to the lipid bilayers that make up their vesicles, transferosomes (Figure 2.8) are morphologically related to liposomes. However, they differ functionally in the flexibility of their membrane, allowing for penetration through pores with a diameter that are 5 to 10 times smaller than their size, without significant losses of the active substance (Fitrya et al., 2020). This ability is a consequence of the combination of the amphiphilic/lipophilic components with surfactants (Antunes, 2016).

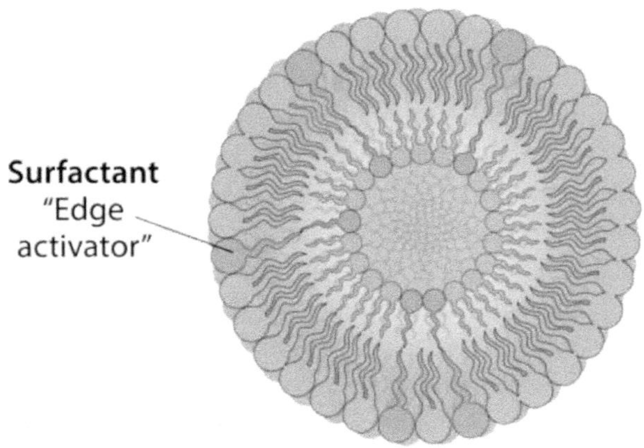

FIGURE 2.8 Schematic representation of transferosome.

Transferosomes have high encapsulation efficacy, are able to protect the encapsulated substance from metabolic degradation, have a slow and gradual release of the active substance, and the flexibility of their membrane minimizes the risk of ruptures of the vesicles on the skin (Jain et al., 2003). They are easily reproducible in a relatively quick process that doesn't use additives (Maghraby et al., 2008). However, due to their predisposition to oxidative degradation, they are chemically unstable and have a high production cost (Fitrya et al., 2020; Hofer et al., 2000).

The *in vitro* release and the skin permeation efficiency in an *ex vivo* model of a formulation containing tetracycline hydrochloride transferosomes was evaluated satisfactorily in a study conducted by Hasanpouri et al. (2018).

Recently, an *in vitro* and *in vivo* study involving transferosomes containing adapalene enriched with vitamin C revealed that this delivery system showed better results in the treatment of acne compared to the commercial product Adiff. In addition, the association with vitamin C played a significant role in improving the quality of treatment (Vasanth et al., 2020).

2.4.1.6 ETHOSOMES (ETOS)

Ethosomes (ETOs) are lipid vesicles that have a composition similar to that of liposomes but are prepared with about 20 to 50% higher concentrations of ethanol and water (Dubey et al., 2007) (Figure 2.9). The fluidizing characteristic of the alcohol on lipids enables ETOs to cross the SC to deeper layers of the skin, in addition to increasing the flexibility of the vesicular membrane, making them also more efficient in the administration of larger quantities of substances through the skin when compared with conventional liposomes (Ramakrishna et al., 2014; Verma & Pathak, 2010).

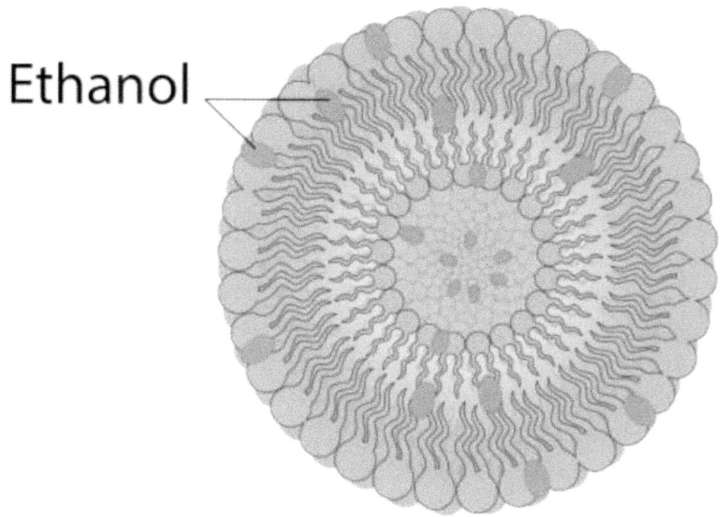

FIGURE 2.9 Schematic representation of ethosome.

Ethosomal systems have several applications in the pharmaceutical and cosmetic industries and can be incorporated into various cosmetic presentations. They have better stability and solubility when compared to other vesicles (Godin & Touitou, 2003). However, the encapsulation efficacy is very low, and portions of the active substance can be lost during the transfer of the organic medium to the aqueous medium, increasing production costs. Additionally, the high concentration of alcohol or other excipients may cause skin irritations (Godin & Touitou, 2003; Park et al., 2014; Shen et al., 2014).

A new formulation developed with ETOs containing azelaic acid showed enhanced anti-acne activity when compared to a conventional gel and a commercial cream containing azelaic acid. The authors concluded, therefore, that the ethosomal formulation is an efficient vesicular carrier system for topical applications (Mistry & Ravikumar, 2016). Another study with ETOs containing azelaic acid demonstrated effective antimicrobial ability *in vitro* against *Proprionibacterium acnes* (Apriani et al., 2019).

The potential anti-acne and skin irritation of the ethosomal gel containing Cryptotanshinone obtained from *Salvia miltiorrhiza* was evaluated in relation to the transdermal permeation and skin deposition *in vitro* and *in vivo* in rabbits. The results showed that the ethosomal gel had better anti-acne effect with mild skin irritation (Yu et al., 2016).

One study demonstrated the incorporation of ethosomal vesicles containing tretinoin in a Carbopol-based gel. The effectiveness of the formulation was evaluated *in vitro* compared to a commercial gel used for the treatment of acne. According to the authors, the results suggest that ETOs are efficient transporters for the dermal and transdermal delivery of tretinoin. They also suggested that the inclusion of ethanol in the ethosome plays an important role in increasing tretinoin permeation (Mishra et al., 2018).

In addition, researchers have also demonstrated that a formulation containing thymoquinone ETOs had a considerable effect on sebaceous gland units, reducing the number and size of the glands. Skin irritation studies revealed that the formulation being tested was a safe, less irritating, and well-tolerable formulation for topical application. The authors concluded, therefore, that the formulation of ETOs loaded with thymoquinone may be an effective treatment for acne vulgaris and other skin disorders (Kausar et al., 2019).

2.4.1.7 NIOSOMES

Niosomes (Figure 2.10) are considered elastic vesicles and are subject to ultra-deformation, so their size, shape, and fluidity can be controlled by changing the composition and production methods (Chen et al., 2019). These vesicles are developed from nonionic surfactants that can attach to the lipids of the corneum layer and act as permeation promoters in the skin. They can encapsulate both hydrophilic and lipophilic compounds, increasing the availability of active ingredients (Kaur & Kumar, 2018; Keservani & Gautam, 2020, 2022; Keservani et al., 2010;).

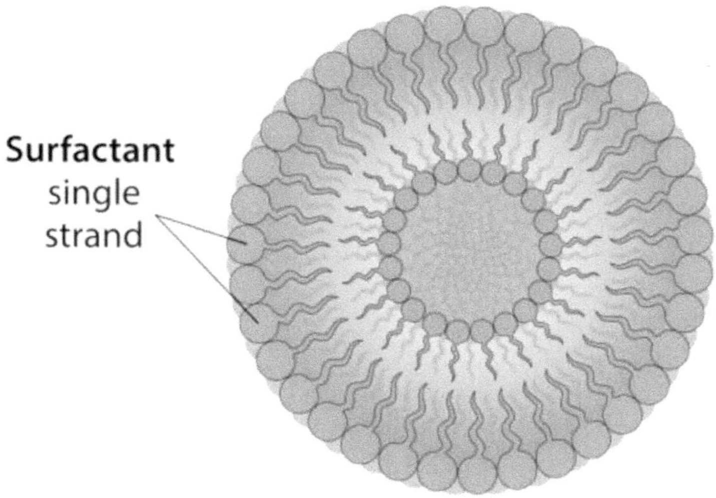

FIGURE 2.10 Schematic representation of noisome.

They are more stable, have lower irritation potential and have lower production costs than other vesicles. In addition, they are commonly applied in cosmetics and in the treatment of skin conditions such as acne vulgaris, dermatitis, psoriasis, and others (Jufri et al., 2017). Their disadvantages include their susceptibility to hydrolysis, fusion, aggregation, and the release of the active substance before reaching the target (Chaikul et al., 2019; Molina, 2018).

One study involved the *in vitro* and *in vivo* analysis of the combination of niosomal formulations containing benzoyl peroxide 1% and clindamycin 1% compared to niosomal clindamycin 1%. Although the statistical difference was not significant, the authors reported that niosomes containing the combination of benzoyl peroxide 1% and clindamycin 1% in the treatment of acne vulgaris showed greater efficacy without increased adverse effects compared to niosomal clindamycin 1% (Mohammadi et al., 2019).

A sequence of studies conducted by Manconi et al. satisfactorily evaluated niosomes containing tretinoin for the treatment of acne vulgaris in three stages: preparation and properties (Manconi et al., 2002) evaluation of photostability (Manconi et al., 2003), and analysis and cutaneous administration *in vitro* (Manconi et al., 2006). The authors highlight that the interactions between the skin and the niosomes containing tretinoin seem to depend on the physicochemical properties of the main component of the vesicular bilayer.

2.4.1.8 MICELLES

Micelles (Figure 2.11) are nanostructures formed from amphiphilic substances, that is, they have a hydrophilic and a hydrophobic part (Bodratti & Alexandridis, 2018). They have a spherical shape and are widely studied as active release nano-systems for topical, oral, and intravenous administration (Montenegro et al., 2016).

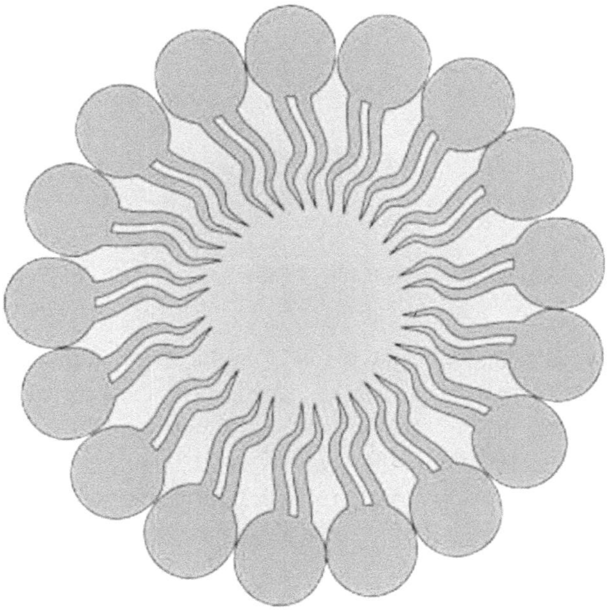

FIGURE 2.11 Schematic representation of micelle.

Micelles can enable the administration of active ingredients in smaller doses and consequently, reduce side effects. They have a high ability to solubilize water-insoluble substances (Gordillo-Galeano & Mora-Huertas, 2018). In addition, they represent a simple membrane model that enables the selective delivery of the substances to the target tissue with lower toxicity and fewer adverse effects (Deng et al., 2017a, b).

Trans-retinoic acid micelles were positively evaluated in the treatment of acne vulgaris. The results revealed that the in the presence of atmospheric oxygen incorporation into micelles significantly reduced the degradation of trans-retinoic acid (Wichit et al., 2012).

Another study involving a micellar formulation of retinoic acid demonstrated satisfactory results *in vitro* and *in vivo*. According to the authors, the formulation under study revealed a higher delivery efficiency at the target site, in addition to providing a more selective and safe topical handling this pathology (Lapteva et al., 2015).

Micelles containing adapalene have also been tested *in vitro* and *in vivo*. In this research, the follicular release in the human skin was studied by using a puncture biopsy technique to extract the intact pilosebaceous unit. The results demonstrated that the micellar solution and gel formulations actually allowed the preferential delivery of adapalene to the pilosebaceous unit (Kandekar et al., 2018).

2.4.1.9 PHYTOSOMES

Phytosomes (Figure 2.12) are molecular complexes formed by phospholipids, such as phosphatidylcholine, and phytocomponents found in natural products (Semalty et al., 2007). They effectively improve the absorption of polar substances insoluble in lipids (Jain et al., 2010) and may be employed in the oral or topical administration of substances (El-Menshawe et al., 2018). This complexation increases the bioavailability of active substances when administered orally and improves the absorption of phytocomponents when applied topically, presenting significantly greater therapeutic benefits (Maramaldi et al., 2016).

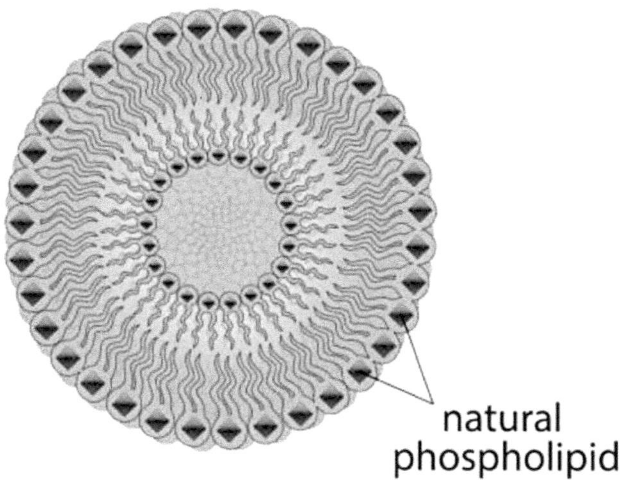

FIGURE 2.12 Schematic representation of phytosome.

The difference between a liposome and a phytosome lies in the fact that liposomes form no bond with the phospholipids and the substances they incorporate (Das & Kalita, 2014; Otlatici et al., 2019).

A study using phytosomal quercetin revealed the potentiated effect that this formulation had on dermal inflammations and the damage caused by UV radiation. These effects are performed due to the antioxidant and anti-inflammatory properties of quercetin, allowing it to sequester free radicals and minimize the oxidative effects produced by UV radiation, thereby reducing lipid peroxidation and inhibiting the production of inflammatory enzymes and other cytokines (Maramaldi et al., 2016).

Phytosomes containing a combination of titrated *Centella asiatica* extract and astaxanthin have also been evaluated to reduce dermal inflammation. The results showed that the combination of titrated *Centella asiatica* extract and astaxanthin in phytosomes was able to inhibit the expression of induced nitric oxide synthase (iNOS) and cyclo-oxygenase type 2 (COX-2); the activity of nuclear transcription factor kappa B (NF-kB); and the release of tumor necrosis factor *alpha* (TNF-α), IL-6 and immunoglobulin E (IgE) (Park et al., 2019).

2.4.1.10 FULLERENES

Fullerenes (Figure 2.13) are compounds based on closed rings of carbon atoms, arranged in a spherical structure (Sharma et al., 2018). The characteristics of this system make it possible to carry substances with therapeutic activities. These characteristics include a reduced size and spherical shape with hollow interior. In addition, they are able to change their hydrophobic nature to a hydrophilic one, facilitating the incorporation of several formulations (Ahmad et al., 2018).

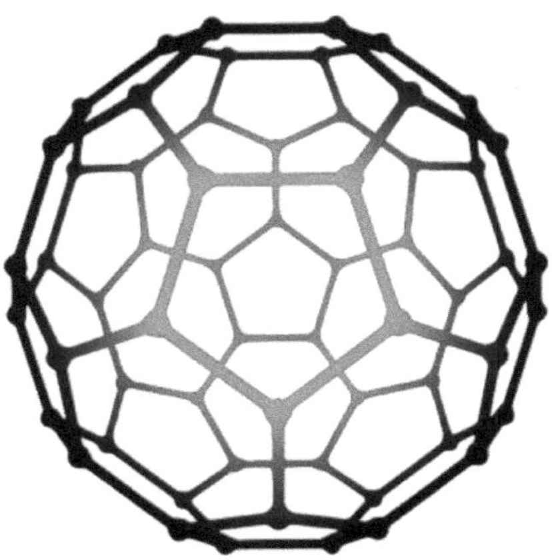

FIGURE 2.13 Schematic representation of fullerene.

Source: designism. https://creativecommons.org/licenses/by-sa/4.0/

Fullerenes have become the target of research for applications in cosmetic formulations because they have an antioxidant effect, protective properties against oxygen free radicals, a depigmenting effect, and a preventive effect against skin lesions caused by UV radiation (Santos et al., 2019). The disadvantages of these systems include the fact that they are not biodegradable and that they cause bioaccumulation because they are fat-soluble. Additionally, their very small size can lead to the unpredictability of toxicological effects (Mousavi et al., 2017; Pulicharla et al., 2016).

Previous research has revealed the antimicrobial activity of fullerene against normal skin microbiota bacteria, including *Propionibacterium acnes* and *Staphylococcus epidermidis* (promoting agents of acne vulgaris). The results have shown that fullerene exhibits antimicrobial activity via inhibition of microbial cell growth and not via bactericidal activity (Aoshima et al., 2009).

Inui et al. (2011) evaluated the topical application of fullerene in patients with acne vulgaris. The results suggested that fullerene suppresses acne by reducing neutrophil infiltration and sebum production.

Other studies, such as Ngan et al. (2014, 2015) have suggested the incorporation of fullerene into cosmetic products. The topical application of fullerene provides protective and regenerative effects against collagen breakdown induced by reactive oxygen species (ROS). Oxidative stress plays an important role in acne formation, and the authors therefore suggest that oxygen radical scavengers are potential therapeutic agents.

2.4.1.11 CYCLODEXTRINS (CDS)

Cyclodextrins (CDs; Figure 2.14) are cyclic oligosaccharides with a hydrophobic internal cavity, an average size of 1.5 nm x 0.7 nm x 0.8 nm and a hydrophilic external surface due to the presence of hydroxyl groups. They can be classified according to the number of glycopyranose units present in their structure (Winter Junior, 2015).

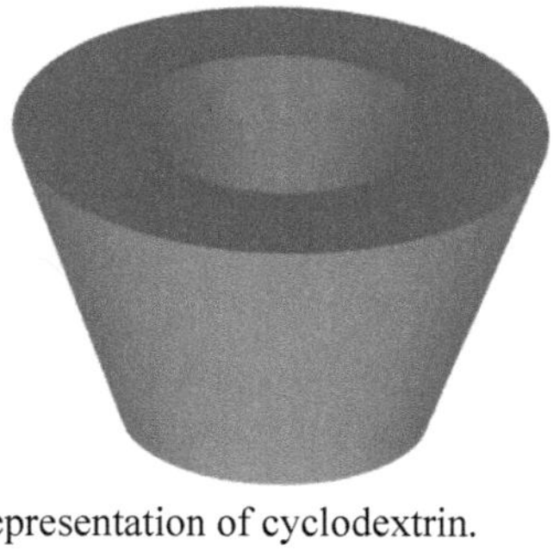

FIGURE 2.14 Schematic representation of cyclodextrin.

In the development of products for topical administration, α-cyclodextrin (α-CD), β-cyclodextrin (β-CD) and γ-cyclodextrin (γ-CD) are applied, in which the active substance can be encapsulated in up to three different areas: on the surface, in the lipophilic ring, or in the aqueous core, depending on the molecule to be complexed (de Miranda et al., 2011). Of these variations, however, β-CD is the most frequently used (Kringel et al., 2017; Santos et al., 2019).

CDs are known in supramolecular chemistry as receptors capable of forming stable inclusion complexes or organized supramolecular nanostructures with a variety of molecules in their hydrophobic cavity via non-covalent bonds, including organic, inorganic, and organometallic compounds (Ferreira, 2009).

Interest in these structures grew in the late 19th century because their complexing properties promote increases in the solubility, dissolution, and bioavailability of poorly soluble substances (Sharma & Baldi, 2016). They are widely applied in the development of cosmetics and medicines for the topical route, especially because they alter physicochemical properties and above all, because they allow hydrophobic substances to cross the SC without affecting its barrier function, delivering substances to the desired target while offering a biocompatible platform, in addition to favoring cell regeneration (Loftsson & Masson, 2001).

CDs can also improve the stability and shelf life of various active ingredients against hydrolysis, oxidation, dehydration, and photodecomposition (Popielec & Loftsson, 2017). The safety aspects and production costs of CDs are conditioned to the administration of high doses (Redenti et al., 2000).

A topical formulation with cyclodextrin complexed to retinoic acid for the treatment of acne vulgaris was evaluated *in vivo*. According to the results, there was an improvement in lesions after 3 months of topical treatment with a good efficacy and tolerability profile, which made it an effective alternative for the treatment of acne vulgaris (Anadolu et al., 2004).

According to previous research, CDs-containing substances such as the essential oil of *Rosmarinus officinalis* L. and quercetin possess antimicrobial activity, antioxidant capacity, and an inhibitory capacity of lipoxygenase and acetylcholinesterase. These characteristics are important for the treatment of dermal alterations, including acne vulgaris (Cutillas et al., 2018; Hong et al., 2018).

CDs with dapsone were formulated to evaluate their anti-acne activity in a gel for topical application. The tests were performed *in vivo* in a mouse model with acne-induced inflammation. CDs with gel dapsone exhibited superior anti-inflammatory and wound healing activities when compared to the reference anti-acne antibiotic Aknemycin® (Shamma et al., 2019).

2.4.1.12 DENDRIMERS

Dendrimers (Figure 2.15) are highly branched globular polymers, with average sizes of 1–10 nm, molecular mass, and well-defined and uniform shapes. These nanostructures are similar to physiological proteins, have low polydispersity and a high degree of functionalization on the surface (Gelfuso et al., 2015; Gautam et al., 2015).

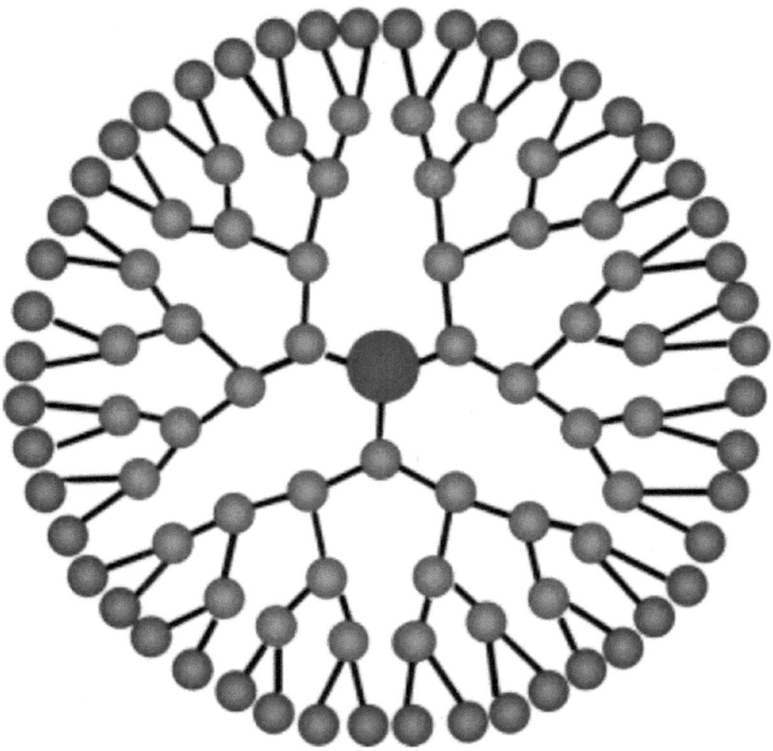

FIGURE 2.15 Schematic representation of dendrimer.

Structurally they consist of three essential components: (i) a central core where active compounds can be incorporated, either in its internal structure or connected or adsorbed on its surface; (ii) branches of repeated units with the number of branches determining their generation and with more branches determining the encapsulation capacity; and (iii) highly functional terminal groups that allow the modification of the role of their surface area (Desai et al., 2011).

The first studies involving dendrimers were reported in 1978. Since then, they have been widely applied as transdermal transport vehicles of active ingredients (Mendes et al., 2017).

Their properties include high hydrosolubility, biocompatibility, encapsulation capacity, absence of immunogenicity, precise molecular weight, small size and polyvalence, which allow for the safe and effective carrying of substances (Mendes et al., 2017; Shaunak, 2015).

As for safety, the possible toxicity may be associated with the polymers used. In general, cationic dendrimers are more toxic and anionic more biocompatible, but they also have high production costs (Desai et al., 2011; Moreira, 2013).

Pharmaceutical applications of dendrimers include non-steroidal anti-inflammatory formulations, antimicrobial, and antiviral substances. Dendrimers containing erythromycin were evaluated *in vitro* in a hydrogel formulation. The results were satisfactory, and the incorporation can be directed to the therapeutic of this pathology (Wróblewska & Winnicka, 2015).

2.5 CONCLUSION

An enormous percentage of people worldwide suffer from acne vulgaris, an inflammatory skin condition, which is subject to multifactorial interpretation and is challenging to classify regarding severity and epidemiology. The therapeutic treatment is greatly affected by these challenges.

Acne vulgaris involves a therapeutic challenge where the study of nanotechnology applied to cosmeceuticals, encouraged by the global market trend of increasingly well-developed products, may be an excellent and innovative therapeutic option of this pathology.

A nanostructure reported in this chapter are characterized by unique and different physical, biology, and chemical properties and include liposomes, niosomes, ETOs, transferosomes, phytosomes, nanoemulsions, polymeric nanoparticles, lipid nanoparticles, micelles, fullerenes, dendrimers, and CDs. When applied to the treatment of acne vulgaris, these nanosystems have proven effective for the targeted and controlled delivery of different compounds and they can offer remarkable advantages, such as biocompatibility, better stability, local specificity, and prolonged action, enabling effective application in the treatment of acne vulgaris.

KEYWORDS

- **acne vulgaris**
- **cyclodextrins**
- **nanocapsules**
- **nanostructures**
- **nanotherapeutics**
- **skin**
- **solid lipid nanoparticles**
- **topical application**

REFERENCES

Abdo, J. M., Sopko, N. A., & Milner, S. M., (2020). The applied anatomy of human skin: A model for regeneration. *Wound Medicine, 28*, 100179. https://doi.org/10.1016/j.wndm.2020.100179.

Ahmad, J., Gautam, A., Komath, S., Bano, M., Garg, A., & Jain, K., (2018). Topical nano-emulgel for skin disorders: Formulation approach and characterization. *Recent Patents on Anti-Infective Drug Discovery, 14*(1), 36–48. https://doi.org/10.2174/1574891x14666181129115213.

Ahmad, S., & Popli, A. H., (2019). A review on efficacy and tolerability of tea tree oil for acne. *Journal of Drug Delivery and Therapeutics Open, 9*(3), 609–612. https://doi.org/https://dx.doi.org/10.22270/jddt.v9i3.2838.

Ahmadi, A. H. R., Bishe, P., Lashgari, N. A., Nilforoushzadeh, M. A., & Zare, S., (2016). Liposomes in cosmetics. *Journal of Skin and Stem Cell, 3*(3). https://doi.org/10.5812/jssc.65815.

Alencar, M. S. De. M., Bochner, R., Dias, M. F. F., & Antunes, A. M. De. S., (2017). Analysis of Brazilian scientific articles about nanotechnology and health. *Revista Eletronica de Comunicação, Informação e Inovação Em Saúde, 11*(1), 1–16.

Algahtani, M. S., Ahmad, M. Z., & Ahmad, J., (2020). Nanoemulgel for improved topical delivery of retinyl palmitate: Formulation design and stability evaluation. *Nanomaterials, 10*(5). https://doi.org/10.3390/nano10050848.

Aljabre, S. H. M., Alakloby, O. M., & Randhawa, M. A., (2015). Dermatological effects of *Nigella sativa. Journal of Dermatology & Dermatologic Surgery, 19*(2), 92–98. https://doi.org/10.1016/j.jdds.2015.04.002.

Al-turfy, I. A., (2015). Cryotherapy for the treatment of acne keloidalis (a clinical interventional therapeutic trial). *Iraqi Postgraduate Medical Journal, 14*(3), 425–428.

Alves, M. P., (2006). *Formas Farmacêuticas Plásticas Contendo Nanocápsulas, Nanoesferas e Nanoemulsões de Nimesulida: Desenvolvimento, Caracterização e Avaliação da*

Permeação Cutânea in Vitro. 2006. 183 f. Tese (Doutorado em Ciências Farmacêuticas) – Universidade Federal do Rio Grande do Sul, Porto Alegre.

Alves, N. C., (2015). Penetração de ativos na pele: Revisão bibliográfica. *Amazônia Science & Health, 3*(4), 36–43. https://doi.org/10.18606/2318-1419/amazonia.sci.health.v3n4p36-43.

Amin, B., & Hosseinzadeh, H., (2016). Black cumin (*Nigella sativa*) and its active constituent, thymoquinone: An overview on the analgesic and anti-inflammatory effects. *Planta Medica, 82*(1, 2), 8–16. https://doi.org/10.1055/s-0035-1557838.

Anadolu, R. Y., Sen, T., Tarimci, N., Birol, A., & Erdem, C., (2004). Improved efficacy and tolerability of retinoic acid in acne vulgaris: A new topical formulation with cyclodextrin complex Ψ. *Journal of the European Academy of Dermatology and Venereology, 18*(4), 416–421. https://doi.org/10.1111/j.1468-3083.2004.00929.x.

Andrade, C. D. S. F. De., Batista, N. F., Lasakosvitsch, P. R., Antunes, V. M. D. S., & Oliveira, C. R., (2018). Avaliação da citotoxicidade do tea tree oil e sua ação antimicrobiana em bactéria *Propionibacterium acnes. Brazilian Journal of Natural Sciences, 1*(3), 13. https://doi.org/10.31415/bjns.v1i3.37.

Andrade, S. F., Cardoso, L. G. V., Carvalho, J. C. T., & Bastos, J. K., (2007). Anti-inflammatory and antinociceptive activities of extract, fractions and populnoic acid from bark wood of *Austroplenckia populnea. Journal of Ethnopharmacology, 109*(3), 464–471. https://doi.org/10.1016/j.jep.2006.08.023.

Antonio, C. R., Trídico, L. A., Marchi, C. M. G., Antonio, J. R., & D'Ávila, S. C. G. P., (2017). High-frequency electrosurgery in ice-pick scars: Pre and post treatment comparative study. *Surgical & Cosmetic Dermatology, 9*(2), 123–126. https://doi.org/10.5935/scd1984-8773.201792917.

Antunes, A. F. V., (2016). *Sistemas Nanoparticulados Aplicados à Dermocosmética*. 2016. 69 f. Dissertação (Mestrado em Ciências Farmacêuticas) – Universidade Lusófona de Humanidades e Tecnologias, Lisboa.

Aoshima, H., Kokubo, K., Shirakawa, S., Ito, M., Yamana, S., & Oshima, T., (2009). Antimicrobial activity of fullerenes and their hydroxylated derivatives. *Biocontrol Sci., 14*(2), 69–72.

Apolinário, A. C., De Pachioni-Vasconcelos, J. A., Pessoa, A., & De Rangel-Yagui, C. O., (2017). Polimerossomos versus lipossomos: A evolução da "bala Mágica." *Quimica Nova, 40*(7), 810–817. https://doi.org/10.21577/0100-4042.20170054.

Apriani, E. F., Rosana, Y., & Iskandarsyah, I., (2019). Formulation, characterization, and *in vitro* testing of azelaic acid ethosome-based cream against *Propionibacterium acnes* for the treatment of acne. *Journal of Advanced Pharmaceutical Technology and Research, 10*(2), 76–80. https://doi.org/10.4103/japtr.JAPTR.

Araviiskaia, E., Lopez, E. J. L., & Pincelli, C., (2021). Dermocosmetics: beneficial adjuncts in the treatment of acne vulgaris. *Journal of Dermatological Treatment, 32*(1), 3–10, DOI: 10.1080/09546634.2019.1628173.

Augusto, M., (2017). Estudo da relação entre a alimentação e a acne vulgar. *Cadernos UniFOA, 35*, 123–133. https://doi.org/ISSN: 1809-9475.

Baby, A. R., Haroutiounian-Filho, C. A., Sarruf, F. D., Tavante-Júnior, C. R., Aparecida, C., Oliveira, S. D., Zague, V., et al., (2008). Estabilidade e estudo de penetração cutânea *in vitro* da rutina veiculada em uma emulsão cosmética através de um modelo de biomembrana alternativo. *Brazilian Journal of Pharmaceutical Sciences, 44*(2), 233–248.

Bailo, G. L., (2018). La regulación de las nanotecnologías en argentina. Sobre polisemia e inestabilidad de los nano-objetos. *Revista de La Facultad de Derecho*, *45*, 1–49. https://doi.org/10.22187/rfd2018n45a1.

Barbero, A. M., & Frasch, H. F., (2017). Effect of stratum corneum heterogeneity, anisotropy, asymmetry, and follicular pathway on transdermal penetration. *Journal of Controlled Release*, *260*, 234–246. https://doi.org/10.1016/j.jconrel.2017.05.034.

Barbosa, V., Scheiffer, G. F. C., Cardozo, A. G. L., Pietruchinski, E., Santos, C. Z., Silveira, D., & Bertocco, A. R. P., (2014). Avaliação da atividade antibacteriana do óleo essencial de *Rosmarinus officinalis* L. E tintura de própolis frente à bactéria causadora da acne *Propionibacterium acnes*. *Revista Brasileira de Plantas Medicinais*, *16*(2), 169–173. https://doi.org/10.1590/S1516-05722014000200001.

Baril, M. B., Franco, G. F., Viana, R. S., & Zanin, S. M. W., (2012). Nanotecnologia aplicada aos cosméticos. *Visão Acadêmica*, *13*(1), 45–54. https://doi.org/10.5380/acd.v13i1.30018.

Baur, J. A., & Sinclair, D. A., (2006). Therapeutic potential of resveratrol: The *in vivo* evidence. *Nature Reviews Drug Discovery*, *5*(6), 493–506. https://doi.org/10.1038/nrd2060.

Bavarsad, N., Akhgari, A., Seifmanesh, S., Salimi, A., & Rezaie, A., (2016). Statistical optimization of tretinoin-loaded penetration-enhancer vesicles (PEV) for topical delivery. *DARU, Journal of Pharmaceutical Sciences*, *24*(1), 1–12. https://doi.org/10.1186/s40199-016-0142-0.

Behera, J., Keservani, R. K., Yadav, A., Tripathi, M., & Chadoker, A., (2010). Methoxsalen loaded chitosan coated microemulsion for effective treatment of psoriasis. *International Journal of Drug Delivery*, *2*(2).

Biedroń, R., Ciszek, M., Tokarczyk, M., Bobek, M., Kurnyta, M., Słominska, E. M., Smoleński, R. T., & Marcinkiewicz, J., (2008). 1-Methylnicotinamide and nicotinamide: Two related anti-inflammatory agents that differentially affect the functions of activated macrophages. *Archivum Immunologiae et Therapiae Experimentalis*, *56*(2), 127–134. https://doi.org/10.1007/s00005-008-0009-2.

Bilal, M., & Iqbal, H. M. N., (2020). New insights on unique features and role of nanostructured materials in cosmetics. *Cosmetics*, *7*(2), 24. https://doi.org/10.3390/cosmetics7020024.

Bochicchio, S., Dalmoro, A., De Simone, V., Bertoncin, P., Lamberti, G., & Barba, A. A., (2020). Simil-microfluidic nanotechnology in manufacturing of liposomes as hydrophobic antioxidants skin release systems. *Cosmetics*, *7*(2), 22. https://doi.org/10.3390/cosmetics7020022.

Bodratti, A. M., & Alexandridis, P., (2018). Amphiphilic block copolymers in drug delivery: Advances in formulation structure and performance. *Expert Opinion on Drug Delivery*, *15*(11), 1085–1104. https://doi.org/10.1080/17425247.2018.1529756.

Boen, M., Brownell, J., Patel, P., & Tsoukas, M. M., (2017). The role of photodynamic therapy in acne: An evidence-based review. *American Journal of Clinical Dermatology*, *18*(3), 311–321. https://doi.org/10.1007/s40257-017-0255-3.

Bonamigo, T., Campos, J. F., Oliveira, A. S., Torquato, H. F. V., Balestieri, J. B. P., Cardoso, C. A. L., Paredes-Gamero, E. J., et al., (2017). Antioxidant and cytotoxic activity of propolis of *Plebeia droryana* and *Apis mellifera* (*Hymenoptera, Apidae*) from the Brazilian Cerrado biome. *PLoS One*, *12*(9). https://doi.org/10.1371/journal.pone.0183983.

Burits, M., & Bucar, F., (2000). Antioxidant activity of *Nigella sativa* essential oil. *Phytotherapy Research*, *14*(5), 323–328. https://doi.org/10.1002/1099-1573(200008)14:5<323::AID-PTR621>3.0.CO;2-Q.

Calixto, J. B., (2005). Twenty-five years of research on medicinal plants in Latin America: A personal view. *Journal of Ethnopharmacology*, *100*(1, 2), 131–134. https://doi.org/10.1016/j.jep.2005.06.004.

Camargo, M., Stella, M., & Raddi, G., (2008). Efeito da quercetina sobre o crescimento e atividade hemolitica de *Staphylococcus aureus*. *Revista Eletrônica de Farmácia*, *V*(3), 71–78.

Campesato, V. R., (2005). *Gravidez E Risco Para Malformações Congênitas*. Universidade Federal do Rio Grande do Su.

Campos, A. C. L., Borges-branco, A., & Groth, A. K., (2007). Wound healing. *Arquivos Brasileiros de Cirurgia Digestiva*, *20*(1), 51–58. https://doi.org/10.1590/S0102-67202007000100010.

Canavez, M. De. J. M., (2011). *O uso da Nanotecnologia nas Empresas: Um Estudo de Caso no Setor de Cosméticos* [2011. 81 f. Dissertação (Mestrado em Ciências Econômicas) – Universidade Federal do Paraná, Curitiba]. https://acervodigital.ufpr.br/handle/1884/25794?show=full (accessed on 1 November 2023).

Cao, H. J., Yang, G. Y., Wang, Y. Y., & Liu, J. P., (2013). Acupoint stimulation for acne: A systematic review of randomized controlled trials. *Medical Acupuncture*, *25*(3), 173–194. https://doi.org/10.1089/acu.2012.0906.

Cao, H., Yang, G., Wang, Y., Liu, J. P., Smith, C. A., Luo, H., & Liu, Y., (2016). *Complementary Therapies for Acne Vulgaris*. 1–138. https://doi.org/10.1002/14651858.CD009436.pub2. Complementary.

Cao, X. P., Chen, Y. F., Zhang, J. L., You, M. M., Wang, K., & Hu, F. L., (2017). Mechanisms underlying the wound healing potential of propolis based on its *in vitro* antioxidant activity. *Phytomedicine*, *34*, 76–84. https://doi.org/10.1016/j.phymed.2017.06.001.

Carvalho, L. P., (2018). *Nanotecnologia Aplicada À Dermocosmética* [2018. 83 f. Dissertação (Mestrado em Ciências Farmacêuticas) – Universidade Lusófona de Humanidades e Tecnologias, Lisboa]. http://recil.grupolusofona.pt/bitstream/handle/10437/8900/TESEFINAL 21_11_2017.pdf?sequence=1 (accessed on 1 November 2023).

Chaieb, K., Kouidhi, B., Jrah, H., Mahdouani, K., & Bakhrouf, A., (2011). Antibacterial activity of Thymoquinone, an active principle of Nigella sativa and its potency to prevent bacterial biofilm formation. *BMC Complementary and Alternative Medicine*, *11*. https://doi.org/10.1186/1472-6882-11-29.

Chaikul, P., Khat-udomkiri, N., Iangthanarat, K., Manosroi, J., & Manosroi, A., (2019). Characteristics and *in vitro* anti-skin aging activity of gallic acid loaded in cationic CTAB niosome. *European Journal of Pharmaceutical Sciences*, *131*, 39–49. https://doi.org/10.1016/j.ejps.2019.02.008.

Chan, M. M. Y., (2002). Antimicrobial effect of resveratrol on dermatophytes and bacterial pathogens of the skin. *Biochemical Pharmacology*, *63*(2), 99–104. https://doi.org/10.1016/S0006-2952(01)00886-3.

Chaudhri, N., Soni, G. C., & Prajapati, S. K., (2015). Nanotechnology: An advance tool for nano-cosmetics preparation. *International Journal of Pharma Research & Review*, *4*(44), 28–40.

Chen, C. C., Tsai, T. H., Huang, Z. R., & Fang, J. Y., (2010). Effects of lipophilic emulsifiers on the oral administration of lovastatin from nanostructured lipid carriers: Physicochemical characterization and pharmacokinetics. *European Journal of Pharmaceutics and Biopharmaceutics*, *74*(3), 474–482. https://doi.org/10.1016/j.ejpb.2009.12.008.

Chen, S., Hanning, S., Falconer, J., Locke, M., & Wen, J., (2019). Recent advances in non-ionic surfactant vesicles (niosomes): Fabrication, characterization, pharmaceutical and cosmetic applications. *European Journal of Pharmaceutics and Biopharmaceutics, 144*, 18–39. https://doi.org/10.1016/j.ejpb.2019.08.015.

Cheng, H. N., Doemeny, L. J., Geraci, C. L., & Schmidt, D. G., (2016). Nanotechnology overview: Opportunities and challenges. *ACS Symposium Series, 1220*, 1–12. https://doi.org/10.1021/bk-2016-1220.ch001.

Chorilli, M., Rimério, T. C., De Oliveira, A. G., & Scarpa, M. V., (2007). Estudo da estabilidade de lipossomas compostos de fosfatidilcolina de soja e fosfatidilcolina de soja hidrogenada adicionados ou não de colesterol por método turbidimétrico. *Latin American Journal of Pharmacy, 26*(1), 31–37.

Coderch, L., Pera, M. De., Perez-Cullell, N., Estelrich, J., Maza, A. De. La., & Parra, J. L., (1999). The effect of liposomes on skin barrier structure. *Skin Pharmacology and Applied Skin Physiology, 12*, 235–246.

Coqueiro, M. E. C., & Santos, J. A. B., (2019). Artigo de revisão benefícios da alta frequência na acne vulgar Grau II: Uma Revisão de Literatura. *Id on Line Revista Multidisciplinar e de Psicologia, 13*(48), 224–242. https://doi.org/10.14295/idonline.v13i48.2120.

Cross, S. E., Russell, M., Southwell, I., & Roberts, M. S., (2008). Human skin penetration of the major components of Australian tea tree oil applied in its pure form and as a 20% solution *in vitro*. *European Journal of Pharmaceutics and Biopharmaceutics, 69*(1), 214–222. https://doi.org/10.1016/j.ejpb.2007.10.002.

Cunha, M. G. Da., Moraes, C., Cebrian, G., Silva, R. F. Da., Reple, S. I. F., Machado, F. C. D. A., & Fonseca, F. L. A., (2020). Dosages of androgenic hormones in adolescent patients with severe acne. *Revista Da Associação Médica Brasileira, 66*(1), 36–41. https://doi.org/10.1590/1806-9282.66.1.36.

Cutillas, A. B., Carrasco, A., Martinez-Gutierrez, R., Tomas, V., & Tudela, J., (2018). Rosmarinus officinalis L. essential oils from Spain: Composition, antioxidant capacity, lipoxygenase and acetylcholinesterase inhibitory capacities, and antimicrobial activities. *Plant Biosystems, 152*(6), 1282–1292. https://doi.org/10.1080/11263504.2018.1445129.

Das, M. K., & Kalita, B., (2014). Design and evaluation of phyto-phospholipid complexes (phytosomes) of Rutin for transdermal application. *Journal of Applied Pharmaceutical Science, 4*(10), 51–57. https://doi.org/10.7324/JAPS.2014.40110.

Daudt, R. M., Emanuelli, J., Külkamp-guerreiro, I. C., Pohlmann, A. R., & Guterres, S. S., (2013). A nanotecnologia como estratégia para o desenvolvimento de cosméticos. *Ciência e Cultura, 65*(3), 28–31.

De Miranda, J. C., Martins, T. E. A., Veiga, F., & Ferraz, H. G., (2011). Cyclodextrins and ternary complexes: Technology to improve solubility of poorly soluble drugs. *Brazilian Journal of Pharmaceutical Sciences, 47*(4), 665–681. https://doi.org/10.1590/S1984-82502011000400003.

Delgado, J. M. F., (2013). *Preparação e Caracterização de Nanotransportadores (Nanocápsulas, Nanoesferas, Lipossomas e Transportadores Lipídicos Nanoestruturados) Sem Substância Ativa [2013. 117 f.* Dissertação (Mestrado em Tecnologia Biomédica) – Instituto Politécnico de Bragança, Bragança]. In: Instituto Politécnico de Bragança. https://bibliotecadigital.ipb.pt/handle/10198/9219 (accessed on 1 November 2023).

Deng, P., Teng, F., Zhou, F., Song, Z., Meng, N., & Feng, R., (2017a). Methoxy poly (ethylene glycol)-b-poly (δ-valerolactone) copolymeric micelles for improved skin delivery of ketoconazole. *Journal of Biomaterials Science, Polymer Edition, 28*(1), 63–78. https://doi.org/10.1080/09205063.2016.1244371.

Deng, P., Teng, F., Zhou, F., Song, Z., Ning, M., Liu, N., & Feng, R., (2017b). Y-shaped methoxy poly (ethylene glycol)-block-poly (epsilon-caprolactone)-based micelles for skin delivery of ketoconazole: *In vitro* study and *in vivo* evaluation. *Materials Science and Engineering C, 78*, 296–304. https://doi.org/10.1016/j.msec.2017.04.089.

Desai, P., Patlolla, R. R., & Singh, M., (2011). Interaction of nanoparticles and cell-penetrating peptides with skin for transdermal drug delivery. *Molecular Membrane Biology, 27*(7), 247–259. https://doi.org/10.3109/09687688.2010.522203.Interaction.

Dessinioti, C., & Dreno, B., (2020). Acne treatments: Future trajectories. *Clinical and Experimental Dermatology, March*, 1–7. https://doi.org/10.1111/ced.14239.

Dhapte-Pawar, V., Kadam, S., Saptarsi, S., & Kenjale, P. P., (2020). Nanocosmeceuticals: Facets and aspects. *Future Science OA*, FSO613. https://doi.org/10.2144/fsoa-2019-0109.

Dikicier, B. S., (2019). Topical treatment of acne vulgaris: Efficiency, side effects, and adherence rate. *Journal of International Medical Research, 47*(7), 2987–2992. https://doi.org/10.1177/0300060519847367.

Dimer, F. A., Friedrich, R. B., Beck, R. C. R., Guterres, S. S., & Pohlmann, A. R., (2013). Impact of nanotechnology on public health: Production of medicines. *Química Nova, 36*(10), 1520–1526. https://doi.org/10.1590/S0100-40422013001000007.

Docherty, J. J., McEwen, H. A., Sweet, T. J., Bailey, E., & Booth, T. D., (2007). Resveratrol inhibition of *Propionibacterium acnes*. *The Journal of Antimicrobial Chemotherapy, 59*(6), 1182–1184. https://doi.org/10.1093/jac/dkm099.

Dréno, B., Pécastaings, S., Corvec, S., Veraldi, S., Khammari, A., & Roques, C., (2018). *Cutibacterium acnes* (*Propionibacterium acnes*) and acne vulgaris: A brief look at the latest updates. *Journal of the European Academy of Dermatology and Venereology, 32*(2), 5–14. https://doi.org/10.1111/jdv.15043.

Dubey, V., Mishra, D., & Jain, N. K., (2007). Melatonin loaded ethanolic liposomes: Physicochemical characterization and enhanced transdermal delivery. *European Journal of Pharmaceutics and Biopharmaceutics, 67*, 398–405. https://doi.org/10.1016/j.ejpb.2007.03.007.

Działo, M., Mierziak, J., Korzun, U., Preisner, M., Szopa, J., & Kulma, A., (2016). The potential of plant phenolics in prevention and therapy of skin disorders. *International Journal of Molecular Sciences, 17*(2), 1–41. https://doi.org/10.3390/ijms17020160.

Edwards, K. A., & Baeumner, A. J., (2006). Analysis of liposomes. *Talanta, 68*(5), 1432–1441. https://doi.org/10.1016/j.talanta.2005.08.031.

Effiong, D. E., Uwah, T. O., Jumbo, E. U., & Akpabio, A. E., (2020). Nanotechnology in cosmetics: Basics, current trends, and safety concerns — A review. *Advances in Nanoparticles, 9*(1), 1–22. https://doi.org/10.4236/anp.2020.91001.

Eid, A. M., Elmarzugi, N. A., Abu, A. L. M., Sawafta, M. N., & Daana, H. I., (2017). A review on the cosmeceutical and external applications of *Nigella sativa*. *Journal of Tropical Medicine, 2017*. https://doi.org/10.1155/2017/7092514.

El-Menshawe, S. F., Ali, A. A., Rabeh, M. A., & Khalil, N. M., (2018). Nanosized soy phytosome-based thermogel as topical anti-obesity formulation: An approach for acceptable level of evidence of an effective novel herbal weight loss product. *International Journal of Nanomedicine, 13*, 307–318. https://doi.org/10.2147/IJN.S153429.

Elmowafy, M., Shalaby, K., Ali, H. M., Alruwaili, N. K., Salama, A., Ibrahim, M. F., Akl, M. A., & Ahmed, T. A., (2019). Impact of nanostructured lipid carriers on dapsone delivery to the skin: *In vitro* and *in vivo* studies. *International Journal of Pharmaceutics*, *572*, 118781. https://doi.org/10.1016/j.ijpharm.2019.118781.

Ereno, D., (2008). Nanotecnologia beleza fundamentada. *Fapesp*, *146*, 6.

Etheridge, M. L., Campbell, S. A., Erdman, A. G., Haynes, C. L., Wolf, S. M., & McCullough, J., (2013). The big picture on nanomedicine: The state of investigational and approved nanomedicine products. *Nanomedicine: Nanotechnology, Biology, and Medicine*, *9*(1), 1–14. https://doi.org/10.1016/j.nano.2012.05.013.

Fabbrocini, G., Staibano, S., De Rosa, G., Battimiello, V., Fardella, N., Ilardi, G., Immacolata La, R. M., et al., (2011). Resveratrol-containing gel for the treatment of acne vulgaris: A single-blind, vehicle-controlled, pilot study. *American Journal of Clinical Dermatology*, *12*(2), 133–141. https://doi.org/10.2165/11530630-000000000-00000.

Faria, E. M. De., Eleamen, G. R. De. A., Silva, A. E., Mendonça, E. A. De. M., & Oliveira, E. E., (2013). Nanotecnologia e meio ambiente: Uma análise sobre os riscos e benefícios dessa tecnologia em um contexto atual. *Revista de Biologia e Farmácia*, *9*(1), 18–26.

Faria-Tischer, P. C. S., & Tischer, C. A., (2012). Nanobiotecnologia: Plataforma tecnológica para biomateriais e aplicação biológica de nanoestruturas. *BBR – Biochemistry and Biotechnology Reports*, *1*(1), 32–53. https://doi.org/10.5433/2316-5200.2012v1n1p32.

Fatima, N., Rehman, S., Nabi, B., Baboota, S., & Ali, J., (2019). Harnessing nanotechnology for enhanced topical delivery of clindamycin phosphate. *Journal of Drug Delivery Science and Technology*, *54*, 101253. https://doi.org/10.1016/j.jddst.2019.101253.

Felippi, C. C., (2008). *Nanopartículas Contendo Isotretinoína: Preparação, Caracterização Físico-Química, Estudo de Estabilidade e Avaliação da Penetração Cutânea*. Universidade Federal do Rio Grande do Sul.

Fernandes, M. F. M., & Filgueiras, C. A. L., (2008). Um panorama da nanotecnologia no Brasil (e seus macro-desafios). *Química Nova*, *31*(8), 2205–2213. https://doi.org/10.1590/S0100-40422008000800050.

Ferreira, F. Da. R., (2009). *Estudo do Encapsulamento de Compostos Antioxidantes em β-ciclodextrina por Métodos Eletroquímicos e Espectroscópicos*. 2009. 100 f. Dissertação (Mestrado em Química e Biotecnologia) – Universidade Federal de Alagoas, Maceió.

Ferreira, H. S., & Rangel, M. D. C., (2009). Nanotecnologia: Aspectos gerais e potencial de aplicação em catálise. *Química Nova*, *32*(7), 1860–1870. https://doi.org/10.1590/S0100-40422009000700033.

Fitrya, F., Fithri, N. A., Winda, M., & Muharni, M., (2020). Ethanol extract of *Parkia speciosa* Hassk. loaded transfersome: Characterization and optimization. *Journal of Pharmacy and Pharmacognosy Research*, *8*(3), 167–176.

Flores-Rojas, C., Cabello-Carlos, S., & Paucar-Lescano, P. K., (2020). Acne in medical students and their associated factors. *Revista Peruana de Investigación En Salud*, *4*(1), 17–23. https://doi.org/10.4314/ajcem.v12i3.

Franco, C. C., Tais, B. M., De Bona Da, S. C., Barin, J. S., Cristiano, E., & De Menezes, R., (2015). Nanoestruturas contendo compostos bioativos extraídos de plantas nanostructures containing bioactive compounds extracted from plants. *Ciência e Natura*, *37*(2), 142–151. https://doi.org/10.5902/2179-460X19743.

Fronza, T., (2006). *Estudo Exploratório de Mecanismos de Regulação Sanitária de Produtos Cosméticos de Base Nanotecnológica no Brasil*. 2006. 92 f. Dissertação (Mestrado em Ciências Farmacêuticas) – Universidade Federal do Rio Grande do Sul, Porto Alegre.

Garvil, M., Arantes, D., & Gouveia, C., (2013). Nanotecnologia em cosméticos e dermocosméticos. *E-RAC*, 1–11. https://doi.org/10.1017/CBO9781107415324.004.

Gautam, S. P., Keservani, R. K., Gautam, T., Gupta, A. K., & Sharma, A. K., (2015). An Alternative Approach for Acetylation of Amine Terminated Polyamidoamine (PAMAM) Dendrimer. *Ars Pharm. 56*(3), 155–159.

Gelfuso, G. M., Matos, B. N., Areda, C. A., Cunha-Filho, M. S., Oliveira, P. M., & Gratieri, T., (2015). Preparações farmacêuticas e cosméticas com uso de nanotecnologia. *Brasília Médica, 52*(1), 8–20. https://doi.org/10.14242/2236-5117.2015v52n1a296p8.

Gentzkow, G. D., (1993). Electrical stimulation to heal dermal wounds. *The Journal of Dermatologic Surgery and Oncology, 19*(8), 753–758. https://doi.org/10.1111/j.1524-4725.1993.tb00420.x.

Godin, B., & Touitou, E., (2003). Ethosomes: New prospects in transdermal delivery. *Critical Reviews in Therapeutic Drug Carrier Systems, 20*(1), 63–102. https://doi.org/10.1615/CritRevTherDrugCarrierSyst.v20.i1.20.

Goh, C. F., Moffat, J. G., Craig, D. Q. M., Hadgraft, J., & Lane, M. E., (2017). Nano-thermal imaging of the stratum corneum and its potential use for understanding of the mechanism of skin penetration enhancer. *Thermochimica Acta, 655*, 278–283. https://doi.org/10.1016/j.tca.2017.07.013.

Gollnick, H., & Schramm, M., (1998). Topical drug treatment in acne. *Dermatology, 196*(1), 119–125. https://doi.org/10.1159/000017844.

Gomathi, K., Gopinath, D., Ahmed, M. R., & Jayakumar, R., (2003). Quercetin incorporated collagen matrices for dermal wound healing processes in rat. *Biomaterials, 24*(16), 2767–2772. https://doi.org/10.1016/S0142-9612(03)00059-0.

González, Y. X. C., Jiménez, D. P., Correa, A. L. V., Cardozo, M. A. R., & Huertas, C. E. M., (2016). Nanopartículas lipídicas a base de propóleos como transportadores de activos de interés cosmético: Desarrollo, caracterización y evaluación de seguridad. *Revista Colombiana de Ciencias Químico-Farmacéuticas, 45*(1), 147–168. https://doi.org/10.15446/rcciquifa.v45n1.58026.

Gordillo-Galeano, A., & Mora-Huertas, C. E., (2018). Solid lipid nanoparticles and nanostructured lipid carriers: A review emphasizing on particle structure and drug release. *European Journal of Pharmaceutics and Biopharmaceutics, 133*, 285–308. https://doi.org/10.1016/j.ejpb.2018.10.017.

Goyal, R., Macri, L. K., Kaplan, H. M., & Kohn, J., (2016). Nanoparticles and nanofibers for topical drug delivery. *Journal of Controlled Release, 240*, 77–92. https://doi.org/10.1016/j.jconrel.2015.10.049.

Gregory, S. R., Piccolo, N., Piccolo, M. T., Piccolo, M. S., & Heggers, J. P., (2002). Comparison of propolis skin cream to silver sulfadiazine: A naturopathic alternative to antibiotics in treatment of minor burns. *Journal of Alternative and Complementary Medicine, 8*(1), 77–83. https://doi.org/10.1089/107555302753507203.

Gupta, M., Agrawal, U., & Vyas, S. P., (2012). Nanocarrier-based topical drug delivery for the treatment of skin diseases. *Expert Opinion on Drug Delivery, 9*(7), 783–804. https://doi.org/10.1517/17425247.2012.686490.

Guterres, S. S., Alves, M. P., & Pohlmann, A. R., (2007). Polymeric nanoparticles, nanospheres and nanocapsules, for cutaneous applications. *Drug Target Insights, 2*, 147–157. https://doi.org/10.1177/117739280700200002.

Hadi, N. A., & Ashor, W., (2010). Nigella sativa oil lotion 20% vs. benzoyl peroxide lotion 5% in the treatment of mild to moderate acne vulgaris. *Iraqi Postgraduate Medical Journal, 9*(4), 20–26.

Hameed, A., Fatima, R., Malik, K., Muqadas, A., & Fazal-Ur-Rehman, M., (2019). Scope of nanotechnology in cosmetics: Dermatology and skin care products. *Journal of Medicinal and Chemical Sciences*, *2*(2), 9–16. http://jmchemsci.com (accessed on 1 November 2023).

Hariharan, P., Paul-Satyaseela, M., & Gnanamani, A., (2016). *In vitro* profiling of anti-methicillin-resistant *Staphylococcus aureus* activity of thymoquinone against selected type and clinical strains. *Letters in Applied Microbiology*, *62*(3), 283–289. https://doi.org/10.1111/lam.12544.

Hart, P. H., Brand, C., Carson, C. F., Riley, T. V., Prager, R. H., & Finlay-Jones, J. J., (2000). Terpinen-4-ol, the main component of the essential oil of *Melaleuca alternifolia* (tea tree oil), suppresses inflammatory mediator production by activated human monocytes. *Inflammation Research*, *49*(11), 619–626. https://doi.org/10.1007/s000110050639.

Hasanpouri, A., Lotfipour, F., Ghanbarzadeh, S., & Hamishehkar, H., (2018). Improvement of dermal delivery of tetracycline using vesicular nanostructures. *Research in Pharmaceutical Sciences*, *13*(5), 385–393. https://doi.org/10.4103/1735-5362.236831.

Helgason, T., Awad, T. S., Kristbergsson, K., McClements, D. J., & Weiss, J., (2009). Effect of surfactant surface coverage on formation of solid lipid nanoparticles (SLN). *Journal of Colloid and Interface Science*, *334*(1), 75–81. https://doi.org/10.1016/j.jcis.2009.03.012.

Hofer, C., Hartung, R., Göbel, R., Deering, P., Lehmer, A., & Breul, J., (2000). New ultradeformable drug carriers for potential transdermal application of interleukin-2 and interferon-α: Theoretic and practical aspects. *World Journal of Surgery*, *24*(10), 1187–1189. https://doi.org/10.1007/s002680010201.

Hong, I. K., Ha, J. H., Han, S., Kang, H., & Park, S. N., (2018). The effect of Alkyl chain number in sucrose surfactant on the physical properties of quercetin-loaded deformable nanoliposome and its effect on *in vitro* human skin penetration. *Nanomaterials*, *8*(8). https://doi.org/10.3390/nano8080622.

Hua, S., (2015). Lipid-based nano-delivery systems for skin delivery of drugs and bioactives. *Frontiers in Pharmacology*, *6*(SEP), 2011–2015. https://doi.org/10.3389/fphar.2015.00219.

Inui, S., Aoshima, H., Nishiyama, A., & Itami, S., (2011). Improvement of acne vulgaris by topical fullerene application: Unique impact on skin care. *Nanomedicine: Nanotechnology, Biology, and Medicine*, *7*(2), 238–241. https://doi.org/10.1016/j.nano.2010.09.005.

Iriguchi, E. K. K., (2012). *Atividade Anti-inflamatória do Extrato Metanólico de Schinus Terebinthifolius Raddi, do Metil Galato e de Derivados Carbohidrazil em Modelos de Inflamação Experimental*. 2012. 92 f. Dissertação (Mestrado em Ciências da Saúde) – Universidade Federal da Grande Dourados, Dourados.

Jain, N., Gupta, B. P., Thakur, N., Jain, R., Banweer, J., Jain, D. K., & Jain, S., (2010). Phytosome: A novel drug delivery system for herbal medicine. *International Journal of Pharmaceutical Sciences and Drug Research*, *2*(4), 224–228. https://doi.org/10.5530/srp.2017.1.2.

Jain, S., Jain, P., Umamaheshwari, R., & Jain, N., (2003). Transfersomes — A novel vesicular carrier for enhanced transdermal delivery: Development, characterization, and performance evaluation. *Drug Development and Industrial Pharmacy*, *29*(9), 1013–1026. https://doi.org/10.1081/DDC-120025458.

Jain, S., Kale, D. P., Swami, R., & Katiyar, S. S., (2018). Codelivery of benzoyl peroxide & adapalene using modified liposomal gel for improved acne therapy. *Nanomedicine*, *13*(12), 1481–1493. https://doi.org/10.2217/nnm-2018-0002.

Janani, S. K., Sureshkumar, R., Upadhyayula, S. S. N., Karthika, C., & Vasanthi, C., (2019). Will the polyphenol and adapalene combination be a good strategy on acne vulgaris? *Medical Hypotheses*, *133*, 109409. https://doi.org/10.1016/j.mehy.2019.109409.

Jrah, H. H., Kouidhi, B., Flamini, G., Bakhrouf, A., & Mahjoub, T., (2011). Chemical composition, antimicrobial potential against cariogenic bacteria and cytotoxic activity of Tunisian *Nigella sativa* essential oil and thymoquinone. *Food Chemistry*, *129*(4), 1469–1474. https://doi.org/10.1016/j.foodchem.2011.05.117.

Jufri, M., Muthaharrah, M., Humairah, E., & Purwaningsih, E. H., (2017). Stability of anti-acne niosome gels containing betel leaf (*Piper betle* L.) essential oil. *International Journal of Applied Pharmaceutics*, *9*, 130–134. https://doi.org/10.22159/ijap.2017.v9s1.72_79.

Kandekar, S. G., Del Río-Sancho, S., Lapteva, M., & Kalia, Y. N., (2018). Selective delivery of adapalene to the human hair follicle under finite dose conditions using polymeric micelle nanocarriers. *Nanoscale*, *10*(3), 1099–1110. https://doi.org/10.1039/c7nr07706h.

Kaul, S., Gulati, N., Verma, D., Mukherjee, S., & Nagaich, U., (2018). Role of nanotechnology in cosmeceuticals: A review of recent advances. *Journal of Pharmaceutics*, *2018*, 1–19. https://doi.org/10.1155/2018/3420204.

Kaur, D., & Kumar, S., (2018). Niosomes: Present scenario and future aspects. *Journal of Drug Delivery and Therapeutics*, *8*(5), 35–43. https://doi.org/10.22270/jddt.v8i5.1886.

Kausar, H., Mujeeb, M., Ahad, A., Moolakkadath, T., Aqil, M., Ahmad, A., & Akhter, M. H., (2019). Optimization of ethosomes for topical thymoquinone delivery for the treatment of skin acne. *Journal of Drug Delivery Science and Technology*, *49*, 177–187. https://doi.org/10.1016/j.jddst.2018.11.016.

Kelidari, H. R., Saeedi, M., Akbari, J., Morteza-Semnani, K., Gill, P., Valizadeh, H., & Nokhodchi, A., (2015). Formulation optimization and *in vitro* skin penetration of spironolactone loaded solid lipid nanoparticles. *Colloids and Surfaces B: Biointerfaces*, *128*, 473–479. https://doi.org/10.1016/j.colsurfb.2015.02.046.

Kelidari, H. R., Saeedi, M., Hajheydari, Z., Akbari, J., Morteza-Semnani, K., Akhtari, J., Valizadeh, H., et al., (2016). Spironolactone loaded nanostructured lipid carrier gel for effective treatment of mild and moderate acne vulgaris: A randomized, double-blind, prospective trial. *Colloids and Surfaces B: Biointerfaces*, *146*, 47–53. https://doi.org/10.1016/j.colsurfb.2016.05.042.

Kerem, Z., Bilkis, I., Flaishman, M. A., & Sivan, L., (2006). Antioxidant activity and inhibition of α-glucosidase by trans-resveratrol, piceid, and a novel trans-stilbene from the roots of Israeli *Rumex bucephalophorus* L. *Journal of Agricultural and Food Chemistry*, *54*(4), 1243–1247. https://doi.org/10.1021/jf052436+.

Keservani, R. K., & Gautam, S. P., (2020). Formulation and evaluation of baclofen liposome vesicles using lecithin. *ARS Pharmaceutica*, *61*(3), 175–180.

Keservani, R. K., & Gautam, S. P., (2022). Skeletal muscle relaxant activity of different formulation of span 60 niosome. *ARS Pharmaceutica*, *63*(91), 32–44.

Keservani, R. K., Kesharwani, R. K., & Sharma, A. K., (2017). Introduction to nanotechnology in drug delivery. In: *Drug Delivery Approaches and Nanosystems* (pp. 1–19). Apple Academic Press. ISBN: 9781771885836.

Keservani, R. K., Sharma, A. K., & Kesharwani, R. K., (2018). Nanoparticulate nanocarriers in drug delivery. In: *Nanobiomaterials* (pp. 3–22). Apple Academic Press. ISBN: 9781771885911.

Keservani, R. K., Sharma, A. K., & Ramteke, S., (2010). Novel vesicular approach for topical delivery of baclofen via niosomes. *Lat. Am. J. Pharm.*, *29*, 1364–1370.

Kim, J., Ochoa, M. T., Krutzik, S. R., Takeuchi, O., Uematsu, S., Legaspi, A. J., Brightbill, H. D., et al., (2002). Activation of toll-like receptor 2 in acne triggers inflammatory cytokine responses. *The Journal of Immunology, 169*(3), 1535–1541. https://doi.org/10.4049/jimmunol.169.3.1535.

Kim, S. Y., Hyun, M. Y., Go, K. C., Zouboulis, C. C., & Kim, B. J., (2015). Resveratrol exerts growth inhibitory effects on human SZ95 sebocytes through the inactivation of the PI3-K/Akt pathway. *International Journal of Molecular Medicine, 35*(4), 1042–1050. https://doi.org/10.3892/ijmm.2015.2098.

Kligman, A., (2005). The future of cosmeceuticals: An interview with albert kligman. *Dermatol Surgery, 31*, 890, 891. https://doi.org/https://doi.org/10.1111/j.1524-4725.2005.31737.

Kou, L., Bhutia, Y. D., Yao, Q., He, Z., Sun, J., & Ganapathy, V., (2018). Transporter-guided delivery of nanoparticles to improve drug permeation across cellular barriers and drug exposure to selective cell types. *Frontiers in Pharmacology, 9*, 1–16. https://doi.org/10.3389/fphar.2018.00027.

Kringel, D. H., Antunes, M. D., Klein, B., Crizel, R. L., Wagner, R., De Oliveira, R. P., Dias, A. R. G., & Zavareze, E. Da. R., (2017). Production, characterization, and stability of orange or eucalyptus essential oil/β-cyclodextrin inclusion complex. *Journal of Food Science, 82*(11), 2598–2605. https://doi.org/10.1111/1750-3841.13923.

Kroes, B. H., Vandenberg, A. J. J., Vanufford, H. C. Q., Vandijk, H., & Labadie, R. P., (1992). Anti-inflammatory activity of gallic acid. *Planta Medica, 58*(6), 499–504. https://doi.org/10.1055/s-2006-961535.

Kumar, P., Naidu, V., & Gupta, P., (2007). Application of hydrolytic kinetic resolution (HKR) in the synthesis of bioactive compounds. *Tetrahedron, 63*(13), 2745–2785. https://doi.org/10.1016/j.tet.2006.12.015.

Kumar, S., (2005). Exploratory analysis of global cosmetic industry: Major players, technology, and market trends. *Technovation, 25*(11), 1263–1272. https://doi.org/10.1016/j.technovation.2004.07.003.

Kushwaha, N., Minocha, N., & Kumar, N., (2020). Use of nanotechnology in cosmeceuticals: A review. *International Journal of Pharmaceutical Science Invention, 9*(I), 43–51.

Kwon, H. H., Yoon, J. Y., Park, S. Y., Min, S., & Suh, D. H., (2014). Comparison of clinical and histological effects between *Lactobacillus*-fermented *Chamaecyparis obtusa* and tea tree oil for the treatment of acne: An eight-week double-blind randomized controlled split-face study. *Dermatology, 229*(2), 102–109. https://doi.org/10.1159/000362491.

Lacatusu, I., Istrati, D., Bordei, N., Popescu, M., Seciu, A. M., Panteli, L. M., & Badea, N., (2020). Synergism of plant extract and vegetable oils-based lipid nanocarriers: Emerging trends in development of advanced cosmetic prototype products. *Materials Science and Engineering C, 108*, 110412. https://doi.org/10.1016/j.msec.2019.110412.

Lacerda, J. R. C., Sousa, J. Da. S., Sousa, L. C. F. S., Borges, M. Da. G. B., Ferreira, R. T. F. V., Salgado, A. B., & Silva, M. J. S. Da., (2013). Popular knowledge on medicinal plants and its applicability in three segments of society in the city of Pombal-PB. *ACSA – Agropecuária Científica No Semi-Árido, 9*(1), 14–23.

Lademann, J., Richter, H., Schanzer, S., Knorr, F., Meinke, M., Sterry, W., & Patzelt, A., (2011). Penetration and storage of particles in human skin: Perspectives and safety aspects. *European Journal of Pharmaceutics and Biopharmaceutics, 77*(3), 465–468. https://doi.org/10.1016/j.ejpb.2010.10.015.

Lange, M. K., Heberlé, G., & Milão, D., (2009). Avaliação da estabilidade e atividade antioxidante de uma emulsão base não-iônica contendo resveratrol. *Brazilian Journal of Pharmaceutical Sciences*, *45*(1), 1–7.

Lapteva, M., Möller, M., Gurny, R., & Kalia, Y. N., (2015). Self-assembled polymeric nanocarriers for the targeted delivery of retinoic acid to the hair follicle. *Nanoscale*, *7*(44), 18651–18662. https://doi.org/10.1039/c5nr04770f.

Lara, V. C. D., (2008). Desenvolvimento de nanocápsulas contendo ácido retinóico para tratamento tópico da acne. *Faculdade de Farmácia de UFMG*, *1*, 1–103.

Lazzaretti, L. L., (2018). *Nanocosméticos: O Olhar Da Ciência Sobre a Toxicidade E O Princípio Da Precaução Para Avaliar Os Potenciais Riscos Desses Produtos*. https://periodicos.feevale.br/seer/index.php/revistaconhecimentoonline/article/view/1604 (accessed on 1 November 2023).

Lee, J. H., Agarwal, V., Bose, A., Payne, G. F., & Raghavan, S. R., (2006). Transition from unilamellar to bilamellar vesicles induced by an amphiphilic biopolymer. *Physical Review Letters*, *96*(4). https://doi.org/10.1103/PhysRevLett.96.048102.

Letchford, K., & Burt, H., (2007). A review of the formation and classification of amphiphilic block copolymer nanoparticulate structures: Micelles, nanospheres, nanocapsules and polymersomes. *European Journal of Pharmaceutics and Biopharmaceutics*, *65*(3), 259–269. https://doi.org/10.1016/j.ejpb.2006.11.009.

Li, Y., Yao, J., Han, C., Yang, J., Chaudhry, M. T., Wang, S., Liu, H., & Yin, Y., (2016). Quercetin, inflammation, and immunity. *Nutrients*, *8*(3), 1–14. https://doi.org/10.3390/nu8030167.

Lima, M. F. Da. S., Barros, V. J. Da. S., & Neto, M. P. L., (2020). Analysis of oral isotretinoin consumption in the specialized component of pharmaceutical assistance in the state of Piauí. *Research, Society and Development*, *9*(2), 1–13. https://doi.org/10.1016/j.solener.2019.02.027.

Lin, T. J., (2010). Evolution of cosmetics: Increased need for experimental clinical medicine. *Journal of Experimental and Clinical Medicine*, *2*(2), 49–52. https://doi.org/10.1016/S1878-3317(10)60009-5.

Loftsson, T., & Masson, M., (2001). Cyclodextrins in topical drug formulations: Theory and practice. *International Journal of Pharmaceutics*, *225*, 15–30. https://doi.org/https://doi.org/10.1016/S0378-5173(01)00761-X.

Lohani, A., Verma, A., Joshi, H., Yadav, N., & Karki, N., (2014). Nanotechnology-based cosmeceuticals. *ISRN Dermatology*, 1–14. https://doi.org/http://dx.doi.org/10.1155/2014/843687 Review.

Lovato, W. E. C., Velasquez, P. A. G., Oliveira, C. D. S., Baruffi, C., Anghinoni, T., Machado, R. C., Lívero, F. A. D. R., et al., (2018). High frequency equipment promotes antibacterial effects dependent on intensity and exposure time. *Clinical, Cosmetic and Investigational Dermatology*, *11*, 131–135. https://doi.org/10.2147/CCID.S156282.

Low, W. L., Martin, C., Hill, D. J., & Kenward, M. A., (2013). Antimicrobial efficacy of liposome-encapsulated silver ions and tea tree oil against pseudomonas aeruginosa, staphylococcus aureus and candida albicans. *Letters in Applied Microbiology*, *57*(1), 33–39. https://doi.org/10.1111/lam.12082.

Lu, K. J., Wang, W., Xu, X. L., Jin, F. Y., Qi, J., Wang, X. J., Kang, X. Q., et al., (2019). A dual deformable liposomal ointment functionalized with retinoic acid and epidermal growth factor for enhanced burn wound healing therapy. *Biomaterials Science*, *7*(6), 2372–2382. https://doi.org/10.1039/c8bm01569d.

Maciel, M. A. M., Pinto, A. C., Veiga, V. F., Grynberg, N. F., & Echevarria, A., (2002). Plantas medicinais: A necessidade de estudos multidisciplinares. *Química Nova, 25*(3), 429–438. https://doi.org/10.1590/s0100-40422002000300016.

Maghraby, G. M. El., Barry, B. W., & Williams, A. C., (2008). Liposomes and skin: From drug delivery to model membranes. *European Journal of Pharmaceutical Sciences, 4*, 203–222. https://doi.org/10.1016/j.ejps.2008.05.002.

Manconi, M., Sinico, C., Valenti, D., Lai, F., & Fadda, A. M., (2006). Niosomes as carriers for tretinoin: III. A study into the *in vitro* cutaneous delivery of vesicle-incorporated tretinoin. *International Journal of Pharmaceutics, 311*(1, 2), 11–19. https://doi.org/10.1016/j.ijpharm.2005.11.045.

Manconi, M., Sinico, C., Valenti, D., Loy, G., & Fadda, A. M., (2002). Niosomes as carriers for tretinoin. I. Preparation and properties. *International Journal of Pharmaceutics, 234*(1, 2), 237–248. https://doi.org/10.1016/S0378-5173(01)00971-1.

Manconi, M., Valenti, D., Sinico, C., Lai, F., Loy, G., & Fadda, A. M., (2003). Niosomes as carriers for tretinoin: II. Influence of vesicular incorporation on tretinoin photostability. *International Journal of Pharmaceutics, 260*(2), 261–272. https://doi.org/10.1016/S0378-5173(03)00268-0.

Maramaldi, G., Togni, S., Pagin, I., Giacomelli, L., Cattaneo, R., Eggenhöffner, R., & Burastero, S. E., (2016). Soothing and anti-itch effect of quercetin phytosome in human subjects: A single-blind study. *Clinical, Cosmetic and Investigational Dermatology, 9*, 55–62. https://doi.org/10.2147/CCID.S98890.

Marcato, P. D., (2009). Preparação, caracterização e aplicações em fármacos e cosméticos de nanopartículas lipídicas sólidas. *Revista Eletrônica de Farmácia, VI*(2), 1–37. https://doi.org/https://doi.org/10.5216/ref.v6i2.6545.

Marianecci, C., Di Marzio, L., Rinaldi, F., Celia, C., Paolino, D., Alhaique, F., Esposito, S., & Carafa, M., (2014). Niosomes from 80s to present: The state of the art. *Advances in Colloid and Interface Science, 205*, 187–206. https://doi.org/10.1016/j.cis.2013.11.018.

Marques, I., Lopes, C., & Souto, E., (2009). Novos sistemas terapêuticos nanotecnológicos. *Revista Da Faculdade de Ciências Da Saúde, 6*, 60–68.

Marson, J. W., & Baldwin, H. E., (2019). An overview of acne therapy, part 1: Topical therapy, oral antibiotics, laser and light therapy, and dietary interventions. *Dermatologic Clinics, 37*(2), 183–193. https://doi.org/10.1016/j.det.2018.12.001.

Martines, M. A. U., Santos, N. D., & Nolasco, L. G., (2016). Propostas estratégicas de gestão de riscos para a nanotecnologia. *Revista Quaestio Iuris, 9*(4), 2450–2488. https://doi.org/10.12957/rqi.2016.22064.

Megersa, M., & Tamrat, N., (2022). *Medicinal Plants Used to Treat Human and Livestock Ailments in Basona Werana District, North Shewa Zone, Amhara Region, Ethiopia.* 2022, Article ID 5242033 | https://doi.org/10.1155/2022/5242033.

Mehnert, W., & Mader, K., (2001). Solid lipid nanoparticles: Production, characterization, and applications. *Advanced Drug Delivery Reviews, 47*, 165–196. https://doi.org/10.1039/9781847550842-00103.

Melo, A. A. M. De., Matsuda, A. H., & Almeida-Muradian, L. B. de. (2012). Identidade e qualidade da própolis proveniente de quatro regiões do Brasil. *Revista Do Instituto Adolfo Lutz, 71*(3), 540–548.

Melo, A., Amadeu, M. S., Lancellotti, M., De Hollanda, L. M., & Machado, D., (2015). The role of nanomaterials in cosmetics: National and international legislative aspects. *Quimica Nova, 38*(4), 599–603. https://doi.org/10.5935/0100-4042.20150042.

Mendes, L. P., Pan, J., & Torchilin, V. P., (2017). Dendrimers as nanocarriers for nucleic acid and drug delivery in cancer therapy. *Molecules*, *22*(9), 1–21. https://doi.org/10.3390/molecules22091401.

Mihranyan, A., Ferraz, N., & Strømme, M., (2012). Current status and future prospects of nanotechnology in cosmetics. *Progress in Materials Science*, *57*(5), 875–910. https://doi.org/10.1016/j.pmatsci.2011.10.001.

Mishra, R., Shende, S., Jain, P. K., & Jain, V., (2018). Formulation and evaluation of gel containing ethosomes entrapped with tretinoin. *Journal of Drug Delivery and Therapeutics*, *8*(5-s), 315–321. https://doi.org/10.22270/jddt.v8i5-s.1982.

Mistry, A., & Ravikumar, P., (2016). Development and evaluation of azelaic acid based ethosomes for topical delivery for the treatment of acne. *Indian Journal of Pharmaceutical Education and Research*, *50*(3), S232–S243. https://doi.org/10.5530/ijper.50.3.34.

Mohammad, A. B., Ghoname, N., Hodeib, A., & Elbadawy, M., (2015). Significance of topical propolis in the treatment of facial acne vulgaris. *Egyptian Journal of Dermatology and Venerology*, *35*(1), 29. https://doi.org/10.4103/1110-6530.162468.

Mohammadi, S., Pardakhty, A., Khalili, M., Fathi, R., Rezaeizadeh, M., Farajzadeh, S., Mohebbi, A., & Aflatoonian, M., (2019). Niosomal benzoyl peroxide and clindamycin lotion versus niosomal clindamycin lotion in treatment of acne vulgaris: A randomized clinical trial. *Advanced Pharmaceutical Bulletin*, *9*(4), 578–583. https://doi.org/10.15171/apb.2019.066.

Mohammed, D., Crowther, J. M., Matts, P. J., Hadgraft, J., & Lane, M. E., (2013). Influence of niacinamide containing formulations on the molecular and biophysical properties of the stratum corneum. *International Journal of Pharmaceutics*, *441*(1, 2), 192–201. https://doi.org/10.1016/j.ijpharm.2012.11.043.

Molina, I. T., (2018). Nano- y micro-sistemas farmacéuticos en la administración ocular de medicamentos. *Anales de La Real Academia de Doctores de España*, *3*, 394–412. https://dialnet.unirioja.es/servlet/articulo?codigo=6858378 (accessed on 1 November 2023).

Moniz, T., Costa, L. S. A., & Reis, S., (2020). Human skin models: From healthy to disease-mimetic systems; characteristics and applications. *British Journal of Pharmacology*, *177*(19), 4314–4329. https://doi.org/10.1111/bph.15184.

Montagner, S., & Costa, A., (2010). Diretrizes modernas no tratamento da acne vulgar: Da abordagem inicial à manutenção dos benefícios clínicos. *Surgical and Cosmetic Dermatology*, *2*(3), 205–213.

Montenegro, L., Lai, F., Offerta, A., Sarpietro, M. G., Micicchè, L., Maccioni, A. M., Valenti, D., & Fadda, A. M., (2016). From nanoemulsions to nanostructured lipid carriers: A relevant development in dermal delivery of drugs and cosmetics. *Journal of Drug Delivery Science and Technology*, *32*, 100–112. https://doi.org/10.1016/j.jddst.2015.10.003.

Moon, S. K., Cho, G. O., Jung, S. Y., Gal, S. W., Kwon, T. K., Lee, Y. C., Madamanchi, N. R., & Kim, C. H., (2003). Quercetin exerts multiple inhibitory effects on vascular smooth muscle cells: Role of ERK1/2, cell-cycle regulation, and matrix metalloproteinase-9. *Biochemical and Biophysical Research Communications*, *301*(4), 1069–1078. https://doi.org/10.1016/S0006-291X(03)00091-3.

Mora-Huertas, C. E., Fessi, H., & Elaissari, A., (2010). Polymer-based nanocapsules for drug delivery. *International Journal of Pharmaceutics*, *385*(1, 2), 113–142. https://doi.org/10.1016/j.ijpharm.2009.10.018.

Moreira, J. R. L., (2013). *A Nanotecnologia na Liberação Controlada de Fármacos no Tratamento do Câncer de Mama*. 2013. 38 f. Monografia (Graduação em Farmácia) – Universidade de Brasília, Brasília.

Morganti, P., Berardesca, E., Guarneri, B., Guarneri, F., Fabrizi, G., Palombo, P., & Palombo, M., (2011). Topical clindamycin 1% vs. linoleic acid-rich phosphatidylcholine and nicotinamide 4% in the treatment of acne: A multicentre-randomized trial. *International Journal of Cosmetic Science*, *33*(5), 467–476. https://doi.org/10.1111/j.1468-2494.2011.00658.x.

Mousavi, S. Z., Nafisi, S., & Maibach, H. I., (2017). Fullerene nanoparticle in dermatological and cosmetic applications. *Nanomedicine: Nanotechnology, Biology, and Medicine*, *13*(3), 1071–1087. https://doi.org/10.1016/j.nano.2016.10.002.

Müller, R. H., Radtke, M., & Wissing, S. A., (2002). Solid lipid nanoparticles (SLN) and nanostructured lipid carriers (NLC) in cosmetic and dermatological preparations. *Advanced Drug Delivery Reviews*, *54*(Suppl.), 131–155. https://doi.org/10.1016/S0169-409X(02)00118-7.

Müller, R. H., Shegokar, R., & Keck, C. M., (2011). 20 years of lipid nanoparticles (SLN & NLC): Present state of development & industrial applications. *Current Drug Discovery Technologies*, *8*(3), 207–227. https://doi.org/10.2174/157016311796799062.

Müller-Goymann, C. C., (2004). Physicochemical characterization of colloidal drug delivery systems such as reverse micelles, vesicles, liquid crystals, and nanoparticles for topical administration. *European Journal of Pharmaceutics and Biopharmaceutics*, *58*(2), 343–356. https://doi.org/10.1016/j.ejpb.2004.03.028.

Nanda, S., Nanda, A., Lohan, S., Kaur, R., & Singh, B., (2016). Nanocosmetics: Performance enhancement and safety assurance. In: *Nanobiomaterials in Galenic Formulations and Cosmetics: Applications of Nanobiomaterials* (Vol. 3, No. 2018, pp. 47–67). Elsevier Inc. https://doi.org/10.1016/B978-0-323-42868-2.00003-6.

Nasir, A., & Friedman, A., (2010). Nanotechnology and the nanodermatology society. *Journal of Drugs in Dermatology*, *9*(7), 879–882.

Ndiaye, M., Philippe, C., Mukhtar, H., & Ahmad, N., (2011). The grape antioxidant resveratrol for skin disorders: Promise, prospects, and challenges. *Archives of Biochemistry and Biophysics*, *508*(2), 164–170. https://doi.org/10.1016/j.abb.2010.12.030.

Ngan, C. L., Basri, M., Tripathy, M., Abedi Karjiban, R., & Abdul-Malek, E., (2015). Skin intervention of fullerene-integrated nanoemulsion in structural and collagen regeneration against skin aging. *European Journal of Pharmaceutical Sciences*, *70*, 22–28. https://doi.org/10.1016/j.ejps.2015.01.006.

Ngan, C. L., Basri, M., Tripathy, M., Karjiban, R. A., & Abdul-Malek, E., (2014). Physicochemical characterization and thermodynamic studies of nanoemulsion-based transdermal delivery system for fullerene. *Scientific World Journal*, *2014*. https://doi.org/10.1155/2014/219035.

Nolasco, L., & Dos, S. N., (2017). Avanços nanotecnológicos e os desafios regulamentares. *Revista Da Faculdade de Direito Da UFMG*, *71*, 375–420. https://doi.org/10.12818/p.0304-2340.2017v71p375.

Oliveira, C. De. L., Ferro, C. D. S., Longati, K., Cunha, S. V. S. Da., Honda, T., Antunes, V. M. De. S., & Oliveira, C. R., (2018). A evolução da molécula de vitamina A utilizada em formulações cosmecêuticas. *Brazilian Journal of Natural Sciences*, *1*(1), 30. https://doi.org/10.31415/bjns.v1i1.13.

Open, T. C., Banerjee, J. R., & Banerjee, R., (2017). Nanocosmetics: The good, the bad and the beautiful. *Journal of Cosmetology & Trichology*, *1*(1), 9–11. https://doi.org/10.17140/TCOJ-1-e005.

Otlatici, G., Yegen, G., Gungor, S., & Aksu, B., (2019). Overview on nanotechnology-based cosmeceuticals to prevent skin aging. *Istanbul Journal of Pharmacy*, *48*(2), 55–62. https://doi.org/10.5152/istanbuljpharm.2018.424278.

Ourique, A. F., Melero, A., Silva, C. D. B. Da., Schaefer, U. F., Pohlmann, A. R., Guterres, S. S., Lehr, C. M., et al., (2011). Improved photostability and reduced skin permeation of tretinoin: Development of a semisolid nanomedicine. *European Journal of Pharmaceutics and Biopharmaceutics*, *79*(1), 95–101. https://doi.org/10.1016/j.ejpb.2011.03.008.

Palmer, B. C., & DeLouise, L. A., (2016). Nanoparticle-enabled transdermal drug delivery systems for enhanced dose control and tissue targeting. *Molecules*, *21*(12), 7–9. https://doi.org/10.3390/molecules21121719.

Pan, S. Y., Litscher, G., Gao, S. H., Zhou, S. F., Yu, Z. L., Chen, H. Q., Zhang, S. F., et al., (2014). Historical perspective of traditional indigenous medical practices: The current renaissance and conservation of herbal resources. *Evidence-Based Complementary and Alternative Medicine*, *2014*. https://doi.org/10.1155/2014/525340.

Pan, W., Qin, M., Zhang, G., Long, Y., Ruan, W., Pan, J., Wu, Z., et al., (2016). Combination of hydrotropic nicotinamide with nanoparticles for enhancing tacrolimus percutaneous delivery. *International Journal of Nanomedicine*, *11*, 4037–4050. https://doi.org/10.2147/IJN.S108545.

Pandey, H., Rani, R., & Agarwal, V., (2016). Liposome and their applications in cancer therapy. *Brazilian Archives of Biology and Technology*, *59*, 1–10. https://doi.org/10.1590/1678-4324-2016150477.

Pardeike, J., Hommoss, A., & Müller, R. H., (2009). Lipid nanoparticles (SLN, NLC) in cosmetic and pharmaceutical dermal products. *International Journal of Pharmaceutics*, *366*(1, 2), 170–184. https://doi.org/10.1016/j.ijpharm.2008.10.003.

Park, J. H., Yeo, I. J., Jang, J. S., Kim, K. C., Park, M. H., Lee, H. P., Han, S. B., & Hong, J. T., (2019). Combination effect of titrated extract of *Centella asiatica* and astaxanthin in a mouse model of phthalic anhydride-induced atopic dermatitis. *Allergy, Asthma & Immunology Research*, *11*(4), 548. https://doi.org/10.4168/aair.2019.11.4.548.

Park, J., & Boo, Y. C., (2013). Isolation of resveratrol from *Vitis viniferae* caulis and its potent inhibition of human tyrosinase. *Evidence-Based Complementary and Alternative Medicine Table*, *2013*, 10–12. https://doi.org/http://dx.doi.org/10.1155/2013/645257.

Park, S. N., Lee, H. J., & Gu, H. A., (2014). Enhanced skin delivery and characterization of rutin-loaded ethosomes. *Korean Journal of Chemical Engineering*, *31*(3), 485–489. https://doi.org/10.1007/s11814-013-0232-3.

Patra, J. K., Das, G., Fraceto, L. F., Campos, E. V. R., Rodriguez-Torres, M. D. P., Acosta-Torres, L. S., Diaz-Torres, L. A., et al., (2018). Nano based drug delivery systems: Recent developments and future prospects. *Journal of Nanobiotechnology*, *16*(1), 1–33. https://doi.org/10.1186/s12951-018-0392-8.

Patwekar, S. L., Pedewad, S. R., & Gattani, S., (2018). Development and evaluation of nanostructured lipid carriers-based gel of isotretinoin. *Particulate Science and Technology*, *36*(7), 832–843. https://doi.org/10.1080/02726351.2017.1305026.

Pettit, R. K., Pettit, G. R., Hamel, E., Hogan, F., Moser, B. R., Wolf, S., Pon, S., Chapuis, J. C., & Schmidt, J. M., (2009). E-Combretastatin and e-resveratrol structural modifications:

Antimicrobial and cancer cell growth inhibitory β-E-nitrostyrenes. *Bioorganic and Medicinal Chemistry*, *17*(18), 6606–6612. https://doi.org/10.1016/j.bmc.2009.07.076.

Popielec, A., & Loftsson, T., (2017). Effects of cyclodextrins on the chemical stability of drugs. *International Journal of Pharmaceutics*, *531*(2), 532–542. https://doi.org/10.1016/j.ijpharm.2017.06.009.

Prairna, Paramanya, A., Sharma, S., Bagdat, R. B., & Ali, A., (2020). Recent practices of medicinal and aromatic plants in nanotechnology. In: *Nanomaterials for Agriculture and Forestry Applications* (pp. 435–467). Elsevier Inc. https://doi.org/10.1016/b978-0-12-817852-2.00018-4.

Prow, T. W., Grice, J. E., Lin, L. L., Faye, R., Butler, M., Becker, W., Wurm, E. M. T., et al., (2011). Nanoparticles and microparticles for skin drug delivery. *Advanced Drug Delivery Reviews*, *63*(6), 470–491. https://doi.org/10.1016/j.addr.2011.01.012.

Pulicharla, R., Zolfaghari, M., Brar, S. K., Cledon, M., Drogui, P., & Surampalli, R. Y., (2016). Cosmetic nanomaterials in wastewater: Titanium dioxide and fullerenes. *Journal of Hazardous, Toxic, and Radioactive Waste*, *20*(1). https://doi.org/10.1061/(ASCE)HZ.2153-5515.0000261.

Purdy, S., & De Berker, D., (2011). Acne vulgaris. *BMJ Clinical Evidence*, *2011*.

Puton, B. M. S., (2019). *Síntese e Avaliação Das Atividades Biológicas e Antioxidante de Galato de Geranila*. 2019. 83 f. Dissertação (Mestrado em Engenharia de Alimentos) – Universidade Regional Integrada do Alto Uruguai e das Missões, Erechim.

Quevedo, J. P. De., (2019). *A Retórica Sobre Inovação, Impactos, Regulação e Riscos na Política Pública de Nanotecnologia do Brasil* [2019. 337 f. Tese (Doutorado em Políticas Públicas) – Universidade Federal do Paraná, Curitiba]. https://doi.org/10.5281/zenodo.1477753.

Rai, V. K., Mishra, N., Yadav, K. S., & Yadav, N. P., (2018). NU SC. *Journal of Controlled Release*, *28*(270), 203–225. https://doi.org/10.1016/j.jconrel.2017.11.049.

Raj, S., Jose, S., Sumod, U. S., & Sabitha, M., (2012). Nanotechnology in cosmetics: Opportunities and challenges. *Journal of Pharmacy and Bioallied Sciences*, *4*(3), 186–193. https://doi.org/10.4103/0975-7406.99016.

Rajesh, S., & Lillard, Jr. J. W., (2000). Nanoparticle-based targeted drug delivery. *Experimental & Molecular Pathology*, *86*(3), 215–223. https://doi.org/10.1016/j.yexmp.2008.12.004. Nanoparticle-based.

Ramakrishna, G. A., Manohar, S. D., & Bhanudas, S. R., (2014). Ethosomes: Carrier for enhanced transdermal drug delivery system. *Journal of Advanced Pharmacy Education & Research*, *4*(4), 380–387.

Ramezanli, T., & Michniak-Kohn, B. B., (2018). Development and characterization of a topical gel formulation of adapalene-tyrospheres and assessment of its clinical efficacy. *Molecular Pharmaceutics*, *15*(9), 3813–3822. https://doi.org/10.1021/acs.molpharmaceut.8b00318.

Ramos, I. M. F. C., (2018). *Nanopartículas Poliméricas Funcionalizadas Para Liberação de Fármaco no Sistema Nervoso Central*. 2018. 241 f. Tese (Doutorado em Engenharia Química) – Universidade Federal do Rio de Janeiro, Rio de Janeiro.

Rattner, H., (2005). Nanotecnologia e a política de ciência e tecnologia. *Passages de Paris*, *2*, 180–188. http://apebfr.org/passagesdeparis/edition2/articles/p180-rattner.pdf (accessed on 1 November 2023).

Redenti, E., Szente, L., & Szejtli, J., (2000). Drug/cyclodextrin/hydroxy acid multicomponent systems. Properties and pharmaceutical applications. *Journal of Pharmaceutical Sciences*, *89*(1), 1–8. https://doi.org/10.1002/(SICI)1520-6017(200001)89:1<1::AID-JPS1>3.0.CO;2-W.

Ribeiro, B. De. M., Almeida, L. M. C., Costa, A., Francesconi, F., Follador, I., & Neves, J. R., (2015). Etiopathogeny of acne vulgaris: A practical review for day-to-day dermatologic practice. *Surgical & Cosmetic Dermatology*, *7*(3), 20–26. https://doi.org/10.5935/scd1984-8773.2015731682.

Riehemann, K., Schneider, S. W., Luger, T. A., Godin, B., Ferrari, M., & Fuchs, H., (2009). Nanomedicine – Challenge and perspectives. *Angewandte Chemie – International Edition*, *48*(5), 872–897. https://doi.org/10.1002/anie.200802585.

Roger, M., Fullard, N., Costello, L., Bradbury, S., Markiewicz, E., O'Reilly, S., Darling, N., et al., (2019). Bioengineering the microanatomy of human skin. *Journal of Anatomy*, *234*(4), 438–455. https://doi.org/10.1111/joa.12942.

Sabouri, M., Samadi, A., Ahmad, N. S., Farboud, E. S., Mirrahimi, B., Hassanzadeh, H., Nassiri, K. M., et al., (2018). Tretinoin loaded nanoemulsion for acne vulgaris: Fabrication, physicochemical and clinical efficacy assessments. *Skin Pharmacology and Physiology*, *31*(6), 316–323. https://doi.org/10.1159/000488993.

Sætern, A. M., Skar, M., Braaten, Å., & Brandl, M., (2005). Camptothecin-catalyzed phospholipid hydrolysis in liposomes. *International Journal of Pharmaceutics*, *288*(1), 73–80. https://doi.org/10.1016/j.ijpharm.2004.09.010.

Sahoo, S. K., & Labhasetwar, V., (2003). Nanotech approaches to drug delivery and imaging. *Drug Discovery Today*, *8*(24), 1112–1120. https://doi.org/10.1016/S1359-6446(03)02903-9.

Sallam, M. A., & Elzoghby, A. O., (2018). Flutamide-loaded zein nanocapsule hydrogel, a promising dermal delivery system for pilosebaceous unit disorders. *AAPS PharmSciTech*, *19*(5), 2370–2382. https://doi.org/10.1208/s12249-018-1087-z.

Sampaio, S. D. A. P., & Bagatin, E., (2008). Experiência de 65 anos no tratamento da acne e de 26 anos com isotretinoína oral. *Anais Brasileiros de Dermatologia*, *83*(4), 361–367. https://doi.org/10.1590/S0365-05962008000400012.

Sánchez-dueñas, L. E., & Tovar-garza, A., (2019). Tratamiento farmacológico tópico en pacientes con acné topical pharmacological treatment in patients with acne. *Dermatología Revista Mexicana*, *63*, 33–40.

Sandru, F., et al., (2019). Treatment of acne vulgaris in relation to its etiopathogenesis. *Romanian Journal of Medical Practice*, *14*(4), 407–412. https://doi.org/10.37897/rjmp.2019.4.13.

Saniee, F., Ghafarian, S. H. R., Kalantari, K. K., Yazdanpanah, P., Soltani, A. R., Dabiri, N., Shirazi, N. G., & Karimpour, F., (2012). Consider of micro-current's effect to variation of facial wrinkle trend, randomized clinical trial study. *Life Science Journal*, *9*(3), 1184–1189.

Santos, A. C., Morais, F., Simões, A., Pereira, I., Sequeira, J. A. D., Pereira-Silva, M., Veiga, F., & Ribeiro, A., (2019). Nanotechnology for the development of new cosmetic formulations. *Expert Opinion on Drug Delivery*, *16*(4), 313–330. https://doi.org/10.1080/17425247.2019.1585426.

Santos, N. C., & Castanho, M. A. R. B., (2002). Liposomes: Has the magic bullet hit the target? *Quimica Nova*, *25*(6B), 1181–1185.

Santos, Z. M. Q. D., Santos, M. Q. D., Zancanaro, V., Bellaver, E. H., Nardi, G. M., Gelinski, J. M. L., & Locatelli, C., (2019). Topical application of phenolic compounds suppresses *Propionibacterium acnes*-induced inflammatory responses in mice with ear edema. *Naunyn-Schmiedeberg's Archives of Pharmacology*, *392*(5), 529–540. https://doi.org/10.1007/s00210-018-01604-z.

Santos, Z. M. Q. D., Velho, M. C., Zan, F. R., Rech, V. C., & Ourique, A. F., (2020). Review of clinical factors that cause acne vulgaris. *International Journal for Innovation Education and Research*, *8*(9), 434–447. https://doi.org/10.31686/ijier.vol8.iss9.2659.

Scalia, S., Franceschinis, E., Bertelli, D., & Iannuccelli, V., (2013). Comparative evaluation of the effect of permeation enhancers, lipid nanoparticles and colloidal silica on *in vivo* human skin penetration of quercetin. *Skin Pharmacology and Physiology*, *26*(2), 57–67. https://doi.org/10.1159/000345210.

Schaffazick, S. R., Guterres, S. S., De Lucca, F. L., & Pohlmann, A. R., (2003). Caracterização e estabilidade físico-química de sistemas poliméricos nanoparticulados para administração de fármacos. *Quimica Nova*, *26*(5), 726–737. https://doi.org/10.1590/s0100-40422003000500017.

Schulz, P. A., (2018). Há mais história lá embaixo – um convite para rever uma palestra. *Revista Brasileira de Ensino de Física*, *40*(4). https://doi.org/10.1590/1806-9126-rbef-2017-0375.

Semalty, A., Semalty, M., & Rawat, M. S. M., (2007). The phyto-phospholipid complexes-phytosomes: A potential therapeutic approach for herbal hepatoprotective drug delivery. *Pharmacognosy Reviews*, *1*(2), 369–374.

Sforcin, J. M., & Bankova, V., (2011). Propolis: Is there a potential for the development of new drugs? *Journal of Ethnopharmacology*, *133*(2), 253–260. https://doi.org/10.1016/j.jep.2010.10.032.

Sforcin, J. M., (2007). Propolis and the immune system: A review. *Journal of Ethnopharmacology*, *113*(1), 1–14. https://doi.org/10.1016/j.jep.2007.05.012.

Shahtalebi, M. A., Bahrinajafi, R., & Nahavandi, S., (2014). Preparation and pharmaceutical evaluation of nicotinamide stick for eradication of *Staphylococcus* epidermidis. *Journal of Research in Medical Sciences*, *19*(7), 654–657.

Shamma, R. N., Salah Ad-din, I., & Abdeltawab, N. F., (2019). Dapsone- gel as a novel platform for acne treatment: *In vitro* evaluation and *in vivo* performance and histopathological studies in acne infected mice. *Journal of Drug Delivery Science and Technology*, *54*, 101238. https://doi.org/10.1016/j.jddst.2019.101238.

Sharma, N., & Baldi, A., (2016). Exploring versatile applications of cyclodextrins: An overview. *Drug Delivery*, *23*(3), 739–757. https://doi.org/10.3109/10717544.2014.938839.

Sharma, N., Singh, S., Kanojia, N., Grewal, A. S., & Arora, S., (2018). Nanotechnology: A modern contraption in cosmetics and dermatology. *Applied Clinical Research, Clinical Trials, and Regulatory Affairs*, *5*(3), 147–158. https://doi.org/10.2174/2213476x05666180528093905.

Shaunak, S., (2015). Perspective: Dendrimer drugs for infection and inflammation. *Biochemical and Biophysical Research Communications*, *468*(3), 435–441. https://doi.org/10.1016/j.bbrc.2015.07.033.

Shelke, S., Shahi, S., Kale, S., Patil, V., & Deshpande, D., (2015). Ethosomes: A novel deformable carrier. *World Journal of Pharmaceutical Sciences*, *3*(9), 1830–1839.

Shen, L. N., Zhang, Y. T., Wang, Q., Xu, L., & Feng, N. P., (2014). Enhanced *in vitro* and *in vivo* skin deposition of apigenin delivered using ethosomes. *International Journal of Pharmaceutics*, *460*(1, 2), 280–288. https://doi.org/10.1016/j.ijpharm.2013.11.017.

Silva, A. M. F. Da., Costa, F. P. Da., & Moreira, M., (2014). Acne vulgar: Diagnóstico e manejo pelo médico de família e comunidade. *Revista Brasileira de Medicina de Família e Comunidade*, *9*(30), 54–63. https://doi.org/10.5712/rbmfc9(30)754.

Silva, C. D. Da., (2009). *Combretum leprosum Mart. (Combretaceae) – Avaliação da Atividade Antiinflamatória Tópica em Modelos de Inflamação de Pele Agudo e Crônico em Camundongos* (Vol. 1) [2009. 97 f. Dissertação (Mestrado em Farmacologia) – Universidade Federal do Paraná, Curitiba]. https://doi.org/10.1017/CBO9781107415324.004.

Silva, G. A., (2004). Introduction to nanotechnology and its applications to medicine. *Surgical Neurology*, *61*(3), 216–220. https://doi.org/10.1016/j.surneu.2003.09.036.

Simões, C. M. O., & Schenkel, E. P., (2002). A pesquisa e a produção brasileira de medicamentos a partir de plantas medicinais: A necessária interação da indústria com a academia. *Revista Brasileira de Farmacognosia*, *12*(1), 35–40. https://doi.org/10.1590/S0102-695X2002000100005.

Soni, K., Kukereja, B. K., Kapur, M., & Kohli, K., (2016). Lipid nanoparticles: Future of oral drug delivery and their current trends and regulatory issues. *International Journal of Current Pharmaceutical Review and Research*, *7*(1), 1–18.

Sonneville-Aubrun, O., Simonnet, J. T., & L'Alloret, (2004). Nanoemulsions: A new vehicle for skincare products. *Advances in Colloid and Interface Science*, *108, 109*(03), 145–149. https://doi.org/10.1016/s0001-8686(03)00146-5.

Souto, E. B., & Müller, R. H., (2008). Cosmetic features and applications of lipid nanoparticles (SLN®, NLC®). *International Journal of Cosmetic Science*, *30*(3), 157–165. https://doi.org/10.1111/j.1468-2494.2008.00433.x.

Souto, E. B., Severino, P., & Santana, M. H. A., (2012). Preparação de nanopartículas poliméricas a partir da polimerização de monômeros – parte I. *Polimeros*, *22*(1), 96–100. https://doi.org/10.1590/S0104-14282012005000006.

Stopar, K., Drobne, D., Eler, K., & Bartol, T., (2016). Citation analysis and mapping of nanoscience and nanotechnology: Identifying the scope and interdisciplinarity of research. *Scientometrics*, *106*(2), 563–581. https://doi.org/10.1007/s11192-015-1797-x.

Sugumar, S., Clarke, S. K., Nirmala, M. J., Tyagi, B. K., Mukherjee, A., & Chandrasekaran, N., (2014). *Nanoemulsion of Eucalyptus Oil and its Larvicidal Activity Against Culex Quinquefasciatus*, 393–402. https://doi.org/10.1017/S0007485313000710.

Surini, S., Mubarak, H., & Ramadon, D., (2018). Cosmetic serum containing grape (*Vitis vinifera* L.) seed extract phytosome: Formulation and *in vitro* penetration study. *Journal of Young Pharmacists*, *10*(2), s51–s55. https://doi.org/10.5530/jyp.2018.2s.10.

Tadros, T., Izquierdo, P., Esquena, J., & Solans, C., (2004). Formation and stability of nano-emulsions. *Advances in Colloid and Interface Science*, *108, 109*, 303–318. https://doi.org/10.1016/j.cis.2003.10.023.

Taleb, M. H., Abdeltawab, N. F., Shamma, R. N., Abdelgayed, S. S., Mohamed, S. S., Farag, M. A., & Ramadan, M. A., (2018). *Origanum vulgare* L. Essential oil as a potential anti-acne topical nanoemulsion—*In vitro* and *in vivo* study. *Molecules*, *23*(9). https://doi.org/10.3390/molecules23092164.

Tanaka, L. S., (2019). Regulación blanda, normas técnicas y armonización regulatoria internacional, para la nanotecnología soft regulation, technical standards, and international regulatory harmonization, for nanotechnology. *Revista Interdisciplinaria En Nanociencias Y Nanotecnología*, *13*(24), 1e-27e. https://doi.org/https://doi.org/10.22201/ceiich.24485691e.2020.24.69621.

Tasoula, E., Gregoriou, S., Chalikias, J., Lazarou, D., Danopoulou, I., Katsambas, A., & Rigopoulos, D., (2012). The impact of acne vulgaris on quality of life and psychic health in young adolescents in Greece: Results of a population survey. *Anais Brasileiros de Dermatologia*, *87*(6), 862–869. https://doi.org/10.1590/s0365-05962012000600007.

Taylor, E. J. M., Yu, Y., Champer, J., & Kim, J., (2014). Resveratrol demonstrates antimicrobial effects against *Propionibacterium acnes in vitro*. *Dermatology and Therapy*, *4*(2). https://doi.org/10.1007/s13555-014-0063-0.

Thiboutot, D., Gollnick, H., Bettoli, V., Dréno, B., Kang, S., Leyden, J. J., Shalita, A. R., et al., (2009). New insights into the management of acne: An update from the global alliance to improve outcomes in acne group. *Journal of the American Academy of Dermatology, 60*(1, 5). https://doi.org/10.1016/j.jaad.2009.01.019.

Tiwari, G., Tiwari, R., Bannerjee, S., Bhati, L., Pandey, S., Pandey, P., & Sriwastawa, B., (2012). Drug delivery systems: An updated review. *International Journal of Pharmaceutical Investigation, 2*(1), 2. https://doi.org/10.4103/2230-973x.96920.

Torchilin, P., (1997). Surface-modified liposomes in gamma- and MR-imaging. *Advanced Drug Delivery Reviews, 24*(96), 301–313.

Tripathi, S. V., Gustafson, C. J., Huang, K. E., & Feldman, S. R., (2013). Side effects of common acne treatments. *Expert Opinion on Drug Safety, 12*(1), 39–51. https://doi.org/10.1517/14740338.2013.740456.

Trivedi, M. K., Bosanac, S. S., Sivamani, R. K., & Larsen, L. N., (2018). Emerging therapies for acne vulgaris. *American Journal of Clinical Dermatology, 19*(4), 505–516. https://doi.org/10.1007/s40257-018-0345-x.

Trommer, H., & Neubert, R. H. H., (2006). Overcoming the stratum corneum: The modulation of skin penetration. A review. *Skin Pharmacology and Physiology, 19*(2), 106–121. https://doi.org/10.1159/000091978.

Tsai, T. H., Chuang, L. T., Lien, T. J., Liing, Y. R., Chen, W. Y., & Tsai, P. J., (2013). *Rosmarinus officinalis* extract suppresses *Propionibacterium acnes* –induced inflammatory responses. *Journal of Medicinal Food, 16*(4), 324–333. https://doi.org/10.1089/jmf.2012.2577.

Tsujimoto, H., & Hara, K., (2018). Development of functional skin care cosmetics using biodegradable PLGA nanospheres. In: *Nanoparticle Technology Handbook* (3rd edn., pp. 445–450). Elsevier B.V. https://doi.org/10.1016/B978-0-444-64110-6.00016-0.

Vasanth, S., Dubey, A., G.S, R., Lewis, S. A., Ghate, V. M., El-Zahaby, S. A., & Hebbar, S., (2020). Development and investigation of vitamin C-enriched adapalene-loaded transfersome gel: A collegial approach for the treatment of acne vulgaris. *AAPS PharmSciTech, 21*(2). https://doi.org/10.1208/s12249-019-1518-5.

Vela-Romera, A., Carriel, V., Martín-Piedra, M. A., Aneiros-Fernández, J., Campos, F., Chato-Astrain, J., Prados-Olleta, N., et al., (2019). Characterization of the human ridged and non-ridged skin: A comprehensive histological, histochemical and immunohistochemical analysis. In: *Histochemistry and Cell Biology* (Vol. 151, No. 1, pp. 57–73). Springer Berlin Heidelberg. https://doi.org/10.1007/s00418-018-1701-x.

Verde, F. R. V., (2017). Nanocosméticos. *Radar Tecnológico*, 17. https://www.gov.br/inpi/pt-br/acesso-a-informacao/pasta-x/radar-tecnologico/arquivos/documentos/n14_radar_tecnologico_nanocosmeticos_versao_estendida_20171116.pdf (accessed on 1 November 2023).

Verma, P., & Pathak, K., (2010). Therapeutic and cosmeceutical potential of ethosomes: An overview. *J Adv Pharm Technol Res, 1*(3), 274–282. https://doi.org/10.4103/0110-5558.72415.

Viegas, C., Bolzani, V. Da. S., & Barreiro, E. J., (2006). Os produtos naturais e a química medicinal moderna. *Quimica Nova, 29*(2), 326–337. https://doi.org/10.1590/s0100-40422006000200025.

Volpi, N., & Bergonzini, G., (2006). Analysis of flavonoids from propolis by on-line HPLC-electrospray mass spectrometry. *Journal of Pharmaceutical and Biomedical Analysis, 42*(3), 354–361. https://doi.org/10.1016/j.jpba.2006.04.017.

Vrignaud, S., Benoit, J. P., & Saulnier, P., (2011). Strategies for the nanoencapsulation of hydrophilic molecules in polymer-based nanoparticles. *Biomaterials*, *32*(33), 8593–8604. https://doi.org/10.1016/j.biomaterials.2011.07.057.

Walocko, F. M., Eber, A. E., Keri, J. E., Al-Harbi, M. A., & Nouri, K., (2017). The role of nicotinamide in acne treatment. *Dermatologic Therapy*, *30*(5), 1–7. https://doi.org/10.1111/dth.12481.

Wang, L., Yang, X., Qin, P., Shan, F., & Ren, G., (2013). Flavonoid composition, antibacterial and antioxidant properties of Tartary buckwheat bran extract. *Industrial Crops and Products*, *49*, 312–317. https://doi.org/10.1016/j.indcrop.2013.04.039.

Wichit, A., Tangsumranjit, A., Pitaksuteepong, T., & Waranuch, N., (2012). Polymeric micelles of PEG-PE as carriers of all-trans retinoic acid for stability improvement. *AAPS PharmSciTech*, *13*(1), 336–343. https://doi.org/10.1208/s12249-011-9749-0.

Winter, Jr. E., (2015). *Zeólita Modificada Com ?-Ciclodextrina: Síntese, Caracterização e Utilização Como Adsorvente, Para a Remediação de Contaminantes e Disruptores Endócrinos*. 2015. 171 f. Tese (Doutorado em Engenharia e Ciências dos Materiais) – Universidade Federal do Paraná, Curitiba.

Wong, X. Y., Sena-Torralba, A., Álvarez-Diduk, R., Muthoosamy, K., & Merkoçi, A., (2020). Nanomaterials for nanotheranostics: Tuning their properties according to disease needs. *ACS Nano*, *14*(3), 2585–2627. https://doi.org/10.1021/acsnano.9b08133.

Wróblewska, M., & Winnicka, K., (2015). The effect of cationic polyamidoamine dendrimers on physicochemical characteristics of hydrogels with erythromycin. *International Journal of Molecular Sciences*, *16*(9), 20277–20289. https://doi.org/10.3390/ijms160920277.

Wu, X., & Guy, R. H., (2009). Applications of nanoparticles in topical drug delivery and in cosmetics. *Journal of Drug Delivery Science and Technology*, *19*(6), 371–384. https://doi.org/10.1016/S1773-2247(09)50080-9.

Wu, Z., Uchi, H., Morino-Koga, S., Shi, W., & Furue, M., (2014). Resveratrol inhibition of human keratinocyte proliferation via SIRT1/ARNT/ERK dependent downregulation of aquaporin 3. *Journal of Dermatological Science*, *75*(1), 16–23. https://doi.org/10.1016/j.jdermsci.2014.03.004.

Xu, J., Lin, R., Wang, J., Wu, Y., Wang, Y., Zhang, Y., Xi, C., & Wu, Q., (2013). Effect of acupuncture anesthesia on acne vulgaris of pricking-bloodletting cupping: A single-blind randomized clinical trail. *Journal of Traditional Chinese Medicine*, *33*(6), 752–756. https://doi.org/10.1016/s0254-6272(14)60007-8.

Yaman, I., Durmus, A. S., Ceribasi, S., & Yaman, M., (2010). Effects of *Nigella sativa* and silver sulfadiazine on burn wound healing in rats. *Veterinarni Medicina*, *55*(12), 619–624.

Yu, Z., Lv, H., Han, G., & Ma, K., (2016). Ethosomes loaded with cryptotanshinone for acne treatment through topical gel formulation. *PLoS One*, *11*(7), 1–11. https://doi.org/10.1371/journal.pone.0159967.

Yukuyama, M. N., Ghisleni, D. D. M., Pinto, T. J. A., & Bou-Chacra, N. A., (2016). Nanoemulsion: Process selection and application in cosmetics: A review. *International Journal of Cosmetic Science*, *38*(1), 13–24. https://doi.org/10.1111/ics.12260.

Zaccaria, V., Curti, V., Di Lorenzo, A., Baldi, A., Maccario, C., Sommatis, S., Mocchi, R., & Daglia, M., (2017). Effect of green and brown propolis extracts on the expression levels of microRNAs, mRNAs and proteins, related to oxidative stress and inflammation. *Nutrients*, *9*(10), 1–17. https://doi.org/10.3390/nu9101090.

Zasada, M., & Budzisz, E., (2019). Retinoids: Active molecules influencing skin structure formation in cosmetic and dermatological treatments. *Postepy Dermatologii i Alergologii, 36*(4), 392–397. https://doi.org/10.5114/ada.2019.87443.

Zhang, X., Guo, Y., Guo, L., Jiang, H., & Ji, Q., (2018). *In vitro* evaluation of antioxidant and antimicrobial activities of melaleuca alternifolia essential oil. *BioMed Research International, 2018*. https://doi.org/10.1155/2018/2396109.

Zidan, A. S., Ahmed, O. A. A., & Aljaeid, B. M., (2016). Nicotinamide polymeric nanoemulsified systems: A quality-by-design case study for a sustained antimicrobial activity. *International Journal of Nanomedicine, 11*, 1501–1516. https://doi.org/10.2147/IJN.S102945.

Zimmerman, E. E., & Crawford, P., (2012). Cutaneous cryosurgery. *American Family Physician, 86*(12), 1118–1124. https://doi.org/10.1201/b17660.

CHAPTER 3

Topical Delivery of Amphotericin B: Focus on Nanocarriers for the Treatment of Cutaneous Leishmaniasis

THAIS TUNES SANTOS,[1] EDUARDO BURGARELLI LAGES,[2,3] MARTA MARQUES GONTIJO DE AGUIAR,[2] GISELE ASSIS CASTRO GOULART,[2] and GABRIEL SILVA MARQUES BORGES[4]

[1]Department of Physiology and Biophysics, Institute of Biological Sciences, Federal University of Minas Gerais, Belo Horizonte, Brazil

[2]Department of Pharmaceutical Products, Faculty of Pharmacy, Federal University of Minas Gerais, Belo Horizonte, Brazil

[3]Vaccine Technology Center (CTVacinas), Federal University of Minas Gerais, Belo Horizonte, Minas Gerais, Brazil

[4]Department of Pharmacy, Faculty of Biological and Health Sciences, Federal University of the Jequitinhonha and Mucuri Valleys, Road MG 367- km 583, Diamantina, Minas Gerais, Brazil.

ABSTRACT

Amphotericin B (AmB) is an antifungal drug that has also been used to treat cutaneous leishmaniasis (CL), a chronic infectious disease caused by protozoa of the genus *Leishmania*. Despite its effectiveness, current AmB therapy requires parenteral administration, which results in compliance problems and severe adverse effects, especially nephrotoxicity. Topical treatment of CL represents an attractive alternative, avoiding the toxicity of parenteral therapy while being administered by a simple painless route.

Novel Nanocarriers forSkin Diseases: Advances and Applications.
Raj K. Keservani and Júlia Scherer Santos (Eds.)

However, the high molecular weight and amphoteric nature of AmB impair its efficient penetration through the skin. In this sense, nanocarriers have been presented as a stimulating strategy to optimize the physicochemical characteristics of AmB and increase its delivery to the deeper layers of the skin. Different types of systems have been investigated, especially liposomes, lipid nanoparticles, and polymeric carriers. In this chapter, we will summarize the main obstacles to the development of formulations for topical delivery of AmB and discuss the potential and advantages of nanomedicine in solving these challenges. In addition, an overview of the performance of nanocarriers for the topical treatment of CL will be provided, focusing on investigations carried out in preclinical models.

3.1 INTRODUCTION

Leishmaniasis is a group of neglected tropical diseases caused by different species of *Leishmania* protozoan parasites that are transmitted by the bite of *Phlebotomine* sandflies (Santos et al., 2012; Ammar et al., 2019). The disease is classified into two main forms: cutaneous leishmaniasis (CL), which initially appears as a localized papule and then progresses to an ulcer upon the loss of the epidermis, resulting in a great impairment of the skin barrier; and visceral leishmaniasis (VL), the fatal form of the disease, where parasites reside in the spleen, liver, and bone marrow (Ammar et al., 2019).

Amphotericin B (AmB) is a polyene antibiotic that was first isolated from *Streptomyces nodosus* in 1955. Initially designed to treat local mycotic infections, the drug was later approved for the treatment of progressive and potentially fatal fungal diseases. AmB also exhibits potent antiparasitic activity for certain protozoan infections, including those caused by species of *Leishmania.* Since its discovery, this broad-spectrum antifungal agent with a favorable resistance profile has been widely used in the clinic (Cavassin et al., 2021; Carolus et al., 2020).

Considering the global burden of Leishmaniasis, about 90% of cases of the disease occur in developing countries, which points to the need for an affordable AmB therapy. In this sense, oral or topical drug delivery routes have important advantages, such as better acceptance given the possibility of self-administration, without the use of injectables, lower cost, and absence of systemic toxicity as normally occurs with parenteral formulations (Chakravarty & Sundar, 2010). Unfortunately, oral administration of AmB results in negligible bioavailability due to poor membrane permeability, low aqueous solubility, and instability at the low pH found in the stomach (Liu et al., 2017;

Serrano & Lalatsa, 2017). After the failure of several clinical trials, it was generally accepted that oral formulations of AmB were unfeasible in clinical practice, although this is starting to change with the increasing advancement of new drug delivery technologies (Liu et al., 2017; Cuddihy et al., 2019; Thanki et al., 2019). Similarly, the high molecular weight and amphoteric nature of AmB also impairs its cutaneous penetration, which severely limits its effectiveness as a topical therapy (Faustino & Pinheiro, 2020; Perez et al., 2016).

Currently, all AmB formulations available to treat CL must be administered intravenously, creating a significant obstacle in patient access to treatment due to pharmacoeconomic considerations. Moreover, AmB toxicity, such as nephrotoxicity, is one of the barriers that prevent its adequate prescription, which can result in the spread of infections and therapeutic failure (Laniado-Laborín & Cabrales-Vargas, 2009; Faustino & Pinheiro, 2020).

Despite the efforts of the World Health Organization (WHO) and the Neglected Diseases Initiative (DND*i*), no effective and safe topical therapeutic alternative is yet available (Eskandari et al., 2019; López et al., 2018; Dar et al., 2020). Interestingly, CL is a particular clinical condition for the evaluation of topical route, as the progression of the disease is characterized by considerable tissue damage. At first, this impairment of the skin barrier may favorize drug permeation, but the re-epithelialization of lesions during treatment may represent an additional challenge for this route effectiveness (Carneiro et al., 2012).

The development of non-invasive formulations of topical AmB, however, is very challenging due to its low aqueous solubility at physiological pH, low permeability through membranes, and tendency to self-aggregation, in addition to its low stability at high temperatures and acidic pH (Liu et al., 2017). Nevertheless, the use of nanotechnology has an encouraging potential in this scenario, not only with the possibility of modulating the physicochemical properties of AmB, but also directly improving its cutaneous penetration (Wang et al., 2021; Torrado et al., 2008). Herein, we will summarize the most important principles of cutaneous administration as well as the applications of nanomedicine as a promising strategy for topical delivery of AmB in CL therapy.

3.2 AMB CHEMISTRY AND MODE OF ACTION

AmB has a highly complex structure characterized by a 38-membered macrolactone ring, composed of a hydrophilic polyhydroxyl chain on one side and a lipophilic polyene hydrocarbon chain on the other side (Figure

3.1). A mycosamine (lactone) residue containing a free amino group rests at one end of the molecule, forming a side chain (Cavassin et al., 2021; Wang et al., 2010) and the positively charged amino group is required for its activity, as well as the polyene subunit (Cuddihy et al., 2019).

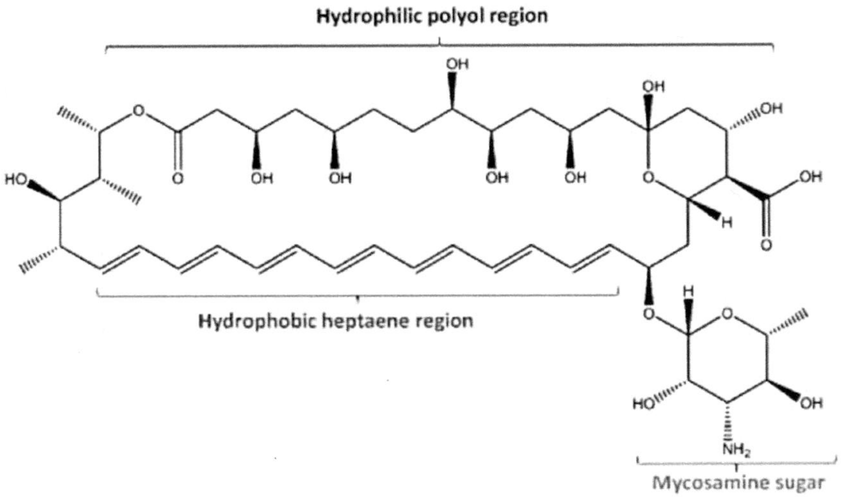

FIGURE 3.1 Chemical structure of AmB.

The classical mechanism of action of AmB involves its preferential binding to ergosterol, the main component of fungal or parasitic cell membranes. The hydrophobic part of the molecule interacts with ergosterol in the lipid bilayer resulting in multimeric transmembrane pores (Figure 3.2). This pores formation allows the extravasation of electrolytes from the intracellular environment, such as potassium, ammonium, and phosphate, in addition to carbohydrates and proteins (Cavassin et al., 2021). These losses, along with a subsequent influx of protons into the pathogenic cell, cause acidification of the intracellular medium with precipitation of the cytoplasm and ultimate cell death (Hamill, 2013; Kamiński, 2014).

Several evidence indicate that ergosterol binding and pore formation may not be the only mechanism leading to cell death. It has been proposed that AmB can also adsorb or sequester ergosterol on the membrane surface, which destabilizes the phospholipid membrane and impairs its functionality and essential cellular processes (Carolus et al., 2020; Faustino & Pinheiro, 2020). In addition, AmB can induce oxidative stress, either directly producing or causing intracellular accumulation of reactive oxygen and nitrogen

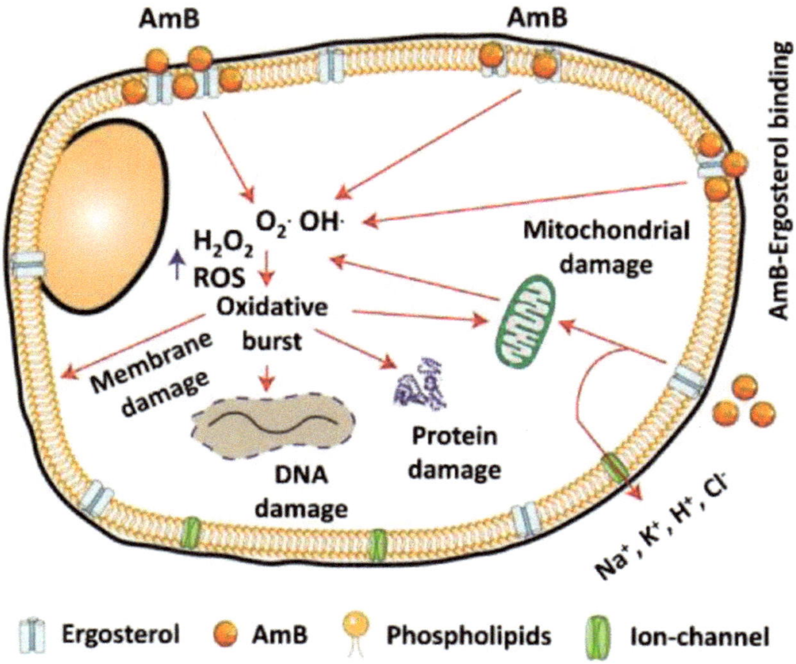

FIGURE 3.2 Mode of action of AmB.

Source: Adapted with permission from: Wang et al. (2021).

species. These molecules have multiple deleterious effects on pathogenic cells, but their specific role in AmB's mode of action is still unclear (Vriens et al., 2017; Mesa-Arango et al., 2014).

3.3 COMMERCIAL FORMULATIONS OF AMB

AmB is an amphiphilic molecule and exhibits very low water solubility and membrane permeability, resulting in negligible absorption when administered orally. Thus, the first marketed formulation of AmB was developed for parenteral use from its combination with sodium deoxycholate, forming a micellar suspension in aqueous medium (Fungizone®, Figure 3.3) (Cavassin et al., 2021).

Despite its efficacy, AmB deoxycholate has several dose-dependent adverse events that limit its use. After dilution in plasma, AmB is rapidly released from the formulation mainly in the form of oligomeric aggregates that lead to toxicity problems, especially nephrotoxicity (Barratt & Bretagne,

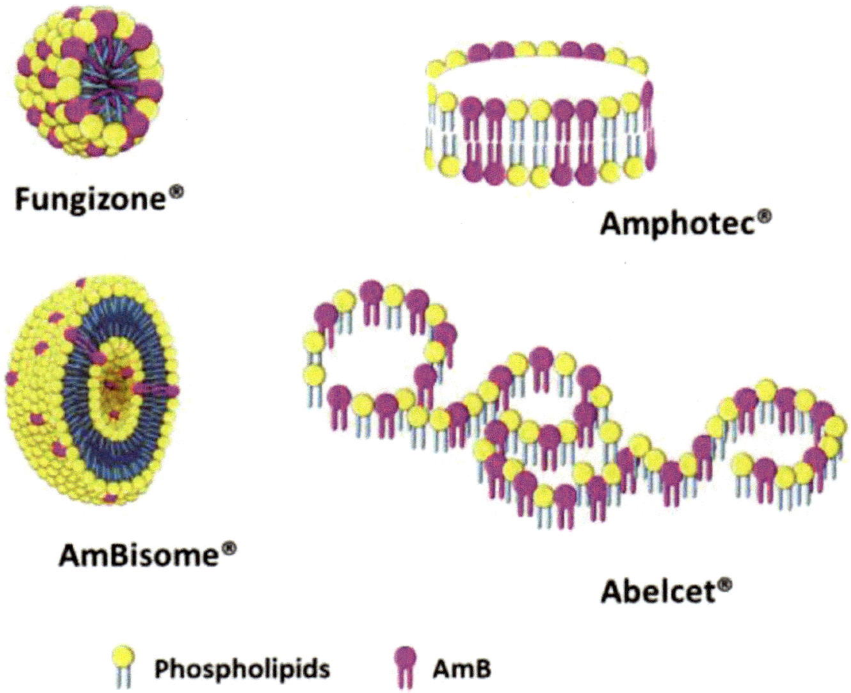

FIGURE 3.3 Commercial formulations of AmB. Amphotec® was discontinued in 2011 because of its high rate of infusion-related events.

Source: Adapted with permission from: Cavassin et al. (2021).

2007). Nephrotoxicity involves vasoconstriction and direct interaction of AmB with epithelial cells, resulting in decreased glomerular filtration rate and tubular dysfunction (Deray, 2002). Additionally, although AmB has a higher affinity for ergosterol, it can also interact with cholesterol present in the lipid bilayer of mammalian cells, which leads to non-selective disruption of cell membranes and is responsible to many of its adverse effects (Cavassin et al., 2021; Laniado-Laborín & Cabrales-Vargas, 2009).

Administration of AmB deoxycholate is also limited by acute infusion-related toxicity, which includes fever, nausea, and vomiting. Due to its microbial origin, AmB stimulates innate immune cells via Toll-like and CD14 receptors, resulting in elevated production of pro-inflammatory cytokines that mediate the onset of these symptoms (Sau et al., 2003; Laniado-Laborín & Cabrales-Vargas, 2009). In addition, AmB deoxycholate has been reported to produce cardiac toxicity, with the development of ventricular arrhythmias and bradycardia (Laniado-Laborín & Cabrales-Vargas, 2009).

In this context, an intense search has been carried out in order to develop formulations capable of immobilizing the monomeric form of AmB, consequently reducing the free amount of AmB in the blood and the toxicity to mammalian cells. These efforts resulted in the development of three lipid formulations in the 1990s (Figure 3.3). In 1995, Abelcet® (amphotericin B lipid complex: ABLC) was launched, a lipid complex consisted of diesteroyl phosphatidylcholine (DSPC) and diesteroyl phosphatidylglycerol (DSPG) forming a multilamellar system characterized as "ribbon-linke." A year later, another nanosystem called Amphotec® (or Amphocil®) was approved by the Food and Drug Administration (FDA) as a colloidal dispersion of AmB into sodium cholesteryl sulfate, forming discoid particles. In 1997, AmBisome® was approved as a liposomal formulation of AmB formed by SUVs of hydrogenated soy phosphatidylcholine, cholesterol, and DSPG (Fernández-García et al., 2017; Torrado et al., 2008; Golenser & Domb, 2006). These formulations exhibit distinct pharmacokinetic profiles and are not interchangeable, with different dosage recommendations (Faustino & Pinheiro, 2020).

Overall, the lipid vehicle enables a more selective and controlled release of AmB to pathogenic cells, which prevents its interaction with cholesterol of the host cells and reduces side effects (Faustino & Pinheiro, 2020). As a result, all these formulations show less nephrotoxicity compared to AmB deoxycholate, while liposomal AmB also exhibit less infusion-related reactions (Lanza et al., 2019; Carolus et al., 2020). In the case of Amphotec®, similar or even more infusion-related reactions were observed due to the up regulation of inflammatory genes and therefore its production was discontinued in 2011 (Hamill, 2013; Cavassin et al., 2021). Despite providing a better safety profile, the high cost of these lipid formulations, especially Ambisome®, and the reduced effectiveness in some cases of co-infection with the human immunodeficiency virus (HIV) are still challenges to be overcome (Guery et al., 2017; Ritmeijer et al., 2011). In addition, the fact that they are still limited to parenteral administration is a major obstacle to their wide use (Faustino & Pinheiro, 2020).

Topical delivery of AmB would be an interesting approach in the management of CL. A topical formulation can provide more efficient delivery of AmB to affected tissues and with fewer adverse effects than parenteral formulations, especially nephrotoxicity. In addition, topical formulations are usually more cost-effective option than parenteral forms and provide greater patient compliance.

3.4 TOPICAL ROUTE OF DRUG ADMINISTRATION

The skin is a multifunctional organ with a complex architecture that performs numerous vital functions and forms a protective barrier against external agents, ultraviolet (UV) radiation, and water loss. It is composed of three different parallel layers, each with specific natures and functions: the outermost layer, the epidermis; the middle layer, the dermis, and the innermost layer, the hypodermis (Figure 3.4) (Alkilani et al., 2015; Prow et al., 2011). Interestingly, while the skin serves as a natural protection against the penetration of external particles, it also provides an accessible and convenient site for drug administration for either local or systemic effects (Benson et al., 2019).

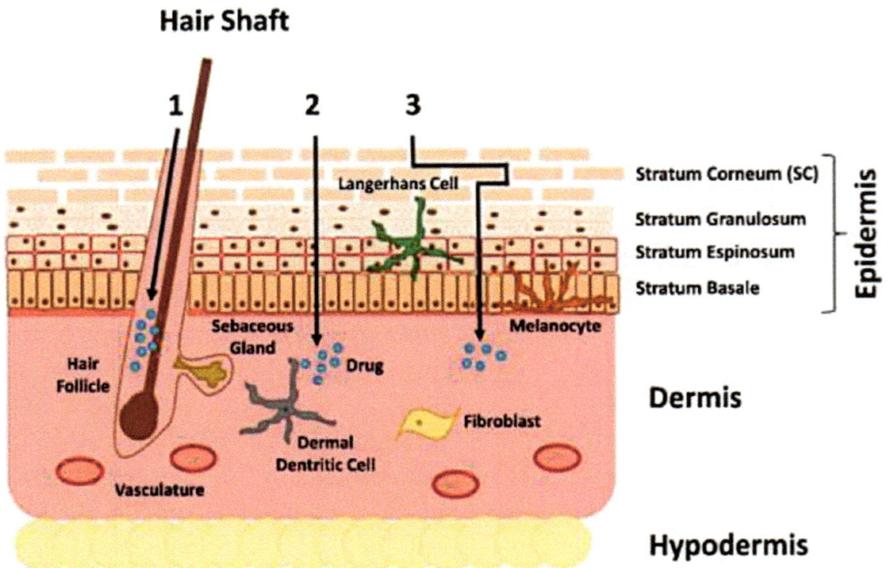

FIGURE 3.4 Representation of skin structures and drug penetration pathways.

Source: Adapted with permission from: Palmer & DeLouise (2016). Topically applied drugs can penetrate the skin in one of three different ways: (1) through the appendageal route; (2) through the intracellular route; or (3) through the intercellular route. Copyright © 2016 by the authors. Licensee MDPI, Basel, Switzerland. http://creativecommons.org/licenses/by/4.0/

The epidermis is the most superficial layer of the skin, in contact with the external environment. It is formed by stratified and keratinized epithelial tissue, without vascularization, being composed of different cell types, including keratinocytes (about 90%), melanocytes, Langerhans cells, and Merkel cells (Honari, 2017). Traditionally, the epidermis is segmented into distinct structural and functional compartments called (from deepest to most superficial): stratum Basale, stratum spinosum, stratum granulosum, and stratum corneum (SC). The SC is considered the main barrier to drug permeation through the skin, preventing the penetration of molecules into the underlying layers (Kapoor et al., 2017). It consists of several layers of dead, flattened, and keratinized cells called corneocytes, which correspond to the last level of keratinocytes differentiation. Corneocytes are intercellularly surrounded by a lipid matrix formed mainly by ceramides, free fatty acids, and cholesterol; and are interconnected by protein structures (Honari, 2017). This organization is characterized as a "brick-and-mortar" system, where corneocytes form the "bricks" and extracellular lipids can be represented as the "mortar" (Menon et al., 2012).

Directly adjacent to the epidermis is the dermis, a fibrous structure composed of collagen, elastic tissue, and other extracellular components, that include vasculature, nerve endings, hair follicles, and glands. In addition to nourishing and sustaining the epidermis, the dermis layer provides a connective tissue framework for strength, flexibility, and protection of deeper anatomical structures (Brown & Krishnamurthy, 2019). Finally, the hypodermis is the deepest layer of the skin and consists of a network of fat cells. It corresponds to the contact layer between the skin and the underlying tissues of the body, such as muscles and bones, and its main function is to provide thermal insulation and protection against external shocks (Alkilani et al., 2015).

Topically applied products can target sites on one or more different layers of the skin, as well as its appendages and underlying tissues. Normally, cutaneous permeation of drugs applied under the skin occurs by passive diffusion through the intact epidermis. The first and most difficult step is to cross the SC due to its barrier properties (Kapoor et al., 2017). Three different permeation pathways through the skin can be identified, as shown in Figure 3.4: (1) the appendageal route, in which permeation can occur through skin appendages such as hair follicles and sebaceous and sweat glands; (2) the intracellular route, in which the drug passes both through the lipid structures of the intercellular region and directly through the corneocytes; and (3) the intercellular route, in which the substance diffuses around corneocytes passing only through the intercellular lipid matrix. While the intra- and intercellular routes involve the passage of drugs through the multiple layers of the epidermis, the appendageal route forms an alternative path allowing direct access to the dermis (Richard et al., 2021; Prow et al., 2011).

In general, transport across intercellular spaces allows for the diffusion of more lipophilic molecules through the continuous lipid matrix. In turn, the intracellular pathway more easily allows the transport of hydrophilic compounds given the highly hydrophilic nature of corneocytes, although it is also necessary for these molecules to cross intercellular lipids to jump from one corneocyte to another (N'Da, 2014). However, all substances cross the skin through a combination of these pathways, and the relative contribution of each may be largely dependent on the physicochemical characteristics of the drug, including solubility, lipophilicity, and molecular weight (Richard et al., 2021).

Favorable physicochemical properties are necessary for molecules to pass through the skin. Ideally, the molecular weight should be less than 500 Da, the log P value should be between 1 and 3, and the melting point should be less than 200°C (Yu et al., 2021). The ability of the molecule to form hydrogen bonds is another influencing factor, as SC is primarily an acceptor of this type of interaction (N'Da, 2014). Furthermore, many drugs are weak acids or bases and can have their degrees of ionization altered by skin pH, which can substantially influence their solubility, chemical stability, and lipophilicity (Zhang et al., 2012).

In the case of CL therapy, the goal of a topical formulation would be to target the dermis, where the parasites accumulate, but avoiding extensive distribution into the systemic circulation (Peralta et al., 2018). However, the topical use of AmB is not largely explored and studies evaluating its efficacy through this route are scarce (Eskandari et al., 2021). This is related to the high molecular weight of AmB (~924 Da) and its poor permeability across biological barriers, which cause it to remain retained in the SC with negligible amounts reaching the dermis layer (Faustino & Pinheiro, 2020; Perez et al., 2016). An important aspect of CL is that the skin of the patients is not always intact, being usually damaged. Therefore, an ideal formulation for the topical treatment of CL should work in all possible situations: intact, partially, or completely damaged skin (Carneiro et al., 2012).

The cream containing 3% AmB (Anfoleish®) is one of the examples of conventional formulations that failed showing efficacy by the topical route when evaluated in a clinical trial (NCT01845727). Although it proved to be safe, the formulation showed low efficacy in patients with CL. After 28 days of treatment with 2 or 3 daily administrations, only about 30% of the patients showed complete healing, with re-epithelialization of the lesions, disappearance of the induration, and absence of recurrence after 6 months. Furthermore, AmB was not present in detectable concentrations in the plasma of treated patients, confirming the low transdermal permeation of the drug (López et al., 2018; Keservani et al., 2020a). Thus, alternative formulations that allow the administration of AmB topically are essential, and in this sense, its insertion in nanocarriers is an attractive and promising approach.

3.5 NANOMEDICINE TO ENHANCE TOPICAL DELIVERY

A wide range of nanocarriers (Keservani et al., 2019), including liposomes, lipid, and polymeric nanoparticles, and cyclodextrin complexes have been developed to enhance drug penetration into the skin (Figure 3.5). Liposomes were the first carriers investigated for this use. They are typically composed of natural phospholipids that have the ability to spontaneously self-assemble in aqueous media and form one or more bilayers delimiting aqueous compartments. Cholesterol is often added to improve the stability of bilayers in the presence of biological fluids, reducing permeability and leakage of encapsulated drugs. Due to the similarity between their lipid composition and SC, these nanocarriers can penetrate more into the epidermal barrier compared to conventional pharmaceutical forms (Zhou et al., 2021; Sala et al., 2018).

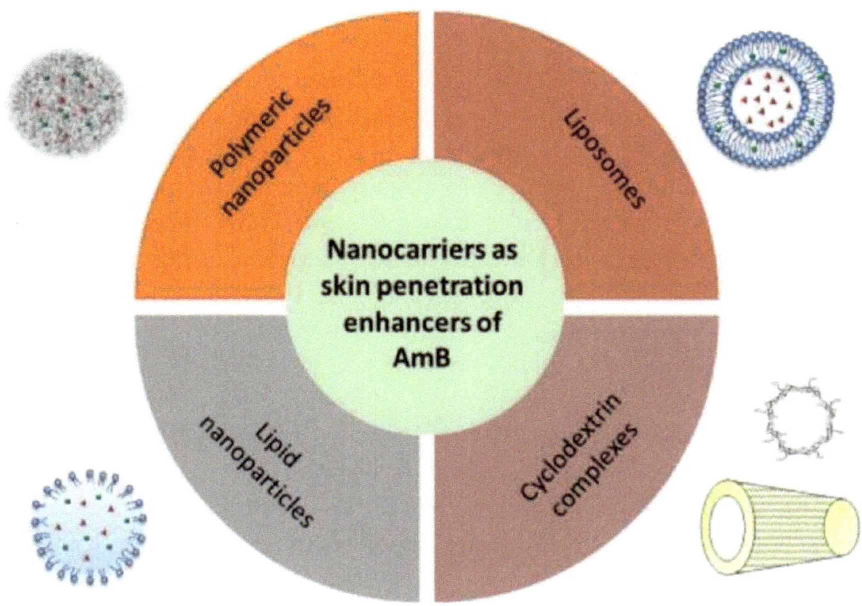

FIGURE 3.5 Schematic representation of AmB-loaded nanocarriers for enhanced skin penetration.

The poor membrane fluidity and elasticity of liposomes, however, make it difficult for them to pass through the SC in an intact form. Thus, they do not exhibit an efficient permeation into the deep layers of the skin and are mainly stopped in the upper layers of the epidermis, where rupture of the vesicles can occur due to their lack of deformability (Sala et al., 2018). This limitation of conventional liposomes has led to changes in their composition and structure to generate new classes of lipid vesicles with flexible and ultra-deformable properties, in particular niosomes (Keservani et al., 2010; Keservani & Gautam, 2020), transfersomes (TRAs), and ethosomes (ETOs) (Hua, 2015; Krishnan & Mitragotri, 2020).

Niosomes (Keservani & Gautam, 2022) are lipid vesicles that have non-ionic surfactants in their composition and a lower amount of cholesterol than that used for liposomes. Although they generally have similar characteristics to liposomes, they are considered more stable and result in higher drug entrapment efficiency, as well as being more cost-effective (Yu et al., 2021). TRAs are a type of vesicle composed of multiple phospholipid bilayers with an additional component, called an edge activator, which is often a single-chain surfactant with a large radius of curvature. The introduction of an edge activator destabilizes the lipid bilayers of the vesicles and increases their deformability by reducing the interfacial tension (Hua, 2015). This allows the vesicles to squeeze through the intercellular regions of the SC under the influence of the transdermal water gradient and deliver the encapsulated drugs deeper into the skin (Krishnan & Mitragotri, 2020). In turn, ETOs are lipid vesicles composed of phospholipids and a large amount of ethanol (20–50%). The inclusion of ethanol can give the vesicles soft and flexible properties, which allow them to more easily penetrate the deeper layers of the skin. Furthermore, ethanol is known to be a skin permeation enhancer, which may provide a synergistic effect to the nanocarrier penetration mechanism (Sala et al., 2018; Hua, 2015).

In addition to these systems, solid lipid nanoparticles (SLNs) (Keservani et al., 2017) are another widely investigated system for topical delivery. They are composed of emulsifiers and solid lipids and adhere to the skin due to their lipid nature forming a monolayer, which creates an occlusive effect to increase water retention within the skin and facilitate its penetration (Krishnan & Mitragotri, 2020). However, low drug loading efficiency and drug leakage during stability are important limitations of SLN. In order to optimize these properties, nanostructured lipid carriers (NLC) were developed as a second generation of nanoparticles in which the lipid matrix is formed by mixing solid and liquid lipids (oils). The addition of a liquid lipid reduces the organization of the lipid matrix and generates defects in the crystal structure, offering more space for drug inclusion; and thus, resulting in higher drug loading and stability compared to SLN (Sala et al., 2018).

Cyclodextrins (CDs) and polymeric nanoparticles (Keservani et al., 2018) are other interesting strategies. CDs are cyclic oligosaccharides with a hydrophilic outer surface and a lipophilic central cavity. They are capable of forming water-soluble inclusion complexes with many lipophilic drugs by hydrogen bonding, van der Waals, and charge-transfer interactions. Cyclodextrin complexes are able to increase drug solubility and affect SC barrier function, which improves drug availability in the skin surface (Cal & Centkowska, 2008; Bíró & Aigner, 2019). In turn, polymeric nanoparticles are colloidal carriers consisting of biodegradable, biocompatible, and non-toxic polymers, which can be of natural or synthetic origin. Chitosan is one of the most used natural polymers, mainly due to its cationic nature that allows it to establish strong interactions with the negatively charged skin surface (Tampucci et al., 2022).

In all these nanosystems (Keservani et al., 2017), permeation through the skin is controlled by many factors, which include both the physicochemical properties of the drug and the formulation characteristics, such as lipid composition and concentration, particle size, and surface charge (Sinico et al., 2005). Among these factors, the influences of size and charge have been widely described. Generally, large particles with a size above 600 nm are not able to reach the deeper layers of the skin and tend to remain in the SC. In contrast, particles smaller than 300 nm can penetrate to some extent in the deeper layers of the skin, while those with size below 70 nm have maximum deposition in the viable layers of the epidermis and dermis (Hua, 2015; Lengert et al., 2020).

The exact mechanisms by which nanocarriers enhance drug penetration through intact skin are not fully understood. The main hypotheses are: (i) the nanocarriers penetrate through skin appendages, including hair follicles and sebaceous glands, and deliver the encapsulated drugs to surrounding tissues; (ii) the nanocarriers disintegrate on the skin surface and formulation components can penetrate the SC with consequent fluidization and modification of SC lipids; (iii) the nanocarriers have adhesive properties on the skin and exert an occlusive effect, which prevents water evaporation and reduces the organization of corneocytes; and (iv) deformable and ultra-deformable nanocarriers can penetrate in their intact form through the SC using the intercellular route (Zhou et al., 2021; Gupta et al., 2012; Sala et al., 2018).

In general, these pathways can occur in a combined manner and are closely linked to the nature of the nanosystem. In the case of conventional liposomes, for example, their lipid composition mainly allows their adsorption on the skin surface and fusion with SC lipids, thus initiating the release of the drug in the tissue. However, they can also exert an occlusive effect on the skin, which is the main mechanism by which SLN and NLC act. Polymeric nanoparticles, in turn, are known to penetrate the skin through an appendageal pathway, accumulating in the hair follicles (Krishnan & Mitragotri, 2020; Sala et al., 2018).

3.6 PERMEATION STUDIES OF AMB-LOADED NANOCARRIERS TO TREAT CUTANEOUS LEISHMANIASIS (CL)

Several drug delivery systems (DDSs) are under development in order to enhance the dispersibility of AmB in aqueous media and promote better permeation across the skin. Some researchers have achieved promising results, like the ones showed by Perez and colleagues (2016) after developing ultra-deformable liposomes containing AmB, with 107 ± 8 nm diameter. The composition of these liposomes has been optimized and Tween80 was found to be the best edge activator, leading to vesicle deformability and maximum AmB content. This formulation allowed higher AmB retention in the SC (around 33%) and in viable epidermis (around 7%) than AmBisome®, that was not found in the SC and less than 2% was quantified in the viable epidermis. When liposomes are exposed to mechanical stress or space confinement in topical route, the presence of an edge activator, like Tween 80, can promote better deformability, leading to the passage through pores smaller than their own size. This shape and volume transformation can be done at lower energy, due their high curvature radius and mobility (Zeb et al., 2016). This could explain the best results found for the formulation developed by Perez et al. (2016).

Another study, published by Peralta and colleagues (2018) also showed that ultra-deformable liposomes (average size of 100 nm) provided better penetration through the skin than conventional liposomes, in a study using human skin in Franz diffusion cells. While AmB penetrated only 12.5% of the skin thickness when loaded in conventional liposomes, from the ultra-flexible vesicles it reached up to 80% of the skin thickness, revealing its penetration in the whole epidermis, reaching the dermis. Curiously, in this study, the penetration of an AmB suspension in HEPES buffer showed the best result.

Nonetheless, an excess of AmB in a solution can lead to precipitation in the form of crystals, which may have low stability and homogeneity, and be irritating, not meeting the requirements of a pharmaceutical formulation. In a complementary study, skin penetration of ultra-deformable liposomes with DiIC18 (fluorescent dye) was assessed *in vivo* in BALB/c mice by confocal fluorescence microscopy. The authors observed that liposomes penetrate mostly through canyons (structures that seems to be invaginations or extensions of the SC) than through cell clusters (Peralta et al., 2018).

Carvalheiro et al. (2021) also explored the deformation property of liposomes with Tween 80 as an edge activator. Liposomes with mean size of 132 ± 2.2 nm were obtained and evaluated through pig skin in Franz diffusion cells. Drug permeation after 24 h was very low for deformable liposomes and free AmB (AmB in hydroalcoholic solution). Retention of free AmB in SC layer was significantly higher (4.0% *vs* 1.2% of applied dose), while the amount of AmB found in the viable epidermis and dermis for liposomes loading AmB (0.3% *vs* 0.2% of applied dose) was significantly higher (Carvalheiro et al., 2021).

Sousa et al. (2017), in turn, optimized a microemulsion containing catolé oil (from a Brazilian palm tree) with a droplet size of 31.02 ± 0.9 nm. *Ex vivo* studies using pig skin without SC, to mimic an injured skin model, showed higher retention of the microemulsion (84.79 ± 2.08 $\mu g*cm^{-2}$) after 24 h than an emulgel and an emulsion containing AmB, 23.83 and 1.26 $\mu g*cm^{-2}$, respectively. For all AmB-loaded formulations retention values were statistically higher than the permeation values. These results are similar to those obtained by Santos et al. (2012); and Matos et al. (2020) for AmB-loaded nanoemulsions.

The low permeation of AmB is a barrier to its topical administration, with its high hydrophobicity and molecular weight being the main constraints, as mentioned above. Another challenge, even for ultra-deformable carriers, is that AmB can decrease membrane deformability due to its interaction with the lipids that form the vesicles and with edge activators (Carvalheiro et al., 2021; Peralta et al., 2018; Perez et al., 2016; Kiryakova et al., 2014). Despite all these obstacles, nanocarriers were found to improve the delivery of AmB to the dermis, where the infected macrophages (target cells) are found. It should be noted that most studies were conducted only in healthy skin. This drawback is important, because skin architecture and permeability are significantly altered under pathological conditions, like CL (Carneiro et al., 2012). For a more complete perspective, some authors evaluated the performance of nanocarriers in experimental models of CL, described in the next section.

3.7 *IN VIVO* STUDIES OF AMB-LOADED NANOCARRIERS TO TREAT CUTANEOUS LEISHMANIASIS (CL)

In this topic, recent studies that evaluated the impact of AmB nanoencapsulation on the effectiveness of CL topical treatment *in vivo* are presented and summarized in Table 3.1.

3.7.1 LIPID NANOCARRIERS

Seeking to provide an efficient AmB topical therapy against CL, researchers have delivered AmB in nanocarriers, with special interest in lipid systems. Some of the lipid systems are capable of deforming and passing through the skin barrier. This ability was explored by Mostafavi et al. (2019) when using niosomes, by Dar et al. (2020) when evaluating ultradeformable liposomes and by Fernández-García et al. (2020) with transferosomes. Allied to this strategy, the authors Mostafavi et al. (2019); and Dar et al. (2020) employed another tactic: the drug combination. Co-incorporating different drugs in the same nanosystem could improve treatment efficacy due to a synergistic effect, especially when they have different mechanisms of action, in addition to delaying the emergence of resistance (Lanza et al., 2019).

Mostafavi et al. (2019) produced niosomes co-encapsulating AmB and Glucantime® (AmB-Glucantime® niosomes). To form a gel, the formulation was incorporated into Carbopol® 934. *In vitro* activity against *Leishmania tropica* showed that the AmB-Glucantime® niosomes were able to inhibit intracellular and extracellular forms of the parasite, leading to the lowest IC_{50} against the amastigote forms and the highest selectivity index. Another interesting result reported by the authors was the increase in the gene expression of metacaspase (marker of apoptosis), IL-12 (indicator of Th1-type response) and a reduction of IL-10 (indicator of Th2-type response) when *Leishmania tropica* promastigotes were treated with AmB-Glucantime® niosomes compared to the control group (untreated). It has been proposed that, for infection control, the predominance of cellular immune response with Th1-type characteristics is necessary, involving cytokines such as IL-12 and IFN-γ, that participate in the resolutive response. This response results in the activation of macrophages, making them capable of eliminating the parasite and controlling the infection, especially through the production of reactive oxygen and nitrogen species (Lipoldová & Demant, 2006). The *in vivo* studies in BALB/c mice inoculated subcutaneously with *Leishmania*

TABLE 3.1 Main Studies of AmB-Loaded Nanocarriers to Treat CL

Type of Nanocarrier	Composition	Animal Model (Dose, Regimen)	In vivo Outcomes	References
Niosome	AmB deoxycholate and Meglumine antimoniate (Glucantime®); Span 40; Tween 40; Cholesterol; Water; Carbopol® 934 and Triethanolamine.	BALB/c mice (uninformed, twice daily for 30 days).	Higher efficacy of the niosomes containing AmB-Meglumine antimoniate in experimental model of CL infected with *Leishmania major* ($n = 6$ per group), evidencing a significant reduction in lesion size compared to placebo (Carbopol® gel without drug) ($p < 0.001$) and compared to Glucantime® intramuscular ($p < 0.05$), although complete healing of the lesion was not observed. Additionally, the group treated with niosomes showed significant less ($p < 0.001$) parasite burden in spleen than placebo group.	Mostafavi et al. (2019)
Ultradeformable liposome	AmB; Miltefosine; Phospholipon 90G; Tween-80; Phosphate buffered saline; Carbopol® 934 and Triethanolamine.	BALB/c mice (AmB 1.5 mg/kg/day, twice daily for 4 weeks).	The treatment with co-loaded AmB-Miltefosine ultra-deformable liposomes resulted in complete lesion resolution with no signs of scaring at the lesion site in BALB/c mice infected with *Leishmania Mexicana* ($n = 5$ per group). Additionally, significant reduction ($p < 0.01$) in the parasite load on the skin was observed for this treated group, compared to all other groups: control group receiving Carbopol® gel, AmB gel or AmB in ultra-deformable liposomes alone.	Dar et al. (2020)
Transfersome	AmB; Sodium deoxycholate; Soya phosphatidylcholine; Phosphate-buffered saline; Ethanol and Mannitol.	BALB/c mice (0.5 mg/mL, 20 mg of formulation/day, once a day for 10 consecutive days).	The experimental model of CL infected with *Leishmania amazonensis* ($n = 4$ per group) showed significant reduction ($p < 0.05$) in lesion size, compared to the control group (untreated) after treatment with transfersome-loaded AmB. The treated groups had an almost complete reduction in parasite load in lesion site.	Fernández-Garciá et al. (2020)
NLC	AmB; Glyceryl monostearate; Isopropyl myristate; Phospholipon 90G; Tween 80; Water; Carbopol® 934; Triethanolamine and Glycerol.	BALB/c mice (50 µL, 0.04% AmB, for 10 consecutive days).	Treatment with NLC delivering AmB led to a significant reduction ($p < 0.05$) of the parasite burden in lesion and lowest percentage increase in mean lesion size (mice infected with *Leishmania major*, $n = 5$ for treatment groups and $n = 4$ for control groups), even though a significant difference was not observed compared with the untreated control group.	Riaz et al. (2020)

TABLE 3.1 *(Continued)*

Type of Nanocarrier	Composition	Animal Model (Dose, Regimen)	In vivo Outcomes	References
Cyclodextrin complex	AmB; γ-cyclodextrin; methyl cellulose and water.	Golden hamster (uninformed, twice daily for 21 consecutive days).	Higher reduction ($p < 0.05$) in lesion size with AmB-Cyclodextrin treatment, compared to the control group (untreated) in an experimental model of CL infected with *Leishmania amazonensis* ($n = 6$ per group).	Ruiz et al. (2014)
Polymeric nanoparticle	AmB deoxycholate; Chitosan; Isobutyl cyanoacrylate and Pluronic F127.	BALB/c mice (uninformed, daily for 3 consecutive weeks).	The treatment with poly(isobutyl cyanoacrylate) nanoparticles coated with chitosan loading AmB showed partial healing of the lesion by histological analyzes after treatment of experimentally infected animals (*Leishmania major*, $n = 6$ per group). The treatment also led to the lowest parasitic load in skin, with significant reduction compared with the nontreated group.	Malli et al. (2019)
Liposome	AmB; Soya phosphatidylcholine; Cholesterol; Dimethyl sulfoxide; Propylene glycol; Oleic acid; Vitamin E; Methylparaben and Propylparaben.	BALB/c mice (50 mg liposomal AmB 0.4%, twice a day, for four weeks).	Higher efficacy of the liposomal formulation containing 0.4% AmB against *Leishmania major* in CL experimental model ($n = 10$ per group), showing significant reduction ($p < 0.001$) in lesion size, together with almost complete elimination of parasites in skin and spleens compared to mice treated with PBS or empty liposomes. No signs of kidney toxicity were observed in histopathological studies and no signs of irritancy was revealed in Draize test (skin and eyes).	Jaafari et al. (2019)

Abbreviations: AmB: amphotericin B; NLC: nanostructured lipid carriers; CL: cutaneous leishmaniasis; and PBS: phosphate-buffered saline.

major promastigotes showed a significant reduction in lesion size for the group treated topically with AmB-Glucantime® niosomes in comparison to placebo (Carbopol® gel without drug) ($p < 0.001$) and to Glucantime® intramuscular, at a dose of 20 mg/kg/day ($p < 0.05$). The lesion size was followed for further 4 weeks after the end of treatment and an increase was observed for the treated groups, but they remained significantly smaller compared to placebo. Regarding the parasite load, the group receiving the niosomal formulation AmB-Glucantime® led to the lowest mean number of parasites/mg of spleen tissue, showing a significant reduction in the parasite load compared to the placebo group ($p < 0.001$). A limitation of this study was the lack of evaluation of the parasite load in the lesion, an important parameter to evaluate the effectiveness of the formulation. Nevertheless, this study is an example of how the association of drugs in nanocarriers can increase the treatment efficacy, even in comparison with the intramuscular route.

In line with this strategy, Dar et al. (2020) developed ultra-deformable liposomes co-encapsulating AmB and Miltefosine (MTF). For skin application, the formulation was also gelled using Carbopol® 934. *In vitro* studies showed a significant decrease in the cytotoxicity of liposomal co-encapsulated drugs in bone marrow-derived macrophages (BMDMs). The lower toxicity, however, was not accompanied by a loss of activity. The authors reported that the co-loaded liposomes were 8.6 and 6.1 times more active (lower IC_{50}) against the amastigote form of *Leishmania mexicana* compared to the solutions of the free drugs, AmB and MTF, respectively. Moreover, high AmB uptake (49% of the initial concentration) by BMDMs was found when using liposomes co-encapsulating MTF. The *in vivo* study with BALB/c mice infected subcutaneously with *Leishmania mexicana* promastigotes showed complete lesion resolution aftertreatment with AmB-MTF co-loaded liposomes. In agreement with this, a significant reduction ($p < 0.01$) in the parasite load was observed in the lesion. The authors suggest that the high efficacy is directly associated with the synergistic effect between MTF and AmB when co-encapsulated in a nanocarrier system. Moreover, significantly higher ($p < 0.01$) production of nitric oxide, interferon-gamma (IFN-γ), and interleukin (IL)-12 was observed, while IL-4 and IL-10 levels were significantly lower ($p < 0.01$). The opposite was observed for the groups treated with free AmB gel and the untreated group.

Still following the deformable vesicle strategy for topical delivery, Fernández-García et al. (2020) developed transfersomes encapsulating AmB (AmB-TF). These nanocarriers showed high activity *in vitro* against *Leishmania amazonensis* and *Leishmania braziliensis* and low toxicity in murine macrophages (J774). The toxicity was also assessed in the skin of healthy mice exposed to AmB-TF and AmB solution (in DMSO) for 6 h. Treated groups showed some inflammatory cells, not observed in the untreated group, and some morphological changes, like compromised junction between the epidermis and the dermis, were more pronounced in AmB-DMSO treatment. *In vivo*, topical pharmacokinetic of AmB-TF revealed that AmB carried in TF was able to reach deeper regions of the skin. The permeation process seemed to increase linearly at shorter times (0.5 h) but saturates over time. They also state that diffusion was easier in the upper layers of the skin, but difficult in deeper skin areas. To assess *in vivo* activity, BALB/c mice were infected subcutaneously with promastigotes of *Leishmania amazonensis* and treated topically with AmB-TF. Animals showed a significant reduction ($p < 0.05$) in lesion size 6 days after the end of the treatment, while mice receiving Glucantime® intralesional (50 mg/kg, once daily, 25 µL) showed significant reduction ($p < 0.05$) during the treatment (on the seventh day), compared to the control group (untreated). Additionally, AmB-TF and Glucantime® intralesional showed high reduction in parasite load on the lesion 98.24 ± 1.54% and 99.78 ± 0.31%, respectively, and no signs of toxicity. Although Glucantime® leads to faster healing of the lesion, the results for topical AmB-TF are encouraging, as this route of administration may favor the patient compliance.

As another alternative to improve the topical permeation of AmB, Riaz & colleagues (2020) developed NLC loaded with AmB (AmB-NLC). To facilitate topical application *in vivo*, the formulation was gelled with Carbopol® 934 (AmB-NLC gel). *In vitro* results showed that AmB-NLC promoted significantly higher growth inhibition of *Leishmania major* and *Leishmania tropica* in promastigote and amastigote forms than an AmB solution. The authors justify this increase in efficacy due to the intrinsic ability of lipid carriers to protect drugs from early degradation. Another feature listed in this study that may have contribute to the higher activity is the controlled drug release from the AmB-NLC, observed in the *in vitro* drug release study, resulting in prolonged exposure of the target cells to AmB and thus, favoring the death of the parasite compared to free AmB. The slower drug release from AmB-NLC may also reduce AmB toxicity, as seen in the MRC-5 (human fetal lung fibroblasts) cytotoxicity assay. *In vivo* studies with BALB/c mice infected by subcutaneous injection of *Leishmania major* promastigotes, the group treated with topical AmB-NLC showed a smaller percentage increase in mean lesion size. Only the groups treated with topical AmB-NLC or intravenous-liposomal AmB (0.025 mg/g weight of mice once every other day) did not show worsening of the lesion for the ulcerative form. Additionally, a significant reduction ($p < 0.05$) in parasite burden per mg of lesion ($\times 10^8$) ± standard error of mean was observed in the groups treated with AmB-NLC and liposomal AmB (65 ± 13 and 58.3 ± 9) compared to the untreated control group (>167.8 ± 11). Free AmB (solution) was not effective in reducing the parasite load. In addition, the skin irritation study showed that the AmB-NLC is safe, with no signs of toxicity (erythema or edema). Thus, this study demonstrated that topically administered nano-encapsulated AmB provided higher inhibition of parasite growth, increased skin permeation and drug deposition compared to free AmB.

3.7.2 CYCLODEXTRINS (CDS) AND POLYMERIC NANOPARTICLES

As previously mentioned, cyclodextrins (CDs) are largely used as nanocarriers and were chosen by Ruiz and colleagues (2014) to deliver AmB, forming an AmB-CD complex. To allow higher residence time on the skin, methyl cellulose was used to form an AmB-CD gel. The *in vitro* activity results showed that the activity of the AmB-CD complex and AmB in deoxycholate were similar against different leishmania species. The *in vivo* study with a golden hamster subcutaneously infected with *Leishmania amazonensis*, showed that AmB-CD gel led to a significant reduction ($p < 0.05$) in lesion size compared to the control (untreated group) at the end of treatment (21 days). However, after discontinuation of treatment, a new progression of inflammation was observed (assessed 5 weeks post-treatment), evidencing the probable presence of remaining parasites. The authors suggest that longer treatment may be needed to achieve higher efficacy. In this study, the parasite load on the lesion was not evaluated, which could be interesting as it would verify the efficiency of AmB-CD gel in reducing the number of parasites after topical application.

Another interesting strategy to increase the activity of nanocarriers is the use of intrinsic bioactive materials. Thus, Malli et al. (2019) developed nanoparticles (Cs-NPs) composed of poly(isobutyl cyanoacrylate), which has antiparasitic activity, and chitosan, a cationic biopolymer that has been associated with wound healing and antibacterial effects. After preparing the Cs-NPs, AmB in deoxycholate (AmB-DOC) was added and the formulation was gelled with Pluronic F127, forming a hydrogel (Cs-NPs/AmB–DOC). The intrinsic activity of the Cs-NPs was evaluated *in vitro*, showing good antileishmanial activity against *Leishmania major* promastigote, axenic amastigote, and intramacrophage forms, but lower than the one found for AmB-DOC. Pluronic F127, Cs-NPs, AmB-DOC, and Cs-NPs/AmB–DOC were evaluated *in vivo*, after infection of BALB/c mice with *Leishmania major* promastigotes. The treatment with Cs-NPs/AmB–DOC led to a lower parasite load compared to the other three groups, showing a possible complementarity between the mechanism of action of Cs-NPs and AmB. The analysis of the skin sections of the treated animals showed the presence of collagen fibers in the hypodermis, indicating tissue repair and skin preserved architecture. The main structural changes were found in the tissues of animals treated with free AmB gel. Thus, the Cs-NPs/AmB–DOC formulation is promising, but more data on lesion size during treatment would be needed to better assess the feasibility of potential clinical use.

3.7.3 SINAAMPHOLEISH®: A NANOCARRIER IN CLINICAL STUDIES

SinaAmpholeish® is the trade name of AmB-loaded liposomes developed by Jaafari et al. (2019 and US2015/0147382A1) in Mashhad University of Medical Sciences, Iran. The optimized formulation showed *in vitro* activity against *Leishmania major* and *Leishmania tropica* and good performance in Franz diffusion cells study, using BALB/c mice skin. Approximately 3.49% of AmB penetrated through the skin and 73.92% was retained into it. Promising results were also reported for the *in vivo* efficacy study in BALB/c mice infected subcutaneously with *Leishmania major* promastigotes. Aftertreatment with the AmB-loaded liposomes, a significantly reduction ($p < 0.001$) in the size of the skin lesion was observed along with a reduction ($p < 0.001$) in the parasite burden of the spleen and lesion, compared to the control groups, which received empty liposomes or PBS. The animals were followed up to 12 weeks post-infection, and by week 12, animals that received AmB-loaded liposomes showed significantly lower lesions compared to the control groups (Figure 3.6). It was also observed almost complete elimination of parasites in the skin and spleen. According to the authors, these positive results can be related to the soya phosphatidylcholine phospholipid, which favors skin hydration, and propylene glycol, DMSO, and oleic acid, that can act as skin permeation facilitators (Jaafari et al., 2019). The spleen was the organ with the highest concentration of AmB, followed by the liver and kidney, 5.0, 3.5, and 2.5 μg/g, respectively. On the other hand, AmB serum concentration was negligible. Histopathological evaluation revealed normal kidney appearance, showing that topical application is a safe alternative capable of reducing AmB-associated nephrotoxicity. These results point to the liposomal formulation loading AmB as a promising alternative in the CL treatment, especially caused by *Leishmania major* and *Leishmania tropica*, once the activity might be variable against different *Leishmania* species (Varikuti et al., 2017). To assess the safety of AmB-loaded liposomes, the researchers carried out a skin and eye irritation study of healthy rabbits (Draize test). Based on the edema and erythema caused at the exposed site, the formulation was considered safe (Eskandari et al., 2018).

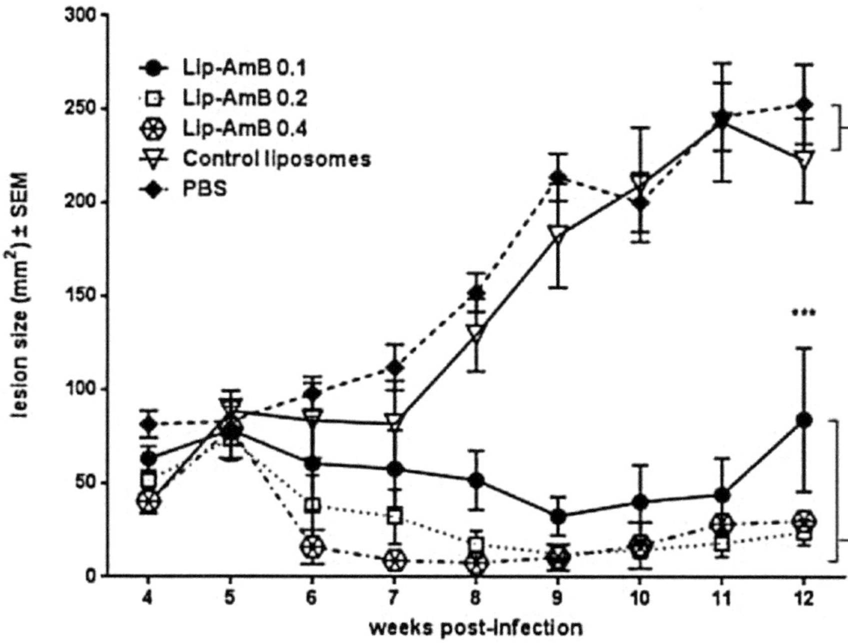

FIGURE 3.6 Lesion size monitored after treatment with topical AmB liposomes in infected BALB/c mice for 12 weeks.

Source: Reproduced with permission from: Jaafari et al. (2019). Values represent means ± standard errors of the means. Treated groups with AmB-loaded liposomes 0.1, 0.2, and 0.4% AmB showed lesion size significantly different from the control groups (mice receiving PBS or empty liposomes) (***, $p < 0.001$).

AmB-loaded liposomes 0.4% were also evaluated in a Phase I clinical trial conducted in a total of 27 healthy volunteers. After application twice a day for one week, no skin reactions were observed and there were no changes in the biophysical characteristics of the skin. However, when Sina-Ampholeish® was used for two weeks (3 times a day) it induced transient severe local skin reactions. For this reason, 2 volunteers had to stop the treatment, and half of the remaining subjects had mild transient reactions. Based on these results, the application twice a day was considered more appropriate and safer (Eskandari et al., 2019).

The activity of SinaAmpholeish® was clinically evaluated, observing similar efficacy between this formulation and intralesional applications of Glucantime® (56.4% versus 67.6%) in reducing lesion size. No serious adverse reactions were observed in any of the treatments (Layegh et al., 2011). Another clinical study is in progress and in this study, patients with CL caused by *Leishmania tropica* are treated with SinaAmpholeish® in combination with intralesional injections of Glucantime®. The objective is to compare the rate of clinical cure in patients receiving topical SinaAmpholeish® and Glucantime® with those receiving Glucantime® alone (Eskandari et al., 2021). If SinaAmpholeish® reaches the commercialization stage, it will represent a major advance in the treatment of leishmaniasis and an example of how nanocarriers can overcome the challenges of AmB topical administration.

3.8 CONCLUSIONS

AmB is one of the most important therapeutic options for the treatment of leishmaniasis. However, its physicochemical characteristics have been a major challenge in the development of formulations for the topical treatment of CL and so far, there are no formulations approved for this route of administration. This chapter showed how nanoencapsulation has provided advances in the development of formulations for topical administration of AmB and how was the performance of these formulations in pre-clinical studies. Regarding clinical trials, a liposomal formulation is being evaluated, representing an advance in the development of topical option for the treatment of CL. Some of the main recent strategies described herein involve the co-encapsulation of different drugs and the use of ultra-deformable carriers. As the topical route is non-invasive route with few toxicity issues, it can provide a greater probability of compliance, resulting in a higher cost-effectiveness rate of resolution of CL.

KEYWORDS

- **amphotericin B (AmB)**
- **antifungal**
- **lipid nanoparticles**
- **liposomes**
- **nanocarriers**
- **nanomedicine**
- **polymeric carriers**

REFERENCES

Alkilani, A. Z., McCrudden, M. T. C., & Donnelly, R. F., (2015). Transdermal drug delivery: Innovative pharmaceutical developments based on disruption of the barrier properties of the stratum corneum. *Pharmaceutics, 7*, 438–470.

Ammar, A. A., Nasereddin, A., Ereqat, S., Dan-Goor, M., Jaffe, C. L., Zussman, E., & Abdeen, Z., (2019). Amphotericin B-loaded nanoparticles for local treatment of cutaneous leishmaniasis. *Drug Delivery and Translational Research, 9*, 76–84.

Barratt, G., & Bretagne, S., (2007). Optimizing efficacy of amphotericin B through nanomodification. *International Journal of Nanomedicine, 2*, 301–313.

Benson, H. A. E., Grice, J. E., Mohammed, Y., Namjoshi, S., & Roberts, M. S., (2019). Topical and transdermal drug delivery: From simple potions to smart technologies. *Current Drug Delivery, 16*, 444–460.

Bíró, T., & Aigner, Z., (2019). Current approaches to use cyclodextrins and mucoadhesive polymers in ocular drug delivery-a mini-review. *Scientia Pharmaceutica, 87*.

Brown, T. M., & Krishnamurthy, K., (2019). *Histology, Dermis*. http://www.ncbi.nlm.nih.gov/pubmed/30570967 (accessed on 1 November 2023).

Cal, K., & Centkowska, K., (2008). Use of cyclodextrins in topical formulations: Practical aspects. *European Journal of Pharmaceutics and Biopharmaceutics, 68*, 467–478.

Carneiro, G., Aguiar, M. G., Fernandes, A. P., & Ferreira, L. A. M., (2012). Drug delivery systems for the topical treatment of cutaneous leishmaniasis. *Expert Opinion on Drug Delivery, 9*, 1083–1097.

Carolus, H., Pierson, S., Lagrou, K., & Van, D. P., (2020). Amphotericin b and other polyenes—Discovery, clinical use, mode of action and drug resistance. *Journal of Fungi, 6*, 321.

Carvalheiro, M., Vieira, J., Faria-Silva, C., Marto, J., & Simões, S., (2021). Amphotericin B-loaded deformable lipid vesicles for topical treatment of cutaneous leishmaniasis skin lesions. *Drug Delivery and Translational Research, 11*, 717–728.

Cavassin, F. B., Baú-Carneiro, J. L., Vilas-Boas, R. R., & Queiroz-Telles, F., (2021). Sixty years of amphotericin B: An overview of the main antifungal agent used to treat invasive fungal infections. *Infectious Diseases and Therapy, 10*, 115–147.

Chakravarty, J., & Sundar, S., (2010). Drug resistance in leishmaniasis. *Journal of Global Infectious Diseases, 2*, 167.

Cuddihy, G., Wasan, E. K., Di, Y., & Wasan, K. M., (2019). The development of oral amphotericin b to treat systemic fungal and parasitic infections: Has the myth been finally realized? *Pharmaceutics, 11*.

Dar, M. J., Khalid, S., McElroy, C. A., Satoskar, A. R., & Khan, G. M., (2020). Topical treatment of cutaneous leishmaniasis with novel amphotericin B-miltefosine co-incorporated second generation ultra-deformable liposomes. *International Journal of Pharmaceutics, 573*.

Deray, G., (2002). Amphotericin B nephrotoxicity. *Journal of Antimicrobial Chemotherapy, 49*, 37–41.

Drugs for Neglected Diseases initiative, (2017). *Topical 3% Amphotericin B Cream for the Treatment of Cutaneous Leishmaniasis in Colombia (Anfoleish)*. ClinicalTrials.gov. Available from: https://clinicaltrials.gov/ct2/show/NCT01845727?term=NCT01845727&draw=2&rank=1 (accessed on 1 November 2023).

Eskandari, S. E., Firooz, A., Nassiri-Kashani, M., Jaafari, M. R., Javadi, A., Miramin, M. A., & Khamesipour, A., (2019). Safety evaluation of topical application of nano-liposomal form of amphotericin B (SinaAmpholeish) on healthy volunteers: Phase I clinical trial. *Iranian Journal of Parasitology, 14*, 197–203.

Eskandari, S. E., Firooz, A., Nassiri-Kashani, M., Jaafari, M. R., Javadi, A., Miramin-Mohammadi, A., Valian-Keshavarz, H., & Khamesipour, A., (2018). Safety evaluation of nano-liposomal formulation of amphotericin B (SinaAmpholeish) in animal model as a candidate for treatment of cutaneous leishmaniasis. *Journal of Arthropod-Borne Diseases, 12*, 269–275.

Eskandari, S. E., Khamesipour, A., Jaafari, M. R., Javadi, A., Mohammadi, A. M., Valian, H. K., Nassiri-Kashani, M., et al., (2021). Combination of topical liposomal amphotericin b and glucantime in comparison with glucantime alone for the treatment of anthroponotic cutaneous leishmaniasis (Acl) caused by leishmania tropica: Study protocol for a randomized, controlled trial. *Iranian Journal of Microbiology, 13*, 718–723.

Faustino, C., & Pinheiro, L., (2020). Lipid systems for the delivery of amphotericin B in antifungal therapy. *Pharmaceutics, 12*, 29.

Fernández-García, R., De Pablo, E., Ballesteros, M. P., & Serrano, D. R., (2017). Unmet clinical needs in the treatment of systemic fungal infections: The role of amphotericin B and drug targeting. *International Journal of Pharmaceutics, 525*, 139–148.

Fernández-García, R., Statts, L., De Jesus, J. A., Dea-Ayuela, M. A., Bautista, L., Simaõ, R., Bolás-Fernández, F., Ballesteros, M. P., Laurenti, M. D., Passero, L. F. D., et al., (2020). Ultradeformable lipid vesicles localize amphotericin B in the dermis for the treatment of infectious skin diseases. *ACS Infectious Diseases, 6*, 2647–2660.

Golenser, J., & Domb, A., (2006). New formulations and derivatives of amphotericin B for treatment of leishmaniasis. *Mini-Reviews in Medicinal Chemistry, 6*, 153–162.

Guery, R., Henry, B., Martin-Blondel, G., Rouzaud, C., Cordoliani, F., Harms, G., Gangneux, J. P., Foulet, F., Bourrat, E., Baccard, M., et al., (2017). Liposomal amphotericin B in travelers with cutaneous and muco-cutaneous leishmaniasis: Not a panacea. *PLoS Neglected Tropical Diseases, 11*.

Gupta, M., Agrawal, U., & Vyas, S. P., (2012). Nanocarrier-based topical drug delivery for the treatment of skin diseases. *Expert Opinion on Drug Delivery, 9*, 783–804.

Hamill, R. J., (2013). Amphotericin B formulations: A comparative review of efficacy and toxicity. *Drugs, 73*, 919–934.

Honari, G., (2017). Skin structure and function. In: *Sensitive Skin Syndrome* (2nd edn., pp. 16–22). CRC Press.

Hua, S., (2015). Lipid-based nano-delivery systems for skin delivery of drugs and bioactives. *Frontiers in Pharmacology, 6*.

Jaafari, M. R., & Khamesipour, A., (2015). *Topical Liposomal Compositions for Delivering Hydrophobic Drugs and Methods Preparing Same*. Publication Number: US 2015/0147382 A1.

Jaafari, M. R., Hatamipour, M., Alavizadeh, S. H., Abbasi, A., Saberi, Z., Rafati, S., Taslimi, Y., et al., (2019). Development of a topical liposomal formulation of amphotericin B for the treatment of cutaneous leishmaniasis. *International Journal for Parasitology: Drugs and Drug Resistance, 11*, 156–165.

Kamiński, D. M., (2014). Recent progress in the study of the interactions of amphotericin B with cholesterol and ergosterol in lipid environments. *European Biophysics Journal, 43*, 453–467.

Kapoor, M. S., Guhasarkar, S., & Banerjee, R., (2017). Stratum corneum modulation by chemical enhancers and lipid nanostructures: Implications for transdermal drug delivery. *Therapeutic Delivery, 8*, 701–718.

Keservani, R. K., & Gautam, S. P., (2020). Formulation and evaluation of baclofen liposome vesicles using lecithin. *ARS Pharmaceutica, 61*(3), 175–180.

Keservani, R. K., & Gautam, S. P., (2022). Skeletal muscle relaxant activity of different formulation of span 60 niosome. *ARS Pharmaceutica, 63*(91), 32–44.

Keservani, R. K., Bandopadhyay, S., Bandyopadhyay, N., & Sharma, A. K., (2020a). Design and fabrication of transdermal/skin drug-delivery system. In: *Drug Delivery Systems* (pp. 131–178). Academic Press.

Keservani, R. K., Kesharwani, R. K., & Sharma, A. K., (2017). Introduction to nanotechnology in drug delivery. In: *Drug Delivery Approaches and Nanosystems* (pp. 1–19). Apple Academic Press. ISBN, 9781771885836.

Keservani, R. K., Sharma, A. K., & Kesharwani, R. K., (2017). *Drug Delivery Approaches and Nanosystems, Two-Volume Set*. CRC Press. ISBN:9781771885850.

Keservani, R. K., Sharma, A. K., & Kesharwani, R. K., (2018). Nanoparticulate nanocarriers in drug delivery. In: *Nanobiomaterials* (pp. 3–22). Apple Academic Press. ISBN, 9781771885911.

Keservani, R. K., Sharma, A. K., & Kesharwani, R. K., (2019). *Nanocarriers for Brain Targeting: Principles and Applications*. CRC Press. ISBN:9781771887304.

Keservani, R. K., Sharma, A. K., &Ramteke, S., (2010). Novel vesicular approach for topical delivery of baclofen via niosomes. *Lat. Am. J. Pharm., 29*, 1364–1370.

Kiryakova, S., Dencheva-Zarkova, M., & Genova, J., (2014). Effect of amphotericin B antibiotic on the properties of model lipid membrane. In: *Journal of Physics: Conference Series* (Vol. 558). of, Institute of Physics Publishing.

Krishnan, V., & Mitragotri, S., (2020). Nanoparticles for topical drug delivery: Potential for skin cancer treatment. *Advanced Drug Delivery Reviews, 153*, 87–108.

Laniado-Laborín, R., & Cabrales-Vargas, M. N., (2009). Amphotericin B: Side effects and toxicity. *Revista Iberoamericana de Micologia, 26*, 223–227.

Lanza, J. S., Pomel, S., Loiseau, P. M., & Frézard, F., (2019). Recent advances in amphotericin B delivery strategies for the treatment of leishmaniases. *Expert Opinion on Drug Delivery, 16*, 1063–1079.

Layegh, P., Rajabi, O., Jafari, M. R., Emamgholi, T. M. P., Moghiman, T., Ashraf, H., & Salari, R., (2011). Efficacy of topical liposomal amphotericin B versus intralesional meglumine antimoniate (glucantime) in the treatment of cutaneous leishmaniasis. *Journal of Parasitology Research, 201*(1), 656523.

Lengert, E. V., Talnikova, E. E., Tuchin, V. V., & Svenskaya, Y. I., (2020). Prospective nanotechnology-based strategies for enhanced intra- and transdermal delivery of antifungal drugs. *Skin Pharmacology and Physiology, 33*, 261–269.

Lipoldová, M., & Demant, P., (2006). Genetic susceptibility to infectious disease: Lessons from mouse models of leishmaniasis. *Nature Reviews Genetics, 7*, 294–305.

Liu, M., Chen, M., & Yang, Z., (2017). Design of amphotericin B oral formulation for antifungal therapy. *Drug Delivery, 24*, 1–9.

López, L., Vélez, I., Asela, C., Cruz, C., Alves, F., Robledo, S., & Arana, B., (2018). A phase II study to evaluate the safety and efficacy of topical 3% amphotericin B cream (Anfoleish) for the treatment of uncomplicated cutaneous leishmaniasis in Colombia. *PLoS Neglected Tropical Diseases, 12*.

Malli, S., Pomel, S., Ayadi, Y., Deloménie, C., Da Costa, A., Loiseau, P. M., & Bouchemal, K., (2019). Topically applied chitosan-coated poly(isobutylcyanoacrylate) nanoparticles are active against cutaneous leishmaniasis by accelerating lesion healing and reducing the parasitic load. *ACS Applied Bio Materials, 2*, 2573–2586.

Matos, A. P. D. S., Lopes D. C. D. X. P., Peixoto, M. L. H., Da Silva, C. V., Vermelho, A. B., Santos-Oliveira, R., Viçosa, A. L., et al., (2020). Development, characterization, and anti-leishmanial activity of topical amphotericin B nanoemulsions. *Drug Delivery and Translational Research, 10*, 1552–1570.

Menon, G. K., Cleary, G. W., & Lane, M. E., (2012). The structure and function of the stratum corneum. *International Journal of Pharmaceutics, 435*, 3–9.

Mesa-Arango, A. C., Trevijano-Contador, N., Román, E., Sánchez-Fresneda, R., Casas, C., Herrero, E., Argüelles, J. C., et al., (2014). The production of reactive oxygen species is a universal action mechanism of amphotericin B against pathogenic yeasts and contributes to the fungicidal effect of this drug. *Antimicrobial Agents and Chemotherapy, 58*, 6627–6638.

Mostafavi, M., Sharifi, I., Farajzadeh, S., Khazaeli, P., Sharifi, H., Pourseyedi, E., Kakooei, S., Bamorovat, M., Keyhani, A., Parizi, M. H., et al., (2019). Niosomal formulation of amphotericin B alone and in combination with glucantime: *In vitro* and *in vivo* leishmanicidal effects. *Biomedicine and Pharmacotherapy, 116*.

N'Da, D. D., (2014). Prodrug strategies for enhancing the percutaneous absorption of drugs. *Molecules, 19*, 20780–20807.

Palmer, B. C., & DeLouise, L. A., (2016). Nanoparticle-enabled transdermal drug delivery systems for enhanced dose control and tissue targeting. *Molecules, 21*, 1719.

Peralta, M. F., Guzmán, M. L., Pérez, A. P., Apezteguia, G. A., Fórmica, M. L., Romero, E. L., Olivera, M. E., & Carrer, D. C., (2018). Liposomes can both enhance or reduce drugs penetration through the skin. *Scientific Reports, 8*.

Perez, A. P., Altube, M. J., Schilrreff, P., Apezteguia, G., Celes, F. S., Zacchino, S., De Oliveira, C. I., et al., (2016). Topical amphotericin B in ultra deformable liposomes: Formulation, skin penetration study, antifungal and antileishmanial activity *in vitro*. *Colloids and Surfaces B: Biointerfaces, 139*, 190–198.

Prow, T. W., Grice, J. E., Lin, L. L., Faye, R., Butler, M., Becker, W., Wurm, E. M. T., Yoong, C., Robertson, T. A., Soyer, H. P., et al., (2011). Nanoparticles and microparticles for skin drug delivery. *Advanced Drug Delivery Reviews, 63*, 470–491.

Riaz, A., Hendricks, S., Elbrink, K., Guy, C., Maes, L., Ahmed, N., Kiekens, F., & Khan, G. M., (2020). Preparation and characterization of nanostructured lipid carriers for improved topical drug delivery: Evaluation in cutaneous leishmaniasis and vaginal candidiasis animal models. *AAPS PharmSciTech, 21*.

Richard, C., Cassel, S., & Blanzat, M., (2021). Vesicular systems for dermal and transdermal drug delivery. *RSC Advances, 11*, 442–451.

Ritmeijer, K., Ter, H. R., Chane, S., Aderie, E. M., Piening, T., Collin, S. M., & Davidson, R. N., (2011). Limited effectiveness of high-dose liposomal amphotericin B (AmBisome) for treatment of visceral leishmaniasis in an ethiopian population with high HIV prevalence. *Clinical Infectious Diseases, 53*.

Ruiz, H. K., Serrano, D. R., Dea-Ayuela, M. A., Bilbao-Ramos, P. E., Bolás-Fernández, F., Torrado, J. J., & Molero, G., (2014). New amphotericin B-gamma cyclodextrin formulation for topical use with synergistic activity against diverse fungal species and *Leishmania* spp. *International Journal of Pharmaceutics, 473*, 148–157.

Sala, M., Diab, R., Elaissari, A., & Fessi, H., (2018). Lipid nanocarriers as skin drug delivery systems: Properties, mechanisms of skin interactions and medical applications. *International Journal of Pharmaceutics, 535*, 1–17.

Santos, C. M., De Oliveira, R. B., Arantes, V. T., Caldeira, L. R., De Oliveira, M. C., Egito, E. S. T., & Ferreira, L. A. M., (2012). Amphotericin B-loaded nanocarriers for topical treatment of cutaneous leishmaniasis: Development, characterization, and *in vitro* skin permeation studies. *Journal of Biomedical Nanotechnology, 8*, 322–329.

Sau, K., Mambula, S. S., Latz, E., Henneke, P., Golenbock, D. T., & Levitz, S. M., (2003). The antifungal drug amphotericin B promotes inflammatory cytokine release by a toll-like receptor- and CD14-dependent mechanism. *Journal of Biological Chemistry, 278*, 37561–37568.

Serrano, D. R., & Lalatsa, A., (2017). Oral amphotericin B: The journey from bench to market. *Journal of Drug Delivery Science and Technology, 42*, 75–83.

Sinico, C., Manconi, M., Peppi, M., Lai, F., Valenti, D., & Fadda, A. M., (2005). Liposomes as carriers for dermal delivery of tretinoin: *In vitro* evaluation of drug permeation and vesicle-skin interaction. *Journal of Controlled Release, 103*, 123–136.

Sousa, G. D., Kishishita, J., Aquino, K. A. S., Presgrave, O. A. F., Leal, L. B., & Santana, D. P., (2017). Biopharmaceutical assessment and irritation potential of microemulsions and conventional systems containing oil from syagrus cearensis for topical delivery of amphotericin b using alternative methods. *AAPS PharmSciTech, 18*, 1833–1842.

Tampucci, S., Paganini, V., Burgalassi, S., Chetoni, P., & Monti, D., (2022). Nanostructured drug delivery systems for targeting 5-α-reductase inhibitors to the hair follicle. *Pharmaceutics, 14*, 286.

Thanki, K., Date, T., & Jain, S., (2019). Improved oral bioavailability and gastrointestinal stability of amphotericin B through fatty acid conjugation approach. *Molecular Pharmaceutics, 16*, 4519–4529.

Torrado, J. J., Espada, R., Ballesteros, M. P., & Torrado-Santiago, S., (2008). Amphotericin B formulations and drug targeting. *Journal of Pharmaceutical Sciences, 97*, 2405–2425.

Varikuti, S., Oghumu, S., Saljoughian, N., Pioso, M. S., Sedmak, B. E., Khamesipour, A., & Satoskar, A. R., (2017). Topical treatment with nanoliposomal amphotericin B reduces early lesion growth but fails to induce cure in an experimental model of cutaneous leishmaniasis caused by *Leishmania mexicana*. *Acta Tropica, 173*, 102–108.

Vriens, K., Kumar, P. T., Struyfs, C., Cools, T. L., Spincemaille, P., Kokalj, T., Sampaio-Marques, B., Ludovico, P., Lammertyn, J., Cammue, B. P. A., et al., (2017). Increasing the fungicidal action of amphotericin B by inhibiting the nitric oxide-dependent tolerance pathway. *Oxidative Medicine and Cellular Longevity, 201*(7), 4064628.

Wang, X., Mohammad, I. S., Fan, L., Zhao, Z., Nurunnabi, M., Sallam, M. A., Wu, J., et al., (2021). Delivery strategies of amphotericin B for invasive fungal infections. *Acta Pharmaceutica Sinica B, 11*, 2585–2604.

Wang, Y. H., Zhang, J. P., Chang, Y., & Hu, C. Q., (2010). A newly identified derivative of amphotericin B: Isolation, structure determination and primary evaluation of the activity and toxicity. *Journal of Antibiotics, 63*, 553–557.

Yu, Y. Q., Yang, X., Wu, X. F., & Fan, Y. B., (2021). Enhancing permeation of drug molecules across the skin via delivery in nanocarriers: Novel strategies for effective transdermal applications. *Frontiers in Bioengineering and Biotechnology, 9*, 646554.

Zeb, A., Qureshi, O. S., Kim, H. S., Cha, J. H., Kim, H. S., & Kim, J. K., (2016). Improved skin permeation of methotrexate via nanosized ultradeformable liposomes. *International Journal of Nanomedicine, 11*, 3813–3824.

Zhang, K., Chen, M., Scriba, G. K. E., Abraham, M. H., Fahr, A., & Liu, X., (2012). Human skin permeation of neutral species and ionic species: Extended linear free-energy relationship analyses. *Journal of Pharmaceutical Sciences, 101*, 2034–2044.

Zhou, H., Luo, D., Chen, D., Tan, X., Bai, X., Liu, Z., Yang, X., & Liu, W., (2021). Current advances of nanocarrier technology-based active cosmetic ingredients for beauty applications. *Clinical, Cosmetic and Investigational Dermatology, 14*, 867–887.

PART II

Novel Nanocarriers for Skin Delivery and Disease

CHAPTER 4

Nanocarriers to Skin Inflammatory Diseases

MANISH GUPTA,[1] HEMANT K. S. YADAV,[1] PRIYA SEN,[1]
GAURAV GUPTA,[1,2,3] ABHAY RAIZADAY,[1] SANTOSH KUMAR SINGH,[1] and AFRASIM MOIN[4]

[1]*School of Pharmacy, Suresh Gyan Vihar University, Jagatpura, Jaipur, Rajasthan, India*

[2]*Department of Pharmacology, Saveetha Dental College, Saveetha Institute of Medical and Technical Sciences, Saveetha University, Chennai, Tamil Nadu, India*

[3]*Uttaranchal Institute of Pharmaceutical Sciences, Uttaranchal University, Dehradun, Uttarakhand, India*

[4]*University of Hail, Saudi Arabia*

ABSTRACT

Nanocarriers for cutaneous drug delivery are interesting area of research because they allow treatments to pass through the skin, which is a highly complicated biological barrier. Skin is the primary interface between the body and the environment. This chapter reviews common inflammatory diseases like dermatitis (atopic dermatitis (AD), seborrheic dermatitis and contact dermatitis), psoriasis, and pruritus. This chapter discusses about the various types of carriers used in skin inflammatory diseases, including polymeric nanocarriers, lipidic nanocarriers, metallic nanocarriers such as gold and silver, and non-metallic nanocarriers such as carbon and graphite. Different methods of preparation of gold nanocarriers are discussed in this

Novel Nanocarriers forSkin Diseases: Advances and Applications.
Raj K. Keservani and Júlia Scherer Santos (Eds.)

chapter like Turkevich method, the Brust method, seeded growth method, synthesis of sliver nanocarriers by using electrochemical method. Advantages of nanocarriers and applications of nanocarriers in drug delivery are discussed. Future aspects of nanocarriers in health care are discussed.

4.1 INTRODUCTION

Nanotechnology may have its roots in the 1950s, when scientist Richard Feynman advocated creating machines that could make compact copies of themselves. At some point, it was discovered that material possessed distinct properties at the nanoscale. Nanoparticles have a greater ability to enter the skins compared to their bulk counterparts related to a variety of factors, such as size and purposeful engineering. Nanotechnology is expected to be the fastest expanding sector for skin care maintenance, and the detection and treatment of skin disease. Nanotechnology (Keservani et al., 2017, 2017a) is a rapidly developing new technique in which the size of a material particle is diminished to that of a single molecule or its aggregates. Nanomedicine is defined as the use of man-made molecular nanodevices and nanostructures for monitoring, repairing, constructing, and controlling human biological systems. It includes topics like nanoparticle medication delivery and molecular nanotechnology and nanovaccinology's potential future applications. Nanoparticle manufacturing technologies have produced a flourishing sector that still needs to be explored and refined. It necessitates near-atom smashing technology, it involves striking large metal marbles of zinc, titanium, or iron at near supersonic speeds to generate tiny metal particles of the required size, homogeneity, and dispersion. It is hoped that these nanoparticles will be effective, targeted, and adaptable therapy alternatives. Nanotechnology-enabled devices and medications are said to be more customizable, adaptable, and can be cost-effective.

Nanostructured carriers (Keservani et al., 2018) are replacing traditional formulations as a preferred route of medicine administration. Targeted drug delivery system (DDS), prolonged release, low toxicity, and protection of labile groups against degradation, and these colloidal particles system with diameters ranging from 0.01 μm to 1 μm have many advantages, including medication adherence to the skin (Keservani et al., 2020a). Drug-delivery nanoparticles (Baig et al., 2018) include nanovesicles, nanospheres, nanocapsules (Sharma et al., 2018), dendrimers (Gautam et al., 2015) and lipidic nanoparticles, metallic nanoparticles, and non-metallic nanoparticles. Zinc oxide (ZnO) particles that are normally opaque and greasy disappear when they are converted to nanoparticles. They also have a pleasant feel. Nanoscale emulsions are less oily, have a superior texture, and penetrate skin and hair more thoroughly when used in emollients and hair conditioners. Stiffness, hydrophobicity, size, and charge are all factors that play into the skin permeation process (Gupta et al., 2013). Nanoparticles are used in medicine as medication carriers. A wide range of materials can be used to make nanocarriers (Keservani et al., 2018, 2019). They can also be used to release medications in a regulated manner. They can target sites of inflammation and provide a therapeutic impact when administered into the human body (Li et al., 2014). Nanocarriers can be engineered to degrade over time and pass through the body via urine or feces (Alexandre et al., 2012).

Largest organ in the human body is skin, performing a wide range of function such as maintaining body temperature, reducing fluid and salt loss, and preventing pathogens such as viruses, bacteria, allergies, and harmful substances from penetrating the body. Several contagious pathogens or inflammatory conditions can cause skin disorders, providing significant issues. Fungal infection, psoriasis, eczema, and allergic contact dermatitis (ACD) are all chronic inflammatory skin disorders characterized by inflammatory T Lymphocytes infiltrating the skin (Sigmundsdottir, 2010).

It also protects against UV light and particulate matter in the outside environment, in addition to serve as a protective border (Jain et al., 2017).

Skin has three layers:

1. **Epidermis:** The epidermis is responsible for our skin color and act as an impermeable barrier. Calcified tissue, hair follicles, and sweat glands are all situated under the epidermis layer.
2. **Hypodermis:** The hypodermis skin layer is made up of fat and connective tissues.
3. **Melanocytes:** These are present in the epidermal layer, are responsible for skin color and produce the pigment melanin.

The Outermost layer (15,000–20,000 nm) of the epidermis is stratum corneum (SC), they act like barrier function of skin. This layer's structure reflects the original skin permeation resistance, which restricts the passage of molecules larger than 500 Dalton. The stratified keratinocytes arranged in layers represent the major portion of epidermis, which consists of SC cells or corneocytes embedded in a protein rich material with a lipid coated and are surrounded by a lipid matrix extracellularly (Monteiro-Riviere, 2010). The horney layer of corneocytes shields the skin's protective layer against harmful substances, microorganisms, and excessive water loss. The dermis is the greatest component of the skin and lies under the epidermis. Lymphatic vessels, sebaceous glands, elastin, hair follicles collagen and sensitive jitters has a diameter of 0.1–0.4 cm. The dermis subcaste's major function is to deliver nutritive support to the viable epidermis as well as structural strength to the skin (Borgheti-Cardoso et al., 2020).

Topical treatments for skin conditions are only as effective as their rectifiers are delivered directly to the damaged skin cells (Bos et al., 2000).

The dermis layer's primary role is to offer nutritional support for the mucosal layer and structural strength for the skin. As a result of its splendid barrier houses, the skin is generally visible as one of the most complicated and tough-to-conquer boundaries within the human frame (Zakrewsky et al., 2015). The skin is often regarded as most complicated barriers that are tough to overcome in the human body due to its extraordinary barrier qualities (Sigmundsdottir, 2010).

4.2 SKIN INFLAMMATORY DISEASES

The skin is the body's organ, made up of water, proteins, fats, and minerals which is constantly exposed to various stimuli identified by the innate immune system (Daniel et al., 2016). Inflammatory skin disease is a common skin disease that can significantly impair the quality of patient's life. Acne and vitiligo patients are primarily concerned by their psychosocial well-being, while patients with psoriasis and atopic dermatitis (AD) are affected both physically and mentally (Ahmed et al., 2013).

Skin diseases can affect 30 to 70% of the worldwide people and have a major impact on their individual person life. It affects persons of all ages, ranging from three-month-old babies to the elderly. Skin illnesses have several origins, including hereditary, inflammatory, and environmental factors, making them difficult to treat despite improvements in dermatology. Fungal skin disease and acne are one of the most common disorders globally, according to 2010 research, with eczema and psoriasis rounds out the top list. Furthermore, skin diseases have been ranked as the 4th major source of non-lethal disease impact (Pradhan et al., 2013).

4.2.1 PSORIASIS

Psoriasis is a persistent papulo cutaneous skin condition that affects people of all ages and causes in both men and women. It is related with depressive symptoms, psoriatic arthritis, and cardiometabolic syndrome, among many other things (Leung et al., 2014).

To treat mild psoriasis, topical medications such as coal tar, vitamin D, retinoids, and topical calcineurin inhibitors are more significant than systemic medications such as methotrexate, cyclosporine, acitretin, hydroxyurea, and laser treatment (Christopher et al., 2021).

4.2.2 DERMATITIS

Dermatitis is a broad term that refers a wide range of skin irritations. It could be caused by number of factors, but the most common are itching, dry skin and rashes. Blisters, oozing, crusting, and flaking of the skin are some common side effects. There are basically three types of dermatitis, which are:

- Atopic dermatitis (eczema);
- Seborrheic dermatitis; and
- Contact dermatitis.

4.2.2.1 ATOPIC DERMATITIS (AD)

Eczema, often known as atopic dermatitis (AD), is a skin condition that may affect both children and adults (Ashlesha et al., 2013). AD is a type of inflammatory skin condition that lasts for years. It frequently occurs before the onset of food allergies and asthma. Recently discovered anomalies in the final differentiation of the epidermal epithelium have been linked to a tropic dermatitis, resulting in defects in the stratum corneum (SC), allowing penetration of allergens and enhanced IgE sensitization. Pathogenic bacteria, especially Staphylococcus aureus and the herpes simplex virus, are more likely to colonized or infect atopic skin. In addition to genetic, environmental, and immunological determinants, the impact of this defective skin barrier is complex (Rebecca et al., 2012). Although topical medications such as ointments and lotions can help manage the symptoms of AD, there is no specific treatment for the condition. AD is characterized by severe itching, which can cause sufferers to have restless nights, worry, and despair. As a result, AD treatment should focus on minimizing the itch-scratch cycle's pruritus and skin inflammation. Emollients and anti-inflammatory corticosteroids are frequently prescribed to individuals suffering from AD, and TCIs such betamethasone valerate and tacrolimus are also often used (Leung et al., 2000).

4.2.2.2 SEBORRHEIC DERMATITIS

The term "seborrheic dermatitis" refers to an oily skin irritation. Face, scalp, and chest are the most general areas for seborrheic dermatitis. Infantile seborrheic dermatitis, sometimes known as diaper rash, is closely related to it. Patients affected with Parkinson's disease or may be of HIV/AIDS are particularly prone to seborrheic dermatitis (Gupta et al., 2004). Recent evidence suggests that *Malassezia* (previously known as Pityrosporum, family Malasseziaceae) and seborrheic dermatitis are linked.

This is due to the fact that antifungals have been demonstrated to be useful in the treatment of SD, and improvement in Seborrheic Dermatitis is associated by a decrease in *Malassezia* levels (Gupta et al., 2004).

Traditionally, keratolytic drugs or corticosteroids were used to treat seborrheic dermatitis (Gupta et al., 2003). Other traditional dose forms for the treatment of scalp seborrheic dermatitis include OTC (over-the-counter) preparations such as coal tar shampoo, tree tea oil shampoo, and so on. Topical antifungal shampoos, such as 1% of Ciclopirox shampoo and 2% of ketoconazole shampoo, and topical corticosteroids, such as 0.12% of Betamethasone Valerate foam and 0.01% of Flucinolone shampoo.

Topical antifungals, such as 0.77% of Ciclopirox gel or cream, 2% of Sertaconazolecream, and others, are used to treat facial and body seborrheic dermatitis in adults. Topical calcineurin inhibitors such as 1% of Pimecrolimuscream and topical corticosteroids such as 0.05% of Desonidecream, 0.01% of Fluocinolone cream, and others are available (Gary et al., 2015).

4.2.2.3 CONTACT DERMATITIS

Inflammatory contact dermatitis is characterized by redness and itchiness on the affected skin following contact with an irritating substance. Irritating contact dermatitis and ACD are the two main forms of contact dermatitis that may occur in people.

Irritant contact dermatitis is characterized by a substance that is not immune-modulate and inducing skin changes (Richard et al., 2010).

ACD is a well-known case of cutaneous hypersensitivity mediated by cells. This happens when xenobiotic substances penetrate the skin and react chemically with self-proteins, triggering a hapten-specific immune response (Gober et al., 2008).

The introduction of corticosteroids transformed in the cure of contact dermatitis and eczematous skin condition in the 1950. Corticosteroids are listed in order of potency for example (Cohen et al., 2004):

- **Super-Potent (Class I):** Clobetasol propionate, halobetasol propionate.
- **Potent (Class II):** Fluocinonide, halcinonide.
- **Upper Mid-Strength (Class III):** Mometasone furoate.
- **Mid-Strength (Class IV):** Desoximetasone.
- **Lower Mid-Strength (Class V):** Hydrocortisone butyrate.
- **Mild (Class VI):** Desonide.
- **Least Potent (Class VII):** Hydrocortisone, dexamethasone.

4.2.3 PRURITUS

Systemic inflammatory skin disorders, illness, neurological problems, and psychogenic disorders can all produce chronic pruritus disorder (itching that lasts longer than 1 month). On a person with unexplained pruritus, a complete blood test and differentiated count, a lung radiograph, and diagnostics of hepatic, kidney, and hypothyroidism should all be conducted. Patients with unidentified itch should be examined on a regular basis. The use of moderate cleansers, emollients, local anesthetics, and cooling agents may help when treating symptoms for the first time. Antihistamines with sedative effects are generally prescribed to patients to aid with sleep. Chronic itching may be alleviated with the use of anticonvulsants, antidepressants, and opioid antagonists (Gil Yosipovitch et al., 2013).

Due to inaccurate drug delivery, traditional approaches to addressing various skin problems demonstrate a lack of efficacy, extended treatment times, recurrence of conditions, systemic adverse effects, or other issues. These drawbacks can be avoided by employing nanomedicine-based techniques that deliver effective site-specific medication delivery to the target site. There is a lot of interest in nanocarriers, such as polymeric and lipidic, and creating new ones like carbon nanotubes (CNTs) for dermatological treatment, in nanocarriers, these nanomedicine-based techniques are developed as prospective therapeutic possibilities (Arya et al., 2020).

4.3 NANOCARRIERS AND THEIR TYPES

Because of their distinct properties, such as the ability to defend therapeutic effects, targeted DDS, because of their high bioavailability, flexibility in adjusting the release profile of active medicines, and customizable surface features, nanoparticles have been widely researched as improved DDSs. Nanoparticles have also been shown to improve drug penetration and permeation through the skin in a number of research. Nanocarriers are an excellent approach for overcoming the restricted skin penetration of unbound medicinal molecules. Their interaction with skin components may be modified to enhance penetration, opening up a wide range of therapeutic possibilities (Fitsum et al., 2017). The selection of drug carrier vehicle is critical for improving the effectiveness and safety of topical therapy. As a result, researchers have concentrated on various formulation techniques to improve medication absorption while lowering undesired side effects while maintaining medicinal efficacy (Jijie et al., 2009).

In addition to the skin's cellular architecture, nanocarriers transport processes must be recognized. Passive diffusion of active substances through the skin occurs predominantly via three pathways: intercellular, transcellular, and follicular. The diffusion process and hence the path of penetration are influenced by physicochemical properties such as the penetrating molecule's molecular weight, solubility, and lipophilicity. The intracellular route is the quickest and direct route for chemical substance to penetrate in the skin; yet it is difficult since the particle must overcome both lipophilic and lipophobicstructures within the skin cells (Schneider et al., 2009). High-affinity amphiphilic nanocarriers may be an effective solution to this issue. When a penetrating particle diffuses across cells to penetrate the SC, this is the most common mode of penetration Particle size and mechanical properties must be taken into account while using this method, since they must be able to bend in the right way (Schneider et al., 2019). The follicular pathway is the most commonly reported method for rigid particles to penetrate the skin. The direct administration of medications through hair follicles and glandular ducts is referred to as this route. As it is, just 0.1 to 0.01% of the skin's surface area is occupied by hair follicles and glandular ducts, respectively, this pathway is severely constrained (Scheuplein, 1967).

4.3.1 POLYMERIC NANOPARTICLES

Small particles diameter in the range of 0.001 μm to 1 μm that can be filled with active chemicals or surface-adsorbed onto the polymeric core are also known as polymeric nanoparticles (NPs). Polymeric NPs have shown a lot of promise in terms of delivering drugs to particular regions for the treatment of diseases (Rancan et al., 2019). Polymeric nanoparticles are classified into nanocapsules, nanosphere, etc.

4.3.1.1 NANOSPHERES AND NANOCAPSULES

Rather of being enclosed inside a polymeric membrane, the medicine is spread throughout the polymer matrix in the form of nanospheres, a polymeric nanoparticle. In the manufacturing of nanoparticles, natural polymers such as gelatin, albumin, and alginate are employed. Synthetic polymers are employed in the production of nanoparticles. Synthetic polymers in the form of premade polymer can be utilized to produce nanoparticles, e.g., polycarpolactone and other polyesters (Maincent et al., 1992).

4.3.1.2 POLYMERIC MICELLES

Polymeric micelles are the amphiphilic polymers that are produced from nanoscopic supramolecular core shell. These are mainly smaller than 0.1 μm in size, and their hydrophilic surface shields them from nonspecific reticuloendothelial absorption. Micelles are spherical aggregates formed in solutions by organizing the component molecules in a spherical shape with a hydrophobic core and a mantle of hydrophilic groups protecting it from water. These are used to transport water-insoluble medications throughout the body. Drugs can be physically confined within the hydrophobic cores or covalently bond attached to micelle component molecules. These have a large loading capacity, are stable under physiological settings, have a slower rate of dissolution, have a high concentration of drug at the target site, and can be functionalized to conjugate targeting ligands (Ferrari et al., 2005). Hydrogels with dexamethasone as the active ingredient, for example, have showed promise in controlled drug delivery for psoriasis treatment (Gupta et al., 2013).

4.3.2 LIPIDIC NANOPARTICLES

Lipid nano-dispersions were originally designed for parenteral administration. Preparations for I.V. injection are the most difficult in terms of system physical stability and patient acceptability because this administration route necessitates full regulation of the dispersion's particle size.

Aside from developing lipid carriers for intravenous route dosage, these systems have piqued attention for obtaining sustained drug release systems targeting brain and liver. Hence, lipid nanoparticles have been shown to be useful for distribution of drugs to the skin (Schaferkorting et al., 2007).

4.3.2.1 LIPOSOMES

Liposomes are composed of spherical synthetic vesicles consist of cholesterol and non-toxic phospholipids. Because of their size, water-repelling (hydrophobic) and water-attracting (hydrophilic), liposomes are desirable drug delivery vehicles (along with biocompatibility; Abolfazl et al., 2013).

4.3.3 METALLIC NANOPARTICLES

Metallic nanoparticles technology has a better track record as medication and biosensor carriers. Nanoparticles of different metals have been created, but silver and gold nanoparticles (AuNPs) are the most important for biomedical applications. A vast range of ligands, including as sugar, peptides, proteins, and DNA, have been coupled to nanoparticles. These nanoparticles feature surface functionalization, making it simple to coat them with ligands. These are employed for active distribution of bioactives, drug discovery, bioassays, detection, imaging, and a variety of other applications due to their functionalization ability (Manivannan et al., 2011).

There are several methods for making metallic nanoparticles, which can be split into two groups: Approaches from the bottom up and top-down (Jamkhande et al., 2019).

4.3.3.1 TOP-DOWN METHODS

This procedure reduces big materials to nano-sized particles. Nanoparticles are made by decreasing the size of the starting material using a variety of physical and chemical techniques (Meyers et al., 2006).

4.3.3.1.1 Mechanical Milling

1. **Ball Milling:** John Benjamin invented this particle size reduction technology in 1970. Ball milling is a potent non-equilibrium processing technology that may produce fine micro-structured dispersion reinforced alloys as well as metastable structured materials.

Mechanical milling is based on the use of high-energy ball milling to minimize particle size. Process factors and milling powder characteristics impact mechanical milling (Mahbub Ulla et al., 2014). Low energy milling and high energy milling are the two varieties depending on the amount of induced mechanical energy delivered to the powder combination. High-energy ball milling is commonly used to generate nanosized particles. This approach is commonly used to make intermetallic nanoparticles.

Bulk powder is combined with multiple hefty balls in this process. A high-speed spinning ball is used to apply high mechanical energy to bulk powder material. Size of particles can be reduced using a variety of high-energy mills, including attrition ball mills, planetary ball mills, and high-energy ball mills (Rajput, 2015), i.e., Maincent (1992) proposed the relationship as a model for grain size reduction during high energy ball milling.

$$D = kt^{2/3}$$

where; 'D' stands for grain diameter; 't' for milling time; and 'k' for constant. This concept was based on the idea that particle size decrease was caused by the creation of shear bands (Meyers et al., 2006).

2. **Mechanochemical Synthesis:** This process works by repeatedly deforming, welding, and fracturing a reactant mixture. Various chemical changes occur at the interface of nano-sized particles during the milling process. The components (such as sodium carbonate and chloride hexahydrate for Fe_3O_2 nanoparticles synthesis) are blended stoichiometrically and milled in the mechanochemical technique of synthesis. The reactants are deformed, fractionated, and welded during the milling process. At the surface interface between the substrate and the reagent, several chemical reactions occur, and reactions that require an elevated temperature would happen at a low temperature without the use of external heat. During the process, a number of displacement reactions occur, as shown below.

$$SxC + yR = xS + RyC$$

where; SxC and yR are reactants; whereas xS is a product; and RyC is a byproduct.

The leftover material is spread in a soluble salt matrix and surrounds the nanoparticles that have been manufactured. After that, the product is removed by washing the particles with a suitable solvent and drying them for 12 hours at 105°C (Jamkhande et al., 2019).

4.3.4 GOLD NANOPARTICLES (AUNPS)

Colloids and surfaces have gained a new subdiscipline in the physics and chemistry of gold nanocarriers. Nanoparticles of gold with unusual optical properties, size-dependent electrochemistry, and high chemical stability have become the new system of choice for a wide range of applications, such as self-assembly, biolabeling, catalysis, electron-transfer theories, phase transfer, DNA melting and assays, and crystal growth, among others. This review focuses on AuNPs, especially those at the very small end of the nanoparticle scale.

Although AuNPs have been employed for a variety of applications, their catalytic activities have been thought to be weak or non-existent for decades. In the heterogeneous low-temperature oxidation of carbon monoxide, Haruta & Hutchings found that gold might be quite active. When put on a metal oxide substrate, such as ferric oxide, AuNPs were shown to be very effective carbon monoxide oxidation catalysts. A novel form of composite oxide catalyst was first blamed for the high activity, but an analysis using electron microscopy revealed that the most active catalysts were tiny gold nanocarriers with a radius of between 2 and 200 nanometers (nm) (Nadagouda et al., 2011).

4.3.4.1 SYNTHESIS OF GOLD NANOPARTICLES (AUNPS)

4.3.4.1.1 Turkevich Method

Turkevich presented his method in 1951. In the 10–20 nm size range, it is one of the most extensively used techniques for creating round AuNPs. For this method to work, gold ions (Au^{3+}) must be reduced to gold atoms (Au0) using catalysts such as citrate, amino acids, ascorbic acid or ultraviolet (UV) light. The Turkevich technique was first restricted by the small number of AuNPs it could generated. In 1973, Frens discovered that by altering the reducing to stabilizing agent ratio, AuNPs of various diameters ranging from 0.016 μm to 0.147 μm could be generated. After a greater understanding of the functions of pH, temperature, and sodium citrate concentration, a particle growth model was established.

4.3.4.1.2 Brust Method

In 1994, the Brust technique was originally described. Using organic solvents and changing the thiol to gold ratio, this approach generates 1.5 nm–5.2 nm AuNPs in a two-phase procedure. Faraday's 2 phase system influenced the Brust technique. A phase transfer agent is used to convert gold salt from an aqueous solution to an organic solvent (e.g., tetraoctylammonium bromide TOAB, toluene). Sodium borohydride is used to decrease the gold in the presence of an alkanethiol after it has been reduced. The alkanethiols stabilize the AuNPs, causing the reaction to shift color from orange to brown. The Schriffin Seeding Growth Method was used to purify AuNPs stabilized with dodecanethiol from TOAB.

4.3.4.1.3 Seeded Growth Method

Gold salts are reduced using a powerful reducing agent, such as sodium borohydride, to form seed particles in this method. Ascorbic acid and a structure-directing agent are added to the metal salt in order to inhibit additional nucleation and to speed up the anisotropy of AuNPs' anisotropy. It is possible to alter the structure of gold nanostructures by altering the concentration of seeds, reducing agents, and structure-directing agents (Monic Shah et al., 2014).

4.3.5 SILVER NANOPARTICLES (AGNPS)

Various sectors, including healthcare, food industry, and consumer products, employ silver nanoparticles (AgNPs) because of their unique physical and chemical characteristics. Optical, electrical, and thermal characteristics, as well as high electrical conductivity and metabolic capacities, are all present. They've been used as antimicrobial agents, in manufacturing, domestic, and healthcare products, consumer goods, medical equipment, surface coating, optical sensors, and cosmetics, as well as in pharmaceuticals, food, diagnostics (Keservani et al., 2016), orthopedics, drug delivery, and antitumor, with the result that the tumor-killing effects of anticancer drugs have been improved drug (Jarouliya et al., 2018; Sardar et al., 2009).

In a variety of applications, silver (Ag) and Ag-based compounds have been widely used to limit bacterial growth. Ag-based compounds, on the other hand, progressively precipitate in solutions and agglomerate and precipitate in emulsions. Because Ag's antibacterial properties are impaired when it is physically isolated from cosmetic components, these occurrences significantly limit its usage as a cosmetic preservative. The usage of Ag nanoparticles can solve a lot of these issues. Reducing particle size also enhances biocompatibility, which has led to a greater focus on nanotechnology's medicinal uses (Xi-Feng et al., 2016).

4.3.5.1 SYNTHESIS FOR SILVER NANOPARTICLES (AGNPS)

4.3.5.1.1 Electrochemical Method

The anode and cathode of this low-cost electrode configuration are made out of bulk silver metal, which will be transformed into colloidal silver particles during the process. Using two polished silver plates, the anode and cathode were vertically positioned 0.01 nm apart. In an electrochemical cell, the electrodes were submerged in 500 mL of distilled water generated using a typical water distiller. During the electrolysis process, the temperature ranged from 20°C to 95°C and the voltage was maintained at 20 V. AgNPs may be synthesized electrochemically if the electrodes' polarity is changed every 30–300s and the electrolysis process is constantly stirred to avoid precipitation. At room temperature, the glass containers containing the silver nanoparticle solutions were used to keep them. Nanoparticle concentrations in liquids were determined using a neutron activation analysis. The nuclear reactor was used to irradiate the samples. For 109Ag (n,c) 110 mAg the half-life of the by-product is 253 days. The gamma radiation intensity emitted by 110 mAg at energies of 0.657 MeV and 0.884 MeV was used to compute the silver content. This was done using a Ge (Li) detector with an energy resolution of 1.33 MeV and an analyzer with 6,144 channels. With the help of DLS experiments performed at 25°C, it was possible to determine the size distribution of AgNPs. Yield emission scanning electron microscopy was used to examine silver powder that was formed on the cathode during the electrochemical process. The size and shape of the nanoparticles in solution were determined using transmission electron microscopy (TEM). An EDS linked with the TEM was utilized to determine the chemical composition of the material. Nanoparticle sizes of greater than 150 nanometers were standardized across many TEM micrographs of the same specimen. This sample's TEM micrographs were used to calculate the average size of more than 150 different nanoparticles. Nanoparticles in aqueous solutions were examined using an AFM in contact mode and mica surfaces as substrates (Kokura et al., 2010).

4.3.6 NON-METALLIC NANOPARTICLES

4.3.6.1 CARBON NANOPARTICLES

In addition to their unique properties, CNTs are also very versatile. Since they have so many unique properties, sensors, actuators, and composites may all benefit from them. Hexagonal carbon networks, 1–100 meters in length, with an average radius of around 0.5 nanometers like a sheet of graphite wound up tightly. There are two fundamental types of nanotubes, SWNTs and MWNTs, which differ in the arrangement of graphene cylinders in their cores. MWNTs have multiple or various layers of graphene cylinders, whereas SWNTs have only one graphene layer (Rashid et al., 2009).

4.3.6.1.1 Synthesis of Carbon Nanoparticles

High-temperature preparation methods such as arc discharge or laser ablation were first used to make CNTs, but low-temperature chemical vapor deposition (CVD) methods (800°C), which allow precise control of CNT orientation, alignment, nanotube length, radius, purity, and size distribution have since taken their place (Sinha et al., 2005). Almost all of these methods need the use of a carrier gas and a vacuum to perform. For applications that need large quantities of nanotubes and industrial-scale production techniques, the gas phase approaches are preferable since they are volumetric. This method's catalytic efficiency is poor due to the short catalyst life and low catalyst number density that result in just a small quantity of catalyst producing nanotubes during gas-phase synthesis (Eatemadi et al., 2014).

CNTs, as well as other carbonaceous particles such as nanocrystalline graphite, amorphous carbon, fullerenes, and other metals (usually Fe, Co, Mo, or Ni) used as catalysts throughout the synthesis, are only negligible amounts in the powders produced by this approach. CNTs are challenging to characterize and use because of the presence of all of these pollutants. For this reason, establishing simple and efficient purification methods is a major challenge in carbon nanotube research. The most popular technique for removing impurities from CNTs is acid treatment.

1. **Plasma-based Synthesis Method or Arc Discharge Evaporation Method:** Arc discharge methods use greater temperatures (above 1,700°C) for carbon nanotube synthesis than other methods, which usually leads in the creation of CNTs with fewer structural defects. The electric arc method, which was first used to generate C_{60} fullerenes, is the most common and arguably easiest method for producing CNTs. In 1991, Iijima used the arc-discharge evaporation technique to find MWCNTs. After that, SWCNTs were developed in 1993 (Jan et al., 2011). An electric arc is created by using two graphite electrodes in this technique, resulting in a high temperature to sublimate carbon. Multi-walled carbon nanotubes (MWCNTs) or single walled carbon nanotubes (SWCNTs) can develop when carbon vapor cools and condenses.

   MWCNTs is generated when no catalyst particles are present between two graphite electrodes, but SWCNTs are formed when Fe, Ni, or Co are used as catalysts. Metal powder can be packed into a hole in the anode to inject catalysts. Along with the graphite, the metal was consumed, resulting in catalyst particles that favored small-diameter SWCNTs (Bethune et al., 1993). The gas pressure in the reaction chamber had a significant impact on the purity and yield of MWCNTs. The final shape of CNTs is greatly influenced by the environment. In helium and methane, they used DC arc discharge of graphite electrodes. Evaporation of methane gas under high pressure and a strong arc current resulted in the formation of thick nanotubes adorned with many carbon nanoparticles. For the anode, a methane gas pressure of 50 Torr and a current of 20 A resulted in 6 mm-diameter MWNTs (Jie et al., 2010). During the evaporation of methane gas, the form of CNTs fluctuated more than in helium gas (Dubrovsky et al., 2003). The formation of SWNTs is possible when a transition metal catalyst is used. A composite anode in a hydrogen or argon environment is used to develop SWNTs in an arc discharge. Co-Ni, Fe-Ni, Fe-No or Co-Cu-Cu-Cu-Cu, Ni-Cu-Cu, Ni-Ti, and so on are examples of anodes consisting of graphite and a metal, such as Ni, Fe, and other elements. It is the metal catalyst that has the most impact on the final product yield. It is essential that the gap distance between the electrodes remain consistent in order to keep the current density and anode consumption rates stable. Unwanted chemicals, such as MWNTs or fullerenes, are often created during this process (Prasek et al., 2011).

2. **Laser Ablation Method:** The laser ablation techniques, graphite target is vaporized in a pressure-controlled oven using helium or argon gas. In that both take advantage of the high temperature created either by laser ablation and utilize the same background gas and catalyst mix, the laser ablation is similar to the arc discharge. The extremely similar reaction circumstances require that the reactions in both laser ablation and electric arc operations are most likely mediated by the same mechanism (Koziol et al., 2010). Without introducing additional heat to the target, SWNTs were made using continuous wave carbon dioxide (CO_2) laser ablation, and it was discovered that the average diameter of SWNTs produced by CO_2 laser rose as laser power increased (Sarangdevot et al., 2015).
3. **Thermal Synthesis Process:** Plasma-based synthesis is based on arc discharge and laser ablation method. Only thermal energy is necessary in thermal synthesis, and the reaction hot zone never reaches 1,200°C. Even in the case of plasma accelerated CVD. In almost all cases, carbon feedstock creates CNTs in the presence of active catalytic species like Fe, Ni, and Co; promoters like Mo and Ru are sometimes added to make the feedstock more active for CNT formation. Thermal synthesis, in fact, is a broad term that refers to a number of CVD processes. The processes of CVD, carbon monoxide synthesis, and flame synthesis are all explained (Golnabi, 2012).
4. **Chemical Vapor Deposition (CVD):** The transition metal catalyst, such as iron, nickel, or cobalt, lowers the temperature required to "break" a gaseous hydrocarbon input into carbon and hydrogen. Coatings, powders, fibers, and monolithic components may all be made using CVD, which is a versatile process. Carbon and silicon may be synthesized into a wide number of different compounds, including carbides, nitrides, oxides, intermetallics, and many more via CVD. A wide range of optical, optoelectronic, and corrosion applications make use of this technology, in addition to its employment in the manufacture of semiconductors and many other electronic components.

A chemical reaction in the vapor phase results in the deposition of a solid on a heated surface, which is known as CVD. It is a type of vapor-transfer method (Varshney, 2014).

To make the CNT samples, researchers used a reactor that included a quartz tube with a diameter of 50 mm, another with a diameter of 40 mm, and an overall length of 1,500 mm. The catalyst ferrocene was placed in a ceramic boat within the central ceramic tube of the first furnace. During the second furnace, CNTs developed and were gathered in ceramic boats in the center of the furnace, which were placed there. The system was initially flushed with Ar to create an oxygen-free atmosphere. In the meanwhile, the second furnace was heated to the required temperature for the reaction. The temperature was maintained at a steady level by keeping the heater on. This process was repeated until the temperature reached 150°C, after which the flow of Ar was switched off. There was an immediate shutdown of the H_2 and C_2H_2 gas lines. There was a time period necessary for this reaction to take place, and it did so. CNT was recovered and weighed separately in the ceramic boats and on the inner walls of the second furnace (Mubarak et al., 2014).

4.4 ADVANTAGES OF NANOCARRIERS

- They are quite stable and have a nanomolar affinity towards antigen.
- They have a high selectivity to their target and a low intrinsic toxicity.
- They combine the features of classical antibodies with the key characteristics of small-molecule medicines.
- They can approach to therapeutic targets that are difficult to detect with conventional antibodies (e.g., active sites of enzymes).
- Apart from intravenous administration, they can be given orally.
- They can be mass-produced at a reasonable cost.
- Their immunostimulatory potential is extremely low.
- They have the ability to penetrate the human blood-brain-barrier to trigger the specific site in the brain.
- Identifying, defining, and characterization of model nanomaterials.
- Measuring and maintaining the level of exposure.
- Analyzing the environment's effect.
- Working on developing a biocompatible hybrid system (Jain, 2005).

4.5 APPLICATION IN DRUG DELIVERY

4.5.1 NANOMATERIALS FOR TISSUE ENGINEERING

Nanoparticles can be used in different types of nanomaterials like tissue healing and replacement, tissue regeneration, implant coatings, structural implant materials, bone healing, bio-resorbable materials, implantable devices (sensory aids, retina implants), and surgical aids (Khambete et al., 2016).

4.5.2 *SITE SPECIFIC DRUG DELIVERY*

For both passive and active medication absorption, liposomes, polymeric micelles, dendrimers (Gautam et al., 2015), iron oxide, and proteins are utilized. The EPR effect of nanoparticles, which takes advantage of nanocarriers and the tumor's leaky vasculature, is used to passively administer drugs to tumors. The site specificity was increased by covalently attaching or adsorbing site-specific ligands to the surface. Drug absorption, dosage frequency, and non-adherence in TB treatment are all improved by active distribution to lung cells (Manivannan et al., 2011).

4.5.3 *IMPLANTABLE DELIVERY SYSTEMS*

Because of their size, regulated and essentially zero order kinetics, nanoparticles can operate as delivery devices; otherwise, as compared to I.V. administration, they may induce toxicity. Liposomes, ethosomes (ETOs), and transferosomes are the different types of carriers. These help to lower the risk of adverse events by limiting peak plasma levels, allowing for more predictable and long-term durations of action, reducing the need for re-dosing, and increasing patient acceptance and compliance (Jain et al., 2002).

4.5.4 *USED AS DIAGNOSTICS AGENT*

In diagnostics (Keservani et al., 2016), AuNPs are the most widely employed nanomaterial. They're also utilized as a connection in the construction of biosensors that detect disease DNA. This approach is substantially more accurate and precise than the fluorescent-molecule assays because several copies of the antibodies and DNA can be coupled to a single nanoparticle. Other advantages of this method include the ease with which gold particles can be synthesized, their low toxicity, and their ability to rapidly connect to molecules of biological relevance (Jain, 2005).

4.5.5 *NANOPARTICLES TO TREAT VARIOUS DISEASES*

Inflammatory disorders are being diagnosed, prevented, and cured using nanotechnology. Developments are being made in the treatment of HIV, hepatitis, and tuberculosis infections, and also in the treatment of melanoma.

4.5.6 NANOPARTICLES IN THE TREATMENT OF INFLAMMATORY DISORDERS

The therapy of bone inflammation is developing because of nanotechnology. Metal nanoparticles provide osteoblasts cells a suitable surface to adhere to the bone. These metallic nanoparticles allow osteoblasts (bone synthesizing cells) to proliferate over a set period of time, allowing for more successful osteo-regeneration. Because of its corrosion resistance and strong biocompatibility, titanium (Ti) is a generally utilized nanomaterial in orthopedics.

Nanotechnology is helping to break down barriers in the treatment of skin infections. Nanomaterials are designed to release therapeutic medicament over time while not repairing any affected skin after the drug has been released. UV radiation is another well-known factor to skin irritation. The SC, or outermost layer of the skin, protects the body from UV rays. Sunscreens are an excellent illustration of how consumers employ nanoparticles to protect themselves from UV radiation. Sunscreen nanoparticles made of ZnO and titanium dioxide (TiO_2) are the most popular. ZnO and TiO_2 nanoparticles absorbed damaging UVA and UVB rays and reflected both heat and visible light back to the atmosphere. By absorption, reflection, and scattering, ZnO and TiO_2 prevent UV rays from reaching living skin cells (Ufuoma et al., 2015).

4.6 MARKETED FORMULATION

- AmBisome® is a brand name of Gilead Science in which the active pharmaceutical ingredient (API) present is Amphotericin B (AmB), in which liposome nanocarriers are used to treat systemic fungal infection and it was approved by the FDA (federal drug approval) in 1997.
- Adagen® (Sigma-Tau pharmaceuticals) was approved by the FDA in 1990 to treat immunodeficiency diseases in which Pegademase Bovine is used as an API and PEGylated adenosine deaminase enzyme is acts a nanocarrier.
- Emend® (Merck) in which Aprepitant used as an API and nanocrystals act as carriers. It was approved by the FDA in 2003 for use as an anti-emetic drug.
- Vitoss® (Stryker) used in the treatment of bone substitute, which was approved by the FDA in 2003, in which Calcium Phosphate is act as an API and Nanocrystals used are as nanocarriers.

- Feridex®/Endorem® (AMAG Pharmaceuticals) was approved by the FDA in 1999 to treat chronic kidney failure in which superparamagnetic iron oxide nanoparticles (SPION) is used as an API and Dextran coated with SPION is act as nanocarriers.
- GastroMARK™ (AMAG Pharmaceuticals) in which SPION used as an API and silicon coated with SPION acts as a nanocarriers. It was approved in 2001 (2009) by the FDA for imaging materials.
- Nanothem® (MagForce) was approved by the FDA in 2010 for the treatment of brain tumors in which iron oxide is used as an API and aminosilane-coated iron nanoparticles act as nanocarriers.

4.7 FUTURE ASPECTS

Nanomedicine is recently one of the most intriguing areas of methodology. More than 1,500 patents have been issued and several clinical studies have been completed as a consequence of extensive research in this area during the last two decades. To provide a precise dose to infected cells such as cancer cells without compromising the normal cell physiology is undoubtedly the new trend in research and innovation that will continue for decades to come (Patra et al., 2018).

AD appears to be a viable target for nanotechnology-based treatments (Damini et al., 2019). Because of the smaller size of the nanocarriers, proteins are able to attach to their surface and form epitopes. NPs are mostly absorbed by cells of any size and employed as protein transporters into cells. NP aggregation occurs as a consequence of the adsorbed proteins behaving in an unexpected way, which enhances their interaction with biological fluids (Ramanunny et al., 2020). The idealistic concept of creating nanorobots (and nanodevices) that can diagnose and heal tissue with full external control has attracted a lot of curiosity. This is still a futuristic research project that humanity may be able to accomplish in the not-too-distant future. Nanomedicines' potential harm to people and the environment, as well as their potential benefits, necessitate long-term research. As a result, a detailed study of new nanomaterials' potential acute and chronic toxic effects on human beings and the environment is required (Patra et al., 2018).

4.8 CONCLUSION

Skin diseases are a category of dermatologic illnesses that cause a significant level of health and economic harm every year. The disadvantage of most commercially available topical therapies is that many of them are linked to systemic circulation side effects that impact the entire body instead of just the skin. As a result, a simple and non-invasive therapeutic strategy is required, as is the development of more target-oriented topical medicines. Novel topically based nanoaggregates for successful therapy have been developed as a result of ongoing research.

However, while several colloidal systems have been predicted to improve topical drug administration, only the most energetic systems will be able to break through the skin barrier and provide personalized pharmacokinetics. These nano-vehicles primarily adjust the flow, adjust the position and size of the drug depot, and even selectively permeabilize the SC.

Nanosystems offer a viable, adaptable platform for biocompatible, safe, and effective topical delivery of pharmaceuticals since they caused no short-term cytotoxicity or morphological alterations in the SC. Preparation of various nanocarrier metallic and non-metallic nanoparticles has shown promising results in medication delivery and in the treatment of skin inflammatory illnesses.

KEYWORDS

- **dermatitis**
- **drug delivery**
- **inflammatory diseases**
- **medication**
- **nanocarrier**
- **nanoparticle**
- **preparation method**
- **site specific drug delivery**

REFERENCES

Ahmed, A., Leon, A., Butler, D. C., & Reichenberg, J., (2013). Quality-of-life effects of common dermatological diseases. *Seminars in Cutaneous Medicine and Surgery., 32*(2), 101–109.

Akbarzadeh, A., Sadabady, R. R., Davaran, S., Sang, W. J., Zarghami, N., Samiei, M., Kouhi, M., & Koshki, K. N., (2013). Liposome: Classification, preparation, and applications. *Nanoscale Research Letter, 8*(1), 102.

Albanese, A., Tang, P. S., & Chan, W. C. W., (2012). The effect of nanoparticle size, shape, and surface chemistry on biological systems. *Annual Review of Biomedical Engineering, 14*, 1–16.

Baig, M. S., Keservani, R. K., Ahmad, M. F., & Baig, M. E., (2018). Smart delivery of nanobiomaterials in drug delivery. In: *Nanobiomaterials* (pp. 241–287). Apple Academic Press. ISBN: 9781771885911.

Berke, R. M., Singh, A., & Guralnick, G., (2012). Atopic dermatitis: An overview. *American Family Physician, 86*(1), 35–42.

Bethune, D. S., Kiang, C. H., Vries, M. S., Gorman, G., Savoy, R., Vasquez, J., et al., (1993). Cobalt-catalyzed growth of carbon nanotubes with single atomic layer walls. *Nature, 363*(6430), 605–607.

Borgheti-Cardoso, L. N., Viegas, J. S. R., Silvestrini, A. V. P., Caron, L. A., Praca, F. G., Kravicz, M., & Bentley, M. (2020). Nanotechnology approaches in the current therapy of skin cancer, *Adv. Drug Deliv. Rev., 153*, 109–136.

Bos, J. D., & Meinardi, M. M. H. M., (2000). The 500 Dalton rule for the skin penetration of chemical compounds and drugs. *Exp. Dermatol., 9*, 165–169.

Cohen, D. E., & Heidary, N., (2004). Treatment of irritant and allergic contact dermatitis. *Dermatologic Therapy, 17*(4), 334–340.

Damiani, G., Eggenhöffner, R., Pigatto, P. D. M., & Bragazzi, N. L., (2019). Nanotechnology meets atopic dermatitis: Current solutions, challenges, and future prospects. Insights and implications from a systematic review of the literature. *Bioactive Materials, 4*, 380–386.

Daniel, C. De. Sa., & Cyro, F. N., (2016). Inflammasomes and dermatology. *An. Bras Dermatol., 91*(5), 566–578.

Dubrovsky, R., & Benzmelnitsyn, V., (2003). Enhanced approach to synthesize carbon allotropes by arc plasma. *Review on Advanced Material Science, 5*, 420–424.

Eatemadi, A., Daraee, H., Karimkhanloo, H., Kouhi, M., Zarghami, N., & Akbarzadeh, A., (2014). Carbon nanotubes: Properties, synthesis, purification, and medical applications. *Nanoscale Reserach Letter, 9*(1), 1–13.

Ferrari, M., (2005). Cancer nanotechnology: Opportunities and challenges. *Nature Reviews Cancer, 5*, 161–171.

Gary, W., Clark, Pope, S. M., & Jaboori, K. A., (2015). Diagnosis and treatment of seborrheic dermatitis. *American Family Physician., 91*(3), 185–190.

Gautam, S. P., Keservani, R. K., Gautam, T., Gupta, A. K., & Sharma, A. K., (2015). An alternative approach for acetylation of amine terminated polyamidoamine (PAMAM) dendrimer. *ARS Pharmaceutica, 56(3)*, 155–159.

Gil, Y. M. D., Jeffrey, D., & Bernhard, M. D., (2013). Chronic pruritus. *New England Journal of Medicine, 368*(17), 1625–1634.

Gober, M., & Gaspari, A., (2008). Allergic contact dermatitis. *Allergic Contact Dermatitis. Dermatologic Immunity*, 1–26.

Golnabi, H., (2012). Carbon nanotube research developments in terms of published papers and patents, synthesis, and production *Scientia Iranica, 19*(6), 2012–2022.

Griffiths, C. E. M., Armstrong, A. W., Gudjonsson, J. E., & Barker, J., (2021). Psoriasis. *Lancet, 397*, 1301–1315.

Gupta, A. K., & Bluhm, R., (2004). Seborrheic dermatitis. *Journal of The European Academy of Dermatology and Vernerology, 18*, 13–26.

Gupta, A. K., Bluhm, R., Cooper, E. A., Summerbell, R., C., & Batra, R., (2003). Seborrheic dermatitis. *Dermatologic Clinics, 21*(3), 401–412.

Gupta, A. K., Madzia, S. E., & Batra, R., (2004). Etiology and management of seborrheic dermatitis. *Dermatology, 208*, 89–93.

Gupta, S., Bansal, R., Gupta, S., Jindal, N., & Jindal, A., (2013). Nanocarriers and nanoparticles for skin care and dermatological treatments. *Indian Dermatol Online Journal, 4*(4), 267–272.

Jain, K. K., (2005). The role of nanobiotechnology in drug discovery. *Drug Discovery Today, 10*(21), 1435-1442.

Jain, S., & Jain, N. K., (2002). Liposomes as drug carrier, In: Jain, N. K., (ed.), *Controlled and Novel Drug Delivery* (2nd edn., pp. 304–352) CBS publisher, New Delhi.

Jain, S., Patel, N., Shah, M. K., Khatri, P., & Vora, N., (2017). Recent advances in lipid-based vesicles and particulate carriers for topical and transdermal application. *Journal of Pharmaceutical Science, 106*, 423–445.

Jamkhande, P. G., Ghule, N. W., Bamer, A. H., & Kalaskar, M. G., (2019). Metal nanoparticles synthesis: An overview on methods of preparation, advantages and disadvantages, and applications. *Journal of Drug Delivery Science and Technology*, 101174.

Jan, P., Jana, D., Jana, C., Hubalek, J., Jasek, O., Adam, V., et al., (2011). Methods for carbon nanotubes synthesis. *J. Mater. Chem., 21,* 15872–15879.

Jarouliya, U., Kesharwani, R. K., & Kesharwani, R. K., (2018). Advances of nanotechnology in cancer therapy. In: *Nanobiomaterials* (pp. 291–328). Apple Academic Press. ISBN: 9781771885911.

Jie, M. A., Wang, J. A., Tsai, C. J., Nussino, R., & Buyong, M. A., (2010). Diameters of single walled carbon nanotubes (SWCNTs) and related nanochemistry and nanobiology. *Front. Mater. Sci. China., 4*(1), 17–28.

Jijie, R., Barras, A., Boukherroub, R., & Szunerits, S., (2017). Nanomaterials for transdermal drug delivery: Beyond the state of the art of liposomal structures. *Journal of Materials Chemistry, 5*(44), 8653–8675.

Keservani, R. K., Bandopadhyay, S., Bandyopadhyay, N., & Sharma, A. K., (2020a). Design and fabrication of transdermal/skin drug-delivery system. In: *Drug Delivery Systems* (pp. 131–178). Academic Press.

Keservani, R. K., Kesharwani, R. K., & Sharma, A. K., (2016). Nanobiomaterials involved in medical imaging technologies. In: *Nanobiomaterials in Medical Imaging* (pp. 303–337). William Andrew Publishing. ISSBN: 978-0-323-41736-5.

Keservani, R. K., Kesharwani, R. K., & Sharma, A. K., (2017a). Introduction to nanotechnology in drug delivery. In: *Drug Delivery Approaches and Nanosystems* (pp. 1–19). Apple Academic Press. ISBN: 9781771885836.

Keservani, R. K., Sharma, A. K., & Kesharwani, R. K., (2017). *Drug Delivery Approaches and Nanosystems, Two-Volume Set.* CRC Press. ISBN:9781771885850.

Keservani, R. K., Sharma, A. K., & Kesharwani, R. K., (2018). Nanoparticulate nanocarriers in drug delivery. In: *Nanobiomaterials* (pp. 3–22). Apple Academic Press. ISBN: 9781771885911.

Keservani, R. K., Sharma, A. K., & Kesharwani, R. K., (2019). *Nanocarriers for Brain Targeting: Principles and Applications*. CRC Press. ISBN:9781771887304.

Khambete, H., Keservani, R. K., Kesharwani, R. K., Jain, N. P., & Jain, C. P., (2016). Emerging trends of nanobiomaterials in hard tissue engineering. In: *Nanobiomaterials in Hard Tissue Engineering* (pp. 63–101). William Andrew Publishing. ISSN: 978-0-323-42862-0.

Khaydarov, R. A., Khaydarov, R. R., Gapurova, O., Estrin, Y., & Scheper, T., (2009). Electrochemical method for the synthesis of silver nanoparticles. *Journal of Nanoparticle Research, 11*(5), 1193–1200.

Kokura, S., Handa, O., Takagi, T., Ishikawa, T., Naito, Y., & Yoshikawa, T., (2010). Silver nanoparticles as a safe preservative for use in cosmetics. *Nanomedicine: Nanotechnology, Biology and Medicine, 6*(4), 570–574.

Koziol, K., Boskovic, B. O., & Yahya, N., (2010). Synthesis of carbon nanostructures by CVD method. *Advanced Structured Materials, 5*, 23–49.

Leung, D. Y. M., & Guttman-Yassky, E., (2014). Deciphering the complexities of atopic dermatitis: Shifting paradigms in treatment approaches. *Journal of Allergy and Clinical Immunology, 134*(4), 769–779.

Leung, D. Y., (2000). Atopic dermatitis: New insights and opportunities for therapeutic intervention. *Journal of Allergy Clin Immunology, 105*(5), 860–876.

Li, H. M., Yu, T., Wang, N., Chang, J., Zhang, D., Du, M., Liu, S., et al., (2014). Tamoxifen embedded in lipid bilayer improves the oncotarget of liposomal daunorubicin *in vivo* *Journal of Materials Chemistry B, 2*, 1619–1625.

Maincent, P., Thouvenot, P., Amicabile, C., Hoffman, M., Kreuter, J., Couvreur, P., & Devissaguet, J., (1992). *Pharmaceutical Research, 9*(12), 1534–1539.

Meyers, M. A., Mishra, A., & Benson, D. J., (2006). Mechanical properties of nanocrystalline materials. *Progress in Material Science., 51*(4), 427–556.

Mikhailova, E. O., (2020). Silver nanoparticles: Mechanism of action and probable bio-application. *Journal of Functional Biomaterials,11*(4), 84.

Monteiro-Riviere, N. A., (2010). *Structure and Function of Skin, Toxicology of the Skin* (pp. 1–18). Informa Healthcare USA, Inc., New York.

Mubarak, N. M., Abdullah, E. C., Jayakumar, N. S., & Sahu, J. N., (2014). An overview on methods for the production of carbon nanotubes. *Journal of Industrial and Engineering Chemistry., 20*(4), 1186–1197.

Nadagouda, M. N., Speth, T. F., & Varma, R. S., (2011). Microwave-assisted green synthesis of silver nanostructures, *Account of Chemical Research, 44*(7) 469–478.

Patra, J. K., Das, G., Fraceto, F. L., Campos, V. R. E., Rodriguez-Torres, M. P., Asosta-Torres, S. L., Diaz-Torres, A. L., et al., (2018). Nanobased drug delivery systems: Recent development and futures prospects. *Journal of Nanobiotrchnology., 16*(1).

Pradhan, M., Singh, D., & Singh, M. R., (2013). Novel colloidal carriers for psoriasis: Current issues, mechanistic insight and novel delivery approaches. *J Control Release, 170*(3), 380–395.

Prasek, J., Drbohlavova, J., Chomoucka, J., Hubalek, J., Jasek, O., Adam, V., et al., (2011). Methods for carbon nanotubes synthesis review. *Journal of Materials Chemistry., 40*(21), 15872–15884.

Rafique, I., Kausar, A., Anwar, Z., & Muhammad, B., (2015). Exploration of epoxy resins, hardening systems, and epoxy/carbon nanotube composite designed for high performance materials: A review. *Polymer-Plastics Technology and Engineering, 55*(3), 312–333.

Rajput, N., (2015). Methods of preparation of nanoparticles: A review. *International Journal of Advanced in Engineering & Technology., 7*(6) 1806.

Ramanunny, A. K., Wadhwa, S., Gulati, M., Singh, S. K., Kapoor, B., Dureja, H., & Chellappan, D. K., (2020). Nanocarriers for treatment of dermatological diseases: Principle, perspective, and practices. *European Journal of Pharmacology*, 173691.

Rancan, F., Volkmann, H., Giulbudagian, M., Schumacher, F., Stanko, J. I., Kleuser, B., & Vogt, A., (2019). Dermal delivery of the high-molecular-weight drug tacrolimus by means of polyglycerol-based nanogels. *Pharmaceutics, 11*(8), 394.

Rangasamy, M., (2011). Nano technology: A review. *Journal of Applied Pharmaceutical Science, 1*(02), 8–16.

Raut, A. S., Prabhu, R. H., & Patravale, V. B., (2013). Psoriasis clinical implications and treatment: A review. *Critical Reviews™ in Therapeutic Drug Carrier Systems., 30*(3), 183–216.

Richard, P., Usatine, Md., & Marcela, R. Md., (2010). Diagnosis and management of contact dermatitis. *American Family Physician, 82*(3), 249–255.

Sahle, F. F., Giulbudagian, M., Bergueiro, J., Lademann, J., & Calderón, M., (2017). Dendritic polyglycerol and *N*-isopropylacrylamide based thermoresponsive nanogels as smart carriers for controlled delivery of drugs through the hair follicle. *Nanoscale, 9*, 172–182.

Sarangdevot, K., & Sonigara, B. S., (2015). The wondrous world of carbon nanotubes: Structure, synthesis, properties, and applications. *Journal of Chemical and Pharmaceutical Research, 7*(6), 916–933.

Sardar, R., Funston, A. M., Mulvaney, P., & Murray, R. W., (2009). Gold nanoparticles: Past, present, and future†. *Langmuir, 25*(24), 13840–13851.

Schaferkorting, M., mehnert, W., & Korting, H., (2007). Lipid nanoparticles for improved topical application of drugs for skin diseases. *Advanced Drug Delivery Reviews, 59*(6), 427–443.

Scheuplein, R. J., (1967). Mechanism of percutaneous absorption. *Journal of Investigative Dermatology, 48*(1), 79–88.

Schneider, M., Stracke, F., Hansen, S., & Schaefer, U. F., (2009). Nanoparticles and their interactions with the dermal barrier. *Dermato-Endocrinology, 1*(4), 197–206.

Shah, M., Badwaik, V., Kherde, Y., Waghwani, H. K., Modi, T., Aguilar, Z. P., Rodgers, H., et al., (2014). Gold nanoparticles: Various methods of synthesis and antibacterial applications. *Frontiers in Bioscience, 19*, 1320-1344.

Sharma, A. K., Keservani, R. K., & Keseharwani, R. K., (2018). *Nanobiomaterials: Applications in Drug Delivery.* CRC Press. ISBN:9781771885911.

Sigmundsdottir, H., (2010). Improving topical treatments for skin diseases. *Trends in Pharmacology Science, 31,* 239–245.

Sinha, N., & Yeow, J. T. W., (2005). Carbon nanotubes for biomedical applications. *IEEE Transactions on Nanobioscience, 4*(2), 180–195.

Ufuoma, I., Haisheng, P., Haichun, L., Cathy, M., Chenxu, Y., & Qun, W., (2015). Nanocarriers in therapy of infectious and inflammatory diseases. *Nanoscale*, 1–40.

Ulla, M., Ali, M. D., & Sharifah, B. A., (2014). Surfactant-assisted ball milling: A noveloute to novel materials with controlled nanostructure: A review. *Review Advanced Material Science, 37,* 1-14.

Varshney, K., (2014). Carbon nanotubes: A review on synthesis, properties, and applications. *International Journal of Engineering Research General Science., 2*(4), 660–677.

Xi-Feng, Z., Zhi-Guo, L., Wei, S., & Sangiliyandi, G., (2016). Silver nanoparticles: Synthesis, characterization, properties, applications, and therapeutic approaches. *International Journal of Molecular Science., 17*(9), 1534.

Zakrewsky, M., Kumar, S., & Mitragotri, S., (2015). Nucleic acid delivery into skin for the treatment of skin disease: Proofs-of-concept, potential impact, and remaining challenges. *Journal of Controlled Release, 219*, 445–456.

CHAPTER 5

Small Interfering RNA Nanocarriers to Skin Delivery

AMIT KUMAR SINGH,[1] AMIT K. SINGH,[1] and SHANTI BHUSHAN MISHRA[2]

[1]*Department of Pharmaceutics, United Institute of Pharmacy, Prayagraj, Uttar Pradesh, India*

[2]*Department of Pharmacognosy, United Institute of Pharmacy, Prayagraj, Uttar Pradesh, India*

ABSTRACT

Gene defect in the skin is one of the major cause of skin disease. The skin diseases that arise due gene defects includes melanoma, alopecia areata (AA), rheumatoid arthritis (RA), pachyonychia congenita (PC), wounds, and psoriasis. These gene defects can be effectively corrected by delivering the specific siRNA to the target region in the skin. The topical delivery of therapeutic moiety in relevant concentration can be promising approach for the management of these skin diseases. In recent year siRNA-based therapy has emerged as a new avenue for the treatment of these skin diseases. However, the use of siRNA as a therapeutic moiety to treat skin disease is limited due to its susceptibility to degradation and inefficient cellular uptake. Further the outer layer of skin that is the stratum corneum (SC), represent the major hurdle for the effective delivery these biomolecules. So, there is an urgent need of an efficient delivery system that not only circumvent the problem associated with sRNA delivery but also target the delivery sRNA to site of action. For this purpose, various delivery system has been investigated by researcher to overcome these barriers among them nanocarrier based formulation has shown ensuring results in preclinical studies. This

Novel Nanocarriers forSkin Diseases: Advances and Applications.
Raj K. Keservani and Júlia Scherer Santos (Eds.)

chapter provides an update on the nanocarriers-based approaches for effective delivery of siRNA for the management of skin disorders.

5.1 INTRODUCTION

5.1.1 SMALL INTERFERING RNA (SIRNA)

In recent decades, the most transformed fields in field of medical science are molecular biology. Major transformation that has been occurred in field of molecular biology is in the field of small non-coding RNA. Small non-coding RNA is the biomolecules that regulates gene expression. Depending upon their role and structure this small non-coding RNA can be categorized into three major categories: miRNAs, siRNAs, and piRNAs (Rao et al., 2009).

Amongst these three types of RNA the siRNA, which is also known as short interfering RNA, is a non-coding double-stranded RNA of 20–23 nucleotide base pairs in length. This size is sufficiently small that it can escape the surveillance of immune system (Leachman et al., 2008) As the name indicates, sRNA is a novel class of RNA that acts by interfering with the expression of the specific gene having a complementary sequence or it can be said that they act by RNA induced silencing complex to specifically degrade target RNA. Silencing the specific genes through sRNA is a potential technique in molecular biology; this technique is a powerful tool for biological investigation and a therapeutic application for many disorders (Kaur & Sharma, 2012). In terms of function, the sRNA is similar to the microRNA, except that the microRNA can regulate the expression of hundreds of genes via imperfect base pairing. While the siRNA acts more specifically by binding more specifically to a single gene at a particular location (Charbe et al., 2020).

In 1988, Fire et al. were the first who observed the RNA interference mechanism mediated by dsRNA in Caenorhabditis elegans (Fire et al., 1988). After that in mammalian cells the effect of RNA inhibition in somatic cells was demonstrated in 2001. Considering the therapeutic potential of sRNA, the first human clinical trial using siRNA as therapeutic entity was conducted in 2004. Till now more than 22 siRNA-based drugs have entered various phases for clinical trials at U.S. Food and Drug Administration (USFDA) (Aljuffali et al., 2016). Recently in 2018 the FDA approved first sRNA-based product Patisiran (ONPATTRO™) for delivery to hepatocytes that witnessed sRNA drug candidates surge in clinical application (Hoy, 2018).

5.2 SIRNA IN SKIN DELIVERY

The robust therapeutic approach of sRNA by means of inhibiting the production of unwanted protein synthesis by the RNA interference make it highly specific and efficient tool to treat various disease and this therapeutic approach render it distinct from other biomolecules (Dharamdasani et al., 2020). Topical delivery of sRNA molecules has emerged as new avenues for the management of various skin disorders. Topical application of sRNA represents a good model for treating various skin diseases due to the avoidance of systemic toxicity. Further the topical application is noninvasive and patient compliance approaches that prevent the metabolism of these biomolecules in gastrointestinal tract and liver. This approach' enables to achieve relevant drug concentration at target site and reduce systemic exposure of the biomolecules (Dharamdasani et al., 2020; Aljuffali & Lin, 2016). Considering the potential of sRNA the various researches has been published in recent decades to treat various skin disorders, such as cutaneous neoplasms (Chen et al., 2014), pachyonychia congenital (PC) (McLean, 2011), allergic skin diseases (Yokozeki et al., 2014), psoriasis (Jakobsen, 2009), atopic dermatitis (AD) (Zhang et al., 2011; Kanazawa et al., 2015), epidermolysis bullosa simplex (Atkinson et al., 2011) and epidermolytic palmoplantar keratoderma (Leslie et al., 2012).

SRNA has shown great potential to treat various skin diseases by inhibiting the over-expression of unwanted gene. The sRNA therapy has been proven to treat various skin disease including alopecia, psoriasis, allergic skin disease, skin cancer, etc. For suppression of specific target gene to treat this skin disease the topical delivery of sRNA could be a considered as a promising approach as the topical delivery avoid the first pass metabolism and thus minimize the side effect associated with systemic administration (Prausnitz et al., 2004; Brown et al., 2006; Liang et al., 2020). However, being have great potential to treat these skin diseases the topical application of these biomolecules is limited. Delivery of siRNA remains a significant hurdle since sRNA is hydrophilic and negatively charged bio-macromolecule with a molecular weight of approximate ~13 kDa these features limit its topical application. siRNAs generally interact poorly with the cell membrane owing its high molecular size and presence of negative charge. Additionally, the stratum corneum (SC), the outer most layer of skin encompasses a major barrier for penetration of these macromolecules. The continuous layer of SC has low permeability, and thus it is difficult to introduce a large hydrophilic molecule through the skin (Geusens et al., 2009; Aljuffaliand, 2016).

To overcome this challenge, the various methods has been reported in literature to promote the internalization of siRNA, like electroporation, lipoplex, and many more. The other approach that has been used to facilitate the permeation of sRNA are used of physical delivery techniques, that includes microneedle patch, sonophoresis, ontophoresis, electroporation, and use of heat-shocks. Despite being an efficient method to overcome the barrier offered by skin and cytoplasm of cells, they have additional limitation of being applied a very small fraction of skin have and self-administration is not possible and thus demands a trained personal to administered it. Additionally, the method employed in this technique are invasive in nature (Kigasawa et al., 2010; Yang et al., 2018; Deng et al., 2016). On the contrary, use of chemical penetration enhancers alone to promote permeation remains ineffective to overcome the barriers encounter in the delivery of siRNA into the viable cell of skin. Further, the continuous usage of these penetration enhancers leads to skin irritation due to cytotoxicity. Although administration of sRNA through intradermal injection offers an efficient method to deliver siRNA into the skin, however its application is limited due to the pain and limited payload capacity (Aljuffali et al., 2016). Therefore, there is utmost need of development of such delivery system that not only overcome the cytoplasmic and skin barriers, but also have flexibility to target desired site or disease site of the skin in a minimally invasive manner.

5.3 SKIN DISEASES TREATED BY SIRNA

In recent decades, a number of small interfering RNA (siRNA) biomolecules has already been approved for the management of various skin disease in animals and human being. To treat these skin diseases the topical route is most preferred route to silence the over-expression of gene of interest that is responsible for disease. This direct application is preferred as to avoid systemic absorption. The oral administration of these biomolecules is not recommended due to presence of unfavorable condition and enzyme in gastrointestinal tract that degrade the gene. Moreover, these macromolecules are difficult to absorb from the bio-membrane of GI. Although the parenteral route can be used to deliver the sRNA, but the pain arises due to injection leads to patient noncompliance. The skin disease which are treated using siRNA are discussed in upcoming section of this chapter.

5.3.1 CUTANEOUS MELANOMA

Cutaneous melanoma is most aggressive type of skin cancer that originates from pigment making cells of skin. It is most common type of melanoma that is triggered by ultraviolet (UV) radiation, and this causes cell death and transformation of healthy cells into malignant cells (Pang et al., 2022). The originating place of cutaneous melanoma is located at epidermal-dermal junction. The current treatment plans for the management of cutaneous melanoma are chemotherapy, immunotherapy, and radiation (Niezgoda et al., 2015) nevertheless these treatment plans are suffered from creation limitation such as non-selectivity, high toxicity and development of drug resistance. The gene therapy with siRNA can be a better alternative to treat cutaneous melanoma with high specificity and lower tissue toxicity. The treatment with siRNA allows specifically target the gene responsible for proliferation of cutaneous melanoma thus slow down the progression of tumor and metastasis of melanoma.

5.3.2 PACHYONYCHIA CONGENITA (PC)

Pachyonychia congenita (PC) is a rare hereditary disorder primarily affecting the nail and skin. The common symptoms of this disease include nail dystrophy, leukokeratosis of the mucous membranes, palmar, and plantar hyperkeratosis, follicular keratosis, and occasionally hyperhidrosis of palms and soles. The patients with pachyonychia congenital experience extreme pain which is associated with palmoplantar hyperkeratosis (Leachman et al., 2008; Feinstein et al., 1988). This rare skin disorder is arisen due to mutation in keratin gene KRT16 and KRT17. Transport of siRNA to keratinocytes could silence the pathological expression of mutant gene that is responsible for skin disorder (Eliason et al., 2012). In a preclinical study using dominant-negative tissue culture model it was shown that that TD101, the siRNA specifically targets the mutant mRNA KRT16 N171K and able to reverse the mutant phenotype of cells and restoring their capability to form a structurally intact keratin intermediate filament network (Hickerson et al., 2008).

5.3.3 PSORIASIS

Psoriasis is an autoimmune, chronic inflammatory skin disorder that is characterized by epidermal hyperproliferation, leukocyte infiltration, sustained skin inflammation and increased vascularity (Billi et al., 2019; Owczarek et al., 2021; Nickoloff et al., 2004). In psoriasis lesion the production of TNF α cytokinin is up regulated. The treatment approach through siRNA basically involves down regulation of TNFα cytokinin production. Besides the over expression of TNFα, the other factor which are also play a key role in pathogenesis of psoriasis are anti-apoptotic protein B-cell lymphoma-extra-large (Bcl-xL) and insulin-like growth factor (IGF) (Jakobsen et al., 2009).

5.3.4 ATOPIC DERMATITIS (AD)

Atopic dermatitis (AD) is a common chronic inflammatory skin disease that is characterized by intense itching, chronically replacing, and recurrent eczematous lesions; its pathological origin of this disease is complex and can co-related with both genetic and environmental factors. The disease not only affect the children but also adult with a prevalence rate varying from 1–20% in different region of world (Leung, 2000; Weidinger et al., 2016). The pathogenesis of pruritus in AD is complex process. The factors responsible for pruritus in AD include a variety of pro-inflammatory cytokines and chemokines that include TNFα, interleukins-1a, interleukins-1b, interleukins-4, interleukins-10 (IL-10) and interleukins-13. Among these cytokines and chemokines IL-10 produced by infiltrating macrophages and lymphocytes. This IL-10 is also produced from keratinocytes on allergen exposure. In pathogenesis of AD nuclear factor κ-light-chain-enhancer of activated B cells also play an important role. In a study conducted by Leung DY and his coworker shows that topical application of RNAi exhibits therapeutic response on AD in NC/Nga mouse (Leung, 2000). Dajee et al. used RNAi based therapy to block NF-κB activity to treat AD in murine model (Dajee et al., 2006).

5.3.5 ALOPECIA AREATA (AA)

Alopecia areata (AA), is a chronic inflammatory and autoimmune disease manifested with hair loss. Although the disease itself is not deadly, but it decreases quality of life of patient. The symptoms of disease include hair loss from scalp and also from any hair bearing skin (Tao et al., 2022; Hordinsky et al., 2015). As stated earlier it is an autoimmune disease that involves CD^{4+} and CD^{8+} T-lymphocytes advocating the participation of Th1 pathways in the development of alopecic lesions. The T-box-21 gene play a major role in cell differentiation and function. In a study conducted using C_3H/HeJ mouse model. The subcutaneous injection of siRNA against T-box 21 lead to elongation of hair soft, revealing its ability to treat r hair loss (Nakamura et al., 2008).

5.3.6 SKIN WOUNDS

The major function of skin is to serves as a protective barrier against environmental invasion. The impairment in protective function of skin and aberrant over-expression of pro-inflammatory molecules play a major role in development of chronic wounds. The inhibition of these pro-inflammatory mediator using siRNA may be an effective therapeutic strategy to promote wound healing. The treatment with siRNA enables us to silence the over-expression of specific gene that are responsible for development of chronic wound may present a safe and effective way to treat these wounds without any side effect (Nelson et al., 2013; Dreifke et al., 2015).

5.4 SIRNA NANOCARRIERS FOR SKIN DELIVERY

In the recent decades, extensive research has been carried out on nanocarriers for delivery of drug molecules and biomolecules as a novel approach because of their size dependent properties. Now a day s nanocarriers are on center of attention in pharmaceutical as well as biological sciences. In past decades nanocarriers has been extensively exploited for biomedical use. Rapid advances in their ability in drug and gene delivery, diagnosis, and bioimaging have led to a revolutionary change in the pharmaceutical and biomedical research arena. Nanocarriers are submicron size carrier molecules which range from 50–1,000 nm. These systems are represented by various carriers like polymeric nanoparticles, liposomes, niosomes, CNTs, nanosuspensions, polymeric micelles, lipid nanoparticle, liquid crystalline nanodispersion, dendrimers, functionalized nanocarriers, solid lipid NPs (SLNs), and nanostructured lipid carriers (NLCs) and many more (Pathak et al., 2017; Singh et al., 2022).

Incorporation of drug and biomolecules into nanocarrier offer various advantages like improved stability of therapeutic moiety, controlled, and sustained drug release from nanoparticles, ability to target the organs of interest and improved bioavailability. Now a day nanoparticulate system has emerged as a novel carrier system for delivery of biomolecules to skin they not only improve absorption through skin, but also facilitate drug targeting to skin and/or its substructures (Schäfer-Korting et al., 2007). Permeation of siRNA into skin can be enhanced by using nanocarrier. The nanometric size of these carriers facilitates close contact with SC thus allowing superficial spreading of incorporated biomolecules. Further these nanoparticles get trap into the hair follicles which also enhance the permeation of biomolecules. Potential of various nanocarrier in delivery of siRNA to skin investigated by various researcher has been summarized in Table 5.1. The various nanocarrier investigated for delivery of siRNA has been discussed in detail in upcoming section of this chapter.

5.4.1 LIPOSOMES

Among the lipid-based system the Liposomes has gained considerable importance in delivery of drug for the topical application for the management of various skin diseases as alone or with penetration enhancer or with some other modification (Keservani & Gautam, 2020; Rahman et al., 2019). Liposomes are composed of an amphiphilic phospholipid bilayer with hydrophilic head and lipophilic tail groups within the lipid structure. The similarity of phospholipid with body lipids makes it biocompatible and ideal carrier for delivery to skin. They have several advantages such as ability to encapsule both hydrophilic and lipophilic materials. The lipophilic drugs encapsulate into lipid bi-layer, and hydrophilic drugs entrap into aqueous compartment. The similarity of composition with cell membrane improves its uptake into cell. Liposomes are preferred for topical application owing to their ability to act as reservoir in SC. The delivery of siRNA through liposomes needs some additional modification. The cationic liposomes are very much desire for delivery of negatively charges sRNA biomolecules. The cationic liposome encapsulates the siRNA by means of electrostatic interaction which further prevent its degradation (Liang et al., 2020). In general, the application of liposomes for delivery of siRNA for skin application is limited due to entanglement of liposomes in superficial layer of skin. However, there are some nanocarrier system that utilizes the nano-liposomes in combination with lipid and other physical carrier systems as studied by Tran et al. (2014) in management of cutaneous melanoma using cationic nano-liposomes with a diameter of almost 50 nm. The study data revealed the ability of liposomes to incorporate, conserve, and release the siRNA into the targeted cells. Further their ability to silence the cells with a high level of Akt3 or V600EB-Raf siRNA were demonstrated specifically to after the application of ultrasound technique. Further the study revealed the safety profile of developed liposomes as there were no sign of toxicity of the targeted cells when delivered the siRNA into the melanoma cells by topical route (Tran et al., 2014).

TABLE 5.1 Nanocarriers Investigated for Topical Delivery of siRNA to Skin

SL. No.	Nanocarrier	Size	Zeta Potential	Target Gene	In-Vitro Study	Animal Model (In Vivo Study)	References
1.	Nanosomes	–	–	DEFB4	–	Skin-humanized mouse model for psoriasis.	Bracke et al. (2014)
2.	Lipid nanoparticles	102 nm	32.14 mv	TNFα and STAT3.	HEK-293 and GFP-tagged HEK cell lines.	Imiquimod-induced psoriasiform mouse model.	Marepally et al. (2014)
3.	Lipid-polymer hybrid nanoparticles 1.	163 nm	35.14 mv	TNFα	Hair less rat skin.	Imiquimod-induced psoriasiform mouse model.	Desai et al. (2013)
4.	Cationic star-shaped polymer based on β-cyclodextrin.	110~268 nm	–	MMP-9	–	Streptozocin-induced diabetic rat.	Li et al. (2014)
5.	Liquid crystalline nanodispersions.	~200 nm	–	GAPDH	Porcine ear skin	Hairless mice	de Carvalho Vicentini et al. (2013)
6.	Carbon nanotubes ~	~1 μm in length	–	BRAF	–	Melanoma-bearing mouse.	Siu et al. (2014)
7.	Gold nanoparticles	27~42 nm	–	EGFR	–	Hairless mouse	Zheng et al. (2012)
8.	Polymeric lipid nanoparticle	142 nm	+25 mv	TNFα	Porcine skin model	Hairless mouse model	Suzuki et al. (2021)
9.	Liposomes	102.5 nm	35.7 mv	GAPDH	Mice skin	Female BALB/C mice	Liang et al. (2020)
10.	Dendrimer and cationic liposomes	99.80 nm (dendrimer) 174.80 (liposomes)	13.40 mv (dendrimer) 29.96 (liposomes)	TNFα	–	Psoriatic plaque mode	Pandi et al. (2018)

TABLE 5.1 *(Continued)*

SL. No.	Nanocarrier	Size	Zeta Potential	Target Gene	In-Vitro Study	Animal Model (In Vivo Study)	References
11.	Liquid nanocrystalline dispersion	202.3–270.3	–11.0 mv to 36.4 mv	GAPDH	Psoriasis skin model	–	Depieri et al. (2016)
12.	Nanostructured lipid carrier	230 nm	10 mv	TNFα	–	Psoriatic animal model	Viegas et al. (2020)
13.	Peptide nanocarrier	–	–	Nuclear 25 factor kappa B (NF-kB).	–	AD model mice	Kanazawa et al. (2015)
14.	Liquid crystalline nanodispersion	147–327 nm	0.076–35 mv	TNFα	L929 cell lines	Hairless mice	Petrilli et al. (2016)
15.	Spherical nucleic acid nanoparticle.	12.38 nm	–28 mv	EGF, EGFR	A431 cell lines	BALBc/mice	Nemati et al. (2017)
16.	Cationic lipid nanocarrier	132.00 ± 6.23 nm	+39.76 mv	IL36α	Dermatomed human skin.	C57BL/6 mice	Boakye et al. (2017)

Recently Liang et al. reported the cationic flexible liposomes (CFL) for topical administration of delivery of siRNA with a combination of sponge *Haliclona* sp. Spicules (SHS). In this study SHS were used to increase the permeation of siRNA by formation of a number of new microchannels in upper part of epidermis. The study revealed that topical application of SHS in combination with CFL leads to improved siRNA permeation many folds compared to the control group (Liang et al., 2020).

5.4.2 DENDRIMERS

The dendrimer which are hyperbranched polymeric structure produced with different chemical composition has gained wider importance for delivery of drug to skin. Dendrimers represent a unique delivery vehicle for skin delivery and has been widely exploited for delivery of a wide range of therapeutic, diagnostic agents and bioactive compounds. The unique chemical composition and flexibility to do some modification make dendrimers as highly promising carriers' system for delivery siRNA. Structurally it consists of a core at the center of structure which is connected to hyperbranched structure. The terminal parts of the this hyperbranched structure contain numerous reactive groups which provide platform for conjunction of drug moieties (Biswas et al., 2013; Tabarzad et al., 2021) Extensive studied has been carried out for delivery of siRNA through dendrimer for this purpose dendrimer with different chemical composition were developed such as poly(amidoamine) dendrimer, carbosilane dendrimer, poly(propyleneimine) dendrimer, poly(L-lysine) dendrimer. Amongst them the poly(amidoamine) dendrimers have gain wider success as it interact with siRNA by electrostatic interaction which is desirable characters for improving the cellular uptake of siRNA (Wu et al., 2013).

A report published by Li et al. confirming the ability of dendrimer to deliver MMM9-siRNA for the management of diabetic wounds. The developed formulation possesses good biocompatibility and exhibits strong complexation ability with siRNA. The wound healing study conducted in diabetic rat revealed that the developed formulation exhibited high transfection efficiency and reduced the expression of MMP-9 gene in skin fibroblast cells. Further the developed formulation exhibited low toxicity on fibroblast thus the study advocating the potential of dendrimer in effective delivery of siRNA (Li et al., 2014).

In a study by Pandi et al. (2018), liposomes and dendrimer were prepared, and comparative study was carried out to access the suitability of nanocarrier for siRNA delivery. In this study dendrimer with different chemical composition namely 1,2-dioleoyl-3-trimethyl ammonium propane (DOTAP) LPM and PAMAM generation-3 (P-G3) dendrimers were formulated and investigated for the topical delivery of siTNF-α. Further *in vivo* efficacy siTNF-α dendriplex is determined and compared with siTNF-α lipoplex using IMQ induced psoriatic plaque model. The author in their research report concluded that both PG3 dendrimers and DOTAP LPM are equally efficacious for topical delivery of TNF-α siRNA in in future they can be explored for delivery of other genes (Pandi et al., 2018).

5.4.3 NANOSTRUCTURED LIPID CARRIER (NLCS)

Nanostructured lipid carrier (NLC) is new generation of lipid nanoparticles, which is an aqueous colloidal dispersion that is composed of blended solid lipids and liquid lipids (oils) (Kong et al., 2014). NLC shows distinct advantages over the conventional drug delivery system (DDS). They are normally composed of biodegradable and biocompatible lipids (Gelfuso et al., 2016). The NLCs are constitute of mixture of solid and liquid lipid that lead to development of imperfection in nanostructure, this imperfection in nanostructure improves the therapeutic loading of drug with improved stability. Furthermore, the NLCs offer close contact with the outer layer of skin due to their nanometric size & lipidic composition that facilitate the drug permeation through skin.

In recent years, Viegas et al. (2020) investigated a multifunctional nanostructured lipid carrier (NLC) for co-delivery tacrolimus and siRNA. The NLCs formulation were characterized for various physicochemical parameter. The data of the characterization studies revealed nano-size range of particle with an average of 230 nm and have a value of zeta potential of + 10 mV. The toxicity study conducted on murine fibroblast presented low toxicity and the result of the *in-vivo* animal model shows the potential of the multifunctional NLC in reduction of the cytokine TNF-α expression about 7-fold that represent a synergistic effect of TAC and TNF-α siRNA. From these studies it was concluded that developed system was huge future potential in the treatment of psoriasis (Viegas et al., 2020).

5.4.4 CARBON NANOTUBE

Carbon nanotube is cylindrical large molecule that is made up of hexagonal hybridized carbon atom and typically in diameter of about nanometer (Alina et al., 2016). Extensive research has been carried out on carbon nanotube for biomedical application. Siu et al. investigated the potential of carbon nanotube in delivery of siRNA for the management of skin melanoma. Despite their ability to enter into the cell effectively they cannot be used as it is; to deliver siRNA. For an efficient delivery of siRNA, the delivery system along with siRNA molecules need certain modification. In this report the researcher designed a non-covalently functionalized single-walled carbon nanotube for topical siRNA delivery by using succinate polyethyleneimine. The developed formulation specifically deliver siRNA to target gene Braf which was proved by both *in-vitro* and *in-vivo* model. *In-vitro* study against B16-F10 cells demonstrated gene silencing induced by IS/C/siRNA complexes. The *in-vivo* study C57BL/6 mice melanoma model exhibited significant uptake of Cy3-labeled siRNA and Braf gene silencing in the tumor tissue. The treatment with melanoma model attenuated the tumor growth for 25-days. The developed non-covalently functionalized carbon nanotube has provided a new viable alternative siRNA delivery in near future (Siu et al., 2014).

5.4.5 NANOSOMES

The classic liposomal formulations that were developed for the dermal delivery of drugs, these liposomes suffer from certain limitation such as they remain confined to the SC owing to rigid structure. Advances in delivery system leads to development of two main classes of liposomes transferosomes and transfersomes (TRAs) that consist of edge activators, surfactant, and ethanol, respectively. Further modification was carried out to increase its applicability for topical formulation and a novel formulation have been developed as novel nanosome-containing siRNA delivery system (SECosome) for human epidermis. The developed system contains surfactant and ethanol and both act as a permeation enhancer. Combining the two enhancers in one liposome particle has synergistic effect on skin penetration capacity (Keran et al., 2014).

Bracke et al. investigated the potential of these novel nanosomes called surfactant-ethanol-cholesterolosomes (SECosomes) for siRNA delivery. The SECosomes were prepared using DOTAP, cholesterol, sodium coholate, and ethanol. The SECosome-siRNA complex (SECoplex) was prepared from SECosomes. The skin penetration study on freshly excised intact human skin revealed that this novel formulation penetrates into the epidermis of and can enter into the keratinocytes. The developed SECoplexes subjected to characterization study the result of these study revealed that the developed formulation possesses mean diameter, 101 nm; surface charge, 56 mV; and 40-fold higher transfection efficiency than free siRNA. Also, SECosomes showed ideal encapsulation efficiency characteristics. The developed SECosome loaded with DFB4 siRNA were able to inhibit the translation of the human defensin-2 peptide and thus result in the normalization of the psoriasis (Bracke et al., 2014).

5.5 CONCLUSION

Topical delivery of siRNA for the treatment of skin diseases offers many potential therapeutic advantages. The siRNA act by inhibiting the expression of target gene, thus suppressive the growth of disease. However, the innate structure of skin makes a big hurdle for entry of siRNA molecules into the skin. Meanwhile, the negative charge of siRNA molecule makes its topical delivery challenging to formulation scientist. The literature has described various newer technique to facilitate its epidermal penetration and cellular transfection of nucleic acids. Here in this chapter, we have discussed a variety of papers showing the potential of nanocarriers in delivery of siRNA. The nanocarrier system such as liposomes, lipid-based polymer hybrid systems, spherical nucleic acid nanoparticles, and cationic cell-penetrating peptide-based systems have been extensively studied for topical delivery of siRNA. Incorporation of siRNA into these nanocarrier has demonstrated high rates of siRNA complexation, protection against degradation, and improved transfection efficiency. The selection of suitable delivery system for siRNA delivery should be based on skin penetration capability, protection of siRNA from degradation, disease site, and delivery of siRNA in the cytoplasm of cells. Skin penetration and cellular penetration are among the significant barriers. It is anticipated that there will be more of progression and development in the field of siRNA-based therapeutic in skin disorders in near future.

ACKNOWLEDGMENT

The authors are thankful to Dr. Prabhat Kumar Upadhyay, Associate Professor, Institute of Pharmaceutical Research, GLA University for their guidance and providing assistance to complete this chapter.

KEYWORDS

- **dendrimers**
- **gene silencing**
- **liposomes**
- **nanostructured lipid carrier**
- **skin**
- **small interfering RNA**
- **topical delivery**

REFERENCES

Alina, M. H., Alexandru, M. G., & Ecaterina, A., (2016). Chapter 10 – inorganic nanoarchitectonics designed for drug delivery and anti-infective surfaces. In: Alexandru, M. G., (eds.), *Surface Chemistry of Nanobiomaterials* (pp. 301–327). William Andrew Publishing.

Aljuffali, I. A., Lin, Y. K., & Fang, J. Y., (2016). Noninvasive approach for enhancing small interfering RNA delivery percutaneously. *Expert. Opin. Drug Deliv.*, *13*(2), 265–280.

Billi, A. C., Gudjonsson, J. E., & Voorhees, J. J., (2019). Psoriasis: Past, present, and future. *J. Invest. Dermatol.*, *139*(11), e133.

Biswas, S., & Torchilin, V. P., (2013). Dendrimers for siRNA delivery. *Pharmaceuticals*, *6*(2), 161–183.

Bracke, S., Carretero, M., Guerrero-Aspizua, S., Desmet, E., Illera, N., Navarro, M., Lambert, J., & Del, R. M., (2014). Targeted silencing of DEFB 4 in a bioengineered skin-humanized mouse model for psoriasis: Development of siRNA SECosome-based novel therapies. *Exp. Dermatol.*, *23*(3), 199–201.

Brown, M. B., Martin, G. P., Jones, S. A., & Akomeah, F. K., (2006). Dermal and transdermal drug delivery systems: Current and future prospects. *Drug Delivery*, *13*(3), 175–187.

Charbe, N. B., Amnerkar, N. D., Ramesh, B., Tambuwala, M. M., Bakshi, H. A., Aljabali, A. A., Khadse, S. C., et al., (2020). Small interfering RNA for cancer treatment: Overcoming hurdles in delivery. *Acta Pharm Sinica B.*, *10*(11), 2075–2109.

Chen, D., Koropatnick, J., Jiang, N., Zheng, X., Zhang, X., Wang, H., Yuan, K., et al., (2014). Targeted siRNA silencing of indoleamine 2, 3-dioxygenase in antigen-presenting cells using mannose-conjugated liposomes: A novel strategy for treatment of melanoma. *J. Immunother.*, *37*(2), 123–134.

Dajee, M., Muchamuel, T., Schryver, B., Oo, A., Alleman-Sposeto, J., De Vry, C. G., Prasad, S., et al., (2006). Blockade of experimental atopic dermatitis via topical NF-κB decoy oligonucleotide. *J. Invest. Dermato.l*, *126*(8), 1792–1803.

De Carvalho, V. F. T., Depieri, L. V., Polizello, A. C., Del, C. J. O., Spadaro, A. C., Fantini, M. C., & Bentley, M. V., (2013). Liquid crystalline phase nanodispersions enable skin delivery of siRNA. *Eur. J. Pharm. and Biopharm.*, *83*(1), 16–24.

Deng, Y., Chen, J., Zhao, Y., Yan, X., Zhang, L., Choy, K., Hu, J., et al., (2016). Transdermal delivery of siRNA through microneedle array. *Scientific Reports*, *6*(1), 1–8.

Depieri, L. V., Borgheti-Cardoso, L. N., Campos, P. M., Otaguiri, K. K., De Carvalho, V. F. T., Lopes, L. B., Fonseca, M. J., & Bentley, M. V., (2016). RNAi mediated IL-6 *in vitro* knockdown in psoriasis skin model with topical siRNA delivery system based on liquid crystalline phase. *Eur. J. Pharm. and Biopharm, 105,* 50–58.

Desai, P. R., Marepally, S., Patel, A. R., Voshavar, C., Chaudhuri, A., & Singh, M., (2013). Topical delivery of anti-TNFα siRNA and capsaicin via novel lipid-polymer hybrid nanoparticles efficiently inhibits skin inflammation *in vivo. J. Controlled Release, 170*(1), 51–63.

Dharamdasani, V., Mandal, A., Qi, Q. M., Suzuki, I., Bentley, M. V., & Mitragotri, S., (2020). Topical delivery of siRNA into skin using ionic liquids. *J. Controlled Release, 323,* 475–482.

Dreifke, M. B., Jayasuriya, A. A., & Jayasuriya, A. C., (2015). Current wound healing procedures and potential care. *Materials Science and Engineering: C., 48*, 651–662.

Eliason, M. J., Leachman, S. A., Feng, B. J., Schwartz, M. E., & Hansen, C. D., (2012). A review of the clinical phenotype of 254 patients with genetically confirmed pachyonychia congenita. *J. Am. Acad. Dermatol., 67*(4), 680–686.

Feinstein, A., Friedman, J., & Schewach-Millet, M., (1988). Pachyonychia congenita. *J. Am. Acad. Dermatol., 19*(4), 705–711.

Fire, A., Xu, S., Montgomery, M. K., et al., (1998). Potent and specific genetic interference by double-stranded RNA in *Caenorhabditis elegans*. *Nature*, *391*, 806–811.

Gelfuso, G. M., Cunha-Filho, M. S., & Gratieri, T., (2016). Nanostructured lipid carriers for targeting drug delivery to the epidermal layer. *Therapeutic Delivery*, *7*(11), 735–737.

Geusens, B., Sanders, N., Prow, T., Van, G. M., & Lambert, J., (2009). Cutaneous short-interfering RNA therapy. *Expert Opin. Drug Deliv.*, *6*(12), 1333–1349.

Hickerson, R. P., Smith, F. J., Reeves, R. E., Contag, C. H., Leake, D., Leachman, S. A., Milstone, L. M., et al., (2008). Single-nucleotide-specific siRNA targeting in a dominant-negative skin model. *J. Invest. Dermatol., 128*(3), 594–605.

Hordinsky, M., & Junqueira, A. L., (2015). Alopecia areata update. *Semin. Cutan. Med. Surg., 34*(2), 72–75.

Hoy, S. M., (2018). Patisiran: First global approval. *Drugs., 78*(15), 1625–1631.

Jakobsen, M., Stenderup, K., Rosada, C., et al., (2009). Amelioration of psoriasis by anti-TNF-α RNAi in the xenograft transplantation model. *Mol Ther., 17,* 1743–1753.

Jakobsen, M., Stenderup, K., Rosada, C., Moldt, B., Kamp, S., Dam, T. N., Jensen, T. G., & Mikkelsen, J. G., (2009). Amelioration of psoriasis by anti-TNF-α RNAi in the xenograft transplantation model. *Molecular Therapy, 17*(10), 1743–1753.

Kanazawa, T., Hamasaki, T., Endo, T., Tamano, K., Sogabe, K., Seta, Y., Ohgi, T., & Okada, H., (2015). Functional peptide nanocarriers for delivery of novel anti-RelA RNA interference agents as a topical treatment of atopic dermatitis. *Int. J. Pharm., 489*(1, 2), 261–267.

Kaur, I. P., & Sharma, G., (2012). siRNA: A new approach to target neuropathic pain. *BioDrugs., 26*(6), 401–412.

Keren, A., David, M., & Gilhar, A., (2014). Novel nanosome delivery system combined with siRNA targeting the antimicrobial gene DFB 4: A new approach for psoriasis management? *Exp. Dermatol., 23*(7), 464, 465.

Kigasawa, K., Kajimoto, K., Hama, S., Saito, A., Kanamura, K., & Kogure, K., (2010). Noninvasive delivery of siRNA into the epidermis by iontophoresis using an atopic dermatitis-like model rat. *Int. J. Pharm., 383*(1, 2), 157–160.

Kong, X., Zhao, Y., Quan, P., & Fang, L., (2016). Development of a topical ointment of betamethasone dipropionate loaded nanostructured lipid carrier. *Asian J. of Pharm. Sci., 11*(2), 248–254.

Leachman, S. A., Hickerson, R. P., Hull, P. R., Smith, F. J., Milstone, L. M., Lane, E. B., Bale, S. J., et al., (2008). Therapeutic siRNAs for dominant genetic skin disorders including pachyonychia congenita. *J. Dermatol. Sci., 51*(3), 151–157.

Leslie, P. D. M., Fu, D. J., Gonzalez-Gonzalez, E., et al., (2012). Generic and personalized RNAi-based therapeutics for a dominant-negative epidermal fragility disorder. *J. Invest. Dermatol., 132,* 1627–1635.

Leung, D. Y., (2000). Atopic dermatitis: New insights and opportunities for therapeutic intervention. *J. Allergy and Clinical Immunol., 105*(5), 860–876.

Li, N., Luo, H. C., Yang, C., Deng, J. J., Ren, M., Xie, X. Y., Lin, D. Z., et al., (2014). Cationic star-shaped polymer as an siRNA carrier for reducing MMP-9 expression in skin fibroblast cells and promoting wound healing in diabetic rats. *Int. J. Nanomed., 9,* 3377.

Liang, X., Zhang, J., Ou, H., Chen, J., Mitragotri, S., & Chen, M., (2020). Skin delivery of siRNA using sponge spicules in combination with cationic flexible liposomes. *Mol. Ther-Nucleic Acids, 20,* 639–648.

Marepally, S., Boakye, C. H., Patel, A. R., Godugu, C., Doddapaneni, R., Desai, P. R., & Singh, M., (2014). Topical administration of dual siRNAs using fusogenic lipid nanoparticles for treating psoriatic-like plaques. *Nanomedicine, 9*(14), 2157–2174.

McLean, W. H., & Moore, C. B., (2011). Keratin disorders: From gene to therapy. *Hum Mol Genet., 20,* 189–197.

Nakamura, M., Jo, J. I., Tabata, Y., & Ishikawa, O., (2008). Controlled delivery of T-box21 small interfering RNA ameliorates autoimmune alopecia (Alopecia Areata) in a C3H/HeJ mouse model. *Am. J. Pathol., 172*(3), 650–658.

Nelson, C. E., Gupta, M. K., Adolph, E. J., Guelcher, S. A., & Duvall, C. L., (2013). siRNA delivery from an injectable scaffold for wound therapy. *Adv. Wound Care, 2*(3), 93–99.

Nemati, H., Ghahramani, M. H., Faridi-Majidi, R., Izadi, B., Bahrami, G., Madani, S. H., & Tavoosidana, G., (2017). Using siRNA-based spherical nucleic acid nanoparticle conjugates for gene regulation in psoriasis. *J. Controlled Release, 268,* 259–268.

Nickoloff, B. J., & Nestle, F. O., (2004). Recent insights into the immunopathogenesis of psoriasis provide new therapeutic opportunities. *J. Clin. Invest., 113*(12), 1664–1675.

Niezgoda, A., Niezgoda, P., & Czajkowski, R., (2015). Novel approaches to treatment of advanced melanoma: A review on targeted therapy and immunotherapy. *BioMed Res. Int.,* 851387.

Owczarczyk-Saczonek, A., Krajewska-Włodarczyk, M., Kasprowicz-Furmańczyk, M., & Placek, W., (2020). Immunological memory of psoriatic lesions. *Int. J. Mol. Sci., 21*(2), 625.

Pandi, P., Jain, A., Kommineni, N., Ionov, M., Bryszewska, M., & Khan, W., (2018). Dendrimer as a new potential carrier for topical delivery of siRNA: A comparative study of dendriplex vs. lipoplex for delivery of TNF-α siRNA. *Int. J. Pharm., 550*(1, 2), 240–250.

Pang, H., Zhou, Y., Wang, J., Wu, H., Cui, C., & Xiao, Z., (2022). SKA3 overexpression predicts poor outcomes in skin cutaneous melanoma patients. *Translational Oncology, 15*(1), 101253.

Pathak, K., Shankar, R., & Joshi, M., (2017). An update of patents, preclinical and clinical outcomes of lipid nanoparticulate systems. *Current Pharmaceutical Design, 23*(43), 6602–6612.

Petrilli, R., Eloy, J. O., Praça, F. S., Del Ciampo, J. O., Fantini, M. A., Fonseca, M. J., & Bentley, M. V., (2016). Liquid crystalline nanodispersions functionalized with cell-penetrating peptides for topical delivery of short-interfering RNAs: A proposal for silencing a pro-inflammatory cytokine in cutaneous diseases. *J. Biomed Nanotechnol., 12*(5), 1063–1075.

Prausnitz, M. R., Mitragotri, S., & Langer, R., (2004). Current status and future potential of transdermal drug delivery. *Nature Rev. Drug Discovery*, *3*(2), 115–124.

Rahman, M., Alam, K., Beg, S., Anwar, F., & Kumar, V., (2019). Liposomes as topical drug delivery systems: State of the arts. In: *Biomedical Applications of Nanoparticles* (pp. 149–161). William Andrew Publishing.

Rao, D. D., Vorhies, J. S., Senzer, N., & Nemunaitis, J., (2009). siRNA vs. shRNA: Similarities and differences. *Adv. Drug Deliv. Rev.*, *61*(9), 746–759.

Schäfer-Korting, M., Mehnert, W., & Korting, H. C., (2007). Lipid nanoparticles for improved topical application of drugs for skin diseases. *Adv. Drug Deliv. Reviews.*, *59*(6), 427–443.

Singh, B., Upadhyay, P. K., & Kumar, M., (2022). Nanocrystal for dermatological application: A comprehensive review. *Current Nanoscience.*, *18*(1), 48–60.

Siu, K. S., Chen, D., Zheng, X., Zhang, X., Johnston, N., Liu, Y., Yuan, K., et al., (2014). Non-covalently functionalized single-walled carbon nanotube for topical siRNA delivery into melanoma. *Biomaterials*, *35*(10), 3435–3442.

Suzuki, I. L., De Araujo, M. M., Bagnato, V. S., & Bentley, M. V., (2021). TNFα siRNA delivery by nanoparticles and photochemical internalization for psoriasis topical therapy. *J. Controlled Release*, *338*, 316–329.

Tabarzad, M., & Ghorbani-Bidkorbeh, F., (2021). Dendrimers formulations to enhance skin drug delivery. In: *Dendrimer-Based Nanotherapeutics* (pp. 399–416). Academic Press.

Tao, Y., & Xu, D., (2022). Combined effects of nonlinear proliferation and logistic damping in a three-component chemotaxis system for alopecia areata. *Nonlinear Analysis: Real World Applications*, *66*, 103517.

Tran, M. A., Gowda, R., Sharma, A., Park, E. J., Adair, J., Kester, M., Smith, N. B., & Robertson, G. P., (2008). Targeting V600EB-Raf and Akt3 using nanoliposomal-small interfering RNA inhibits cutaneous melanocytic lesion development. *Cancer Research*, *68*(18), 7638–7649.

Viegas, J. S., Praca, F. G., Caron, A. L., Suzuki, I., Silvestrini, A. V., Medina, W. S., Del Ciampo, J. O., et al., (2020). Nanostructured lipid carrier co-delivering tacrolimus and TNF-α siRNA as an innovate approach to psoriasis. *Drug Deliv Translational Res.*, *10*(3), 646–660.

Weidinger, S., & Novak, N., (2016). Atopic dermatitis. *Lancet*, *387*(10023), 1109–1122.

Wu, J., Huang, W., & He, Z., (2013). Dendrimers as carriers for siRNA delivery and gene silencing: A review. *The Scientific World Journal*, 630654.

Yang, G., Zhang, Y., & Gu, Z., (2018). Punching and electroporation for enhanced transdermal drug delivery. *Theranostics*, *8*(13), 3688.

Yokozeki, H. A., (2014). Nucleic acid-based medication for allergic skin diseases. *J. Dermatol. Sci.*, *75*, 75–81.

Zhang, B., Alysandratos, K. D., Angelidou, A., et al., (2011). Human mast cell degranulation and preformed TNF secretion require mitochondrial translocation to exocytosis sites: Relevance to atopic dermatitis. *J. Allergy Clin. Immunol.*, *127*, 1522–1531.

Zheng, D., Giljohann, D. A., Chen, D. L., Massich, M. D., Wang, X. Q., Iordanov, H., Mirkin, C. A., & Paller, A. S., (2012). Topical delivery of siRNA-based spherical nucleic acid nanoparticle conjugates for gene regulation. *Proc. Nat. Acad. Sci.*, *109*(30), 11975–11980.

CHAPTER 6

Improvement of Skin Cancer by Transdermal Drug Delivery System

BHUSHAN R. RANE,[1] NIDHI S. KATE,[1] SAMALI S. RAUT,RAJ K. KESERVANI,[2] and ASHISH S. JAIN[1]

[1]Shri D.D. Vispute College of Pharmacy and Research Center, Devad-Vichumbe, Panvel, Navi Mumbai, Maharashtra, India

[2]Faculty of B. Pharmacy, CSM Group of Institutions, Prayagraj, Uttar Pradesh, India

ABSTRACT

This review article combines research on medication delivery systems, most notably the transdermal method. TDDS have been employed as medication delivery devices that are both safe and effective. Their potential for sustained delivery is being explored globally by scientists with a high rate of achievement. Because of the various benefits of the TDDS, numerous studies are being conducted now to add newer medications into the system. Transdermal drug administration is the non-invasive distribution of drugs to the circulatory system from the surface of the skin. TDDS has numerous advantages over traditional injectable and oral techniques. Skin cancer is a rising problem in Western countries. Melanoma is most common in those who have fair skin and have been exposed to the sun for a long time, although other variables also play a role. The depletion of the ozone layer has led to an increase in UV-induced skin cancers. Other factors like environmental, genetic, and immunological problems add to the rising scale of this cancer. The risk of developing skin cancer, including both melanoma and nonmelanoma skin cancers, is linked to exposure to the sun. Use of sunscreen appropriately, limiting sun exposure, and avoiding tanning beds are all preventative methods.

Novel Nanocarriers forSkin Diseases: Advances and Applications.
Raj K. Keservani and Júlia Scherer Santos (Eds.)

6.1 INTRODUCTION

One of the most difficult delivery methods has been payload transfer over the epidermal barrier to the systemic circulation. Necessary skin needs and facilitated skin layer cross-over distribution attempts have resulted in the development of several non-invasive, non-oral methods, equipment, and systems that have been standardized, concurrently employed, and are undergoing continual upgrading and improvement. Transdermal delivery methods include iontophoresis, electroporation, sonophoresis, magnetophoresis, dermal patches, nanocarriers, needled and needle-free shots, and injectors. The current review examines the current state of the art, as well as the benefits and drawbacks of systems, devices, and transdermal delivery patches, including passage facilitation techniques for drugs and other payloads, permeation, and absorption feasibility studies, and physicochemical properties affecting delivery through various transdermal modes, as well as examples of drugs, vaccines, genes, and other payloads (Akhtar et al., 2020). The fact that most of skin malignancies are nonmelanomatous in nature. Keratinized epithelial cells give rise to malignant nonmelanoma skin tumors. Basal cell carcinoma (BCC) and squamous cell carcinoma (SCC) are two of these malignancies. Melanoma makes up roughly 2% of all malignant skin cancers, yet it is responsible for the majority of deaths. In 2010, more than 2 million instances of skin cancer were reported in the United States. The most frequent type of BCC is slow-growing and locally invasive. SCC is the second most frequent type of nonmelanomatous skin cancer, accounting for 20% to 30% of all occurrences (Linares et al., 2015).

6.1.1 TRANSDERMAL DRUG DELIVERY SYSTEM (DDS)

Transdermal drug delivery systems (DDSs) are topically administered medications in self-contained, discrete dosage forms that, when applied to the skin, deliver the drug to systemic circulation at a predetermined and controlled rate over a prolonged period of time to increase therapeutic efficacy and reduce drug toxicity. TDDS retains drug concentrations within the therapeutic window for an extended period of time, ensuring that levels do not fall below the minimum effective concentration or exceed the maximum effective concentration (Bala et al., 2014; Keservani et al., 2020a). Transdermal DDS prioritizes over other conventional delivery routes because it is a painless, non-invasive means of drug delivery (Akhtar et al., 2020). TDDS has been extensively researched over the last few decades due to advantages such as greater patient compliance, better drug release, tissue targeting, preventing pre-systemic metabolism in the liver, and many others. The stratum corneum (SC), on the other hand, is a rate-limiting barrier to drug absorption through the skin, that has been a never-ending issue in TDDS. Although the skin appears to be a suitable route of administration for local and systemic therapy, it is a challenging barrier to penetrate for most substances. The epidermis, dermis, and hypodermis are the three primary layers, with a total thickness range from 0.5 to 4 mm, depending on body regions, age, and sex (Roohnikan et al., 2019). The epidermis is a non-vascularized, multi-layered stratum in which cells receive nutrients by diffusion from the lower layers, with the SC, the outermost layer, acting as the significant obstacle to drug passage (Eckhart et al., 2013). The various types of nanoparticles and nanoemulsions currently being investigated for TDDS applications, desirable physicochemical characteristics of all these systems, their routes of permeation through the skin, and current advancements using these systems to treat conditions like alopecia, wound healing, psoriasis, and melanoma (Carter et al., 2019). Transdermal delivery has made a significant contribution to clinical practice, which is yet to completely realize its potential as a substitute for oral administration and parenteral routes. The clinical usage of first-generation transdermal delivery systems for the delivery of smaller, lipophilic, low-dose pharmaceuticals has increased steadily. Clinical products have also been developed employing second-generation delivery techniques such as chemical enhancers, noncavitational ultrasound, and iontophoresis; the ability of iontophoresis to control delivery rates promptly adds functionality. Microneedles, thermal ablation, microdermabrasion, electroporation, and transdermal delivery is positioned to greatly boost its influence on medicines by implementing these emerging second and third-generation enhancement techniques (Prausnitz et al., 2008). The ability of transdermal DDSs to cure cancer has been proven. They can lessen the side effects and toxicity linked with anticancer agents by increasing drug bioavailability by site-specific drug delivery (Kriplani et al., 2021). Nanoparticles such as lipid-based nanoparticles, liposomes, niosomes (Keservani et al., 2010, 2020, 2022), transfersomes (TRAs), ethosomes (ETOs), dendrimers (Gautam et al., 2018), micellar nanoparticles, polymeric, metallic, and magnetic nanostructures have all been studied for transdermal administration of drugs (Jijie et al., 2017).

6.1.2 ADVANTAGES OF TRANSDERMAL DELIVERY SYSTEMS

Because the transdermal route is convenient and safe, it is an appealing choice for delivery. The following are the advantages of delivering medications through the skin to attain systemic effects (Verma et al., 2017):

- Activity that is predictable and lasts a long time reducing unfavorable side effects.
- Avoiding drug level fluctuations.
- Boosting physiological and pharmacological actions.
- Enables the use of drugs with a short half-life and a restricted therapeutic window.
- First-pass metabolism is avoided.
- Increased patient compliance as a result of the elimination of numerous dosage regimens.
- It is simple to discontinue therapy at any moment.
- Maintain drug plasma concentrations.
- Make it possible for self-administration.
- Improve therapeutic efficacy.
- Preventing gastro-intestinal incompatibility.
- The ability to administer a drug to a certain place more selectively to sites of skin cancer.

6.1.3 PHYSIOLOGY OF SKIN

Skin contributes about 10% of the total body weight (Jiang et al., 2020). It is the first barrier from external microbial invasions and helps to prevent water loss. The thickness of the skin is 0.1 mm–1.5 mm (Lawton et al., 2019). The skin consists of three main layers: epidermis, dermis, and hypodermis.

The epidermis is the outermost layer of the skin, and it is keratinized or cornified. The SC layer of this epidermis consists of dead flattened corneocytes which are 10–15 layers and is surrounded by the lipid matrix (Jiang et al., 2020). This layer consists of keratinocytes which is a fundamental epidermal cell. Keratinocytes allow the continuous replenishing of the epidermis (Dehdashtian et al., 2018). Along with keratinocytes, it contains cells like melanocytes which are responsible for skin color. This layer also contains Langerhans cells and Merkel cells that are responsible for protection from UV radiation, Antigen representing cells (APCs), etc. (Jiang et al., 2020; Dehdashtian et al., 2018). As the epidermis is avascular that is, it does not have any blood vessels, the absorption of the active moiety depends upon the underneath layers. Hence this layer is the first barrier to absorption. Underneath the SC, we have a viable epidermis (Chen et al., 2018), this layer has a good hydration degree and hence provides faster and easier diffusion rates (Jiang et al., 2020).

The dermis is the next layer that is beneath the epidermis, it has a greater thickness as compared to the epidermis of 1–5 mm (Lawton et al., 2019). This layer consists of sweat glands, sebaceous glands, blood capillaries, hair follicles, lymphatic vessels, nerve endings, and connective tissues (Jiang et al., 2020). This layer receives an abundance of blood supply and consists of features like the apocrine gland, eccrine gland, and hair follicles. In place of keratinocytes, it contains mast cells, fibroblasts, and dendritic cells (Dehdashtian et al., 2018; Chen et al., 2018; Ramadon et al., 2021). The fibroblast is a major cell and is responsible for the synthesis of elastin, collagen, and viscous gel. The collagen makes up about 70% of the dermis, it toughens and strengthens the dermis layer. Elastin fibers help to provide elasticity to this layer. Both types of these cells are affected by age and UV radiation which causes the stretching or sagging of the skin. Mast cells are involved in inflammatory processes and mediate immune responses. The main functions of this layer are – (i) cushioning the deeper structures from mechanical injury; (ii) providing nourishment to the epidermis; (iii) wound healing; and (iv) protection (Lawton, 2019; Ramadon et al., 2021). The dermis consists of the capillary network which gives rise to the microcirculation system of nutrients, temperature regulation, and the systemic absorption of the drug (Jiang et al., 2020). The dermis is divided into two parts: (a) superficial dermis; and (b) deep dermis (Dehdashtian et al., 2018; Lawton, 2019).

Hypodermis lies below the dermis and has a high content of fat (Lawton, 2019). It is also called superficial fascia or the subcutaneous layer. The functions of hypodermis are: (i) to provide protection; (ii) to work as a connecting tissue between the skin, muscles, and bones; (iii) thermoregulation; and (iv) sense of touch or sensation (Lawton, 2019; Ramadon et al., 2021). As thus later mainly contains adipose tissues it helps in thermal insulation (Ramadon et al., 2021).

6.2 CHANCES OF SKIN CANCER AND ALLERGENS RESPONSIBLE

Skin carcinoma is not that common in India. India acquires the position of 32nd worldwide for skin melanoma. According to the WHO estimation, the number of new cases for the year 2020 was estimated at 3,916 which was 0.30% more than the previous year's estimation. The mortality rate was increased by 0.27% with cases of about 2,296.

For the year 2020, Australia along with Sweden and Finland are the leading countries according to the WHO estimation. Australia ranks third for emerging new cases of skin melanoma with an 8.1% increase in the incidence cases. Sweden ranks 5th with a 6.8% rise in the new cases also Finland ranks 5th with a 5.9% increase in the incidence cases.

6.2.1 FACTORS ASSOCIATED WITH SKIN CANCER

Numerous factors are involved in cancer. The major two factors are the biological and non-biological factors that are related to the pathogenesis of cutaneous cancers.

6.2.1.1 BIOLOGICAL FACTORS

These factors are called non-modifiable factors. The skin is the outermost layer of the body and is the largest organ. The main function of the skin is to protect from the external harmful environment. Some examples of harmful external factors are UV radiation, infectious microorganisms, toxic chemicals, and also mechanical stress. Skin is also responsible for exhibiting immune responses. Biological factors which cause the onset of action for skin cancers are responsible for the alteration of the protein synthesis. This shows a negative effect on the skin cells and impacts the proliferation of the skin, and this results in the rising of skin cancer like melanoma and non-melanoma skin cancers (Khan et al., 2022).

6.2.1.2 NON-BIOLOGICAL FACTORS

These factors are also called modifiable factors. The reasons associated with these factors are mainly environmental effects like exposure to harmful light, pollutants, etc., the skin helps in protecting against the environmental stresses which are chemical, biological, and physical. Hence again it shows negative effects on the skin cells giving rise to skin cancer (Khan et al., 2022). The most prevalent cause of skin melanoma is being exposed to harmful UV radiation for a prolonged period (Jordan et al., 2022). There are three types of UV radiation. UVA (ultraviolet A) produces reactive oxygen species (ROS), which when interacting with the lipids and proteins give rise to some intermediated capable of interacting with the DNA and resulting in the breakdown of the DNA. The most carcinogenic radiation is the UVB (ultraviolet B) radiation which causes structural damage to the DNA and RNA. Lastly, UVC (ultraviolet C) radiation's effects on the DNA are repairable. UVC rarely causes skin cancer (Khan et al., 2022).

6.2.2 THE OTHER FACTORS INCLUDE

6.2.2.1 GENETIC FACTORS

The phenotype of the skin, i.e., the color of the skin is very important. Also, the color associated with hair and freckles is an important phenotype feature. Xeroderma pigmentosa is a rare autosomal recessive DNA repair disorder in which the ability to repair the damage produced by UV radiation is impaired. This increases the risk of freckling, sunburn, and early childhood skin cancers in individuals. A mutation in the CDKN2A gene is the most common cause of hereditary melanoma. Women with mutations in the MDM2 gene are more likely to develop melanoma at a younger age (Craythorne et al., 2017).

6.2.2.2 OBESITY

The correlation between obesity and skin cancer is not yet clear. But some studies have shown a positive relationship between the two. It is seen that obesity gives rise to the formation of ROS which leads to the breakdown of the DNA molecule (Karimi et al., 2017).

6.2.2.3 ENVIRONMENTAL FACTORS

There are many factors contributing, and one cannot point to a single factor to be a major contributor. The factors listed include smoking, passive smoking, hair dyes, and hormone therapy. According to some evidence, using sunbeds or tanning salons can raise the risk of melanoma (Marks et al., 1995; Lai et al., 2018).

6.2.2.4 CHRONIC INFLAMMATION

Scars, burns, chronic ulcers, sinus tracts, or inflammatory diseases that cause persistent inflammation predispose to the development of SCC. In chronically inflamed conditions SCC is denoted as Marjolin ulcer. Approximately

1 of the skin cancers arise due to inflamed skin and 90 of the lesions present on the skin are due to SCC (Lai et al., 2018).

6.2.2.5 HUMAN PAPILLOMA VIRUS (HPV)

The relation between skin melanoma especially SCC is not very clear, but studies have shown that β-HPV type is associated with the cancerous activity. α-HPV has shown significant association in cancers like cervical but in contrast to that, the presence of β-HPV DNA does not appear to be required for the malignant phenotype to persist (Lai et al., 2018; Apalla et al., 2017).

6.2.2.6 TRANSPLANT/IMMUNOSUPPRESSION

The risk of developing cancer is seen to be more in patients with low or weak immunity also patients requiring high immunosuppression dose during transplants are likely to develop skin cancer specifically SCC (Rizvi et al., 2017; Carr et al., 2020). Immunosuppressants like cyclosporine and sirolimus have shown a contribution to increasing the risk of melanoma. For early identification of skin cancer, patients who had a transplant or have taken immunosuppressants should have a yearly checkup (Rizvi et al., 2017; Ascha et al., 2017).

6.3 SITES OF SKIN CANCER

The main risk factor for skin cancer is exposure to UV light. The most common types of cancer are basal cell and squamous cell cancers, which are linked to cumulative UV exposure over time. Melanoma, the most dangerous type, is more closely linked to prolonged sun exposure and sunburn. Melanoma can develop anywhere on the skin, not just where it has been sunburned. Always examine your entire body for anomalies in your skin, especially moles, but the most prevalent skin cancer areas are listed in subsections (Lewis et al., 2021).

6.3.1 FACE

It should come as no surprise that the most common site for skin cancer to occur is on your face. Nearly every single day of our life, our face is subjected to sunlight. And the most visible region of your face, your nose, is the most commonly affected by skin cancer. The good thing is that these tumors, which are mostly basal cell and squamous cell cancers, are frequently detected early and are quite easy to cure.

6.3.2 SCALP

The majority of scalp skin malignancies arise in balding men. Even if you have got a head of full hair, your scalp is nevertheless susceptible to infection. On the scalp, both melanomas, as well as nonmelanoma skin cancers, are frequent. So, keep watch on any patches on your scalp.

6.3.3 EARS

According to a recent study, the ear seems to be the third most prevalent site for basal cell skin carcinoma. Men's ears are highly susceptible, owing to shorter haircuts. To protect your ears, apply sunscreen to them every day and wear hats with at least a three-inch brim. Baseball caps and brimless hats will expose them.

6.3.4 NECK

Melanoma is frequently found in men's necks. Nonmelanoma skin cancers are significantly more common in these areas than melanomas, which account for one-third of all melanomas. Since your neck is exposed almost every day, make sure your daily facial sunscreen also covers your neck.

6.3.5 HANDS

The most frequent type of skin cancer that develops on the hands is SCC. Squamous cell skin tumors on the hand might be difficult to identify. Minor firm nodules, scaly or crusty skin, small wounds, or ulcers can all be symptoms of these malignancies. So don't dismiss a cut that isn't healing or a dry area that won't go away. Take precautions and have it tested.

6.3.6 THE BACK AND THE CHEST

Men's melanomas are mostly found on the trunk. While it is simple to check your chest for skin cancer, keeping an eye on your back may be more difficult. Use a well-lit mirror or enlist the help of another individual. Examine any new or changing areas that are becoming larger, darker, or uneven in any way.

6.3.7 LEGS

Melanoma is most commonly found in women's legs, particularly the lower legs. Melanoma is extremely treatable if detected in its early stages and detected frequently. So, inspect the backs of your legs, as well as your ankles and feet. Remember to apply sunscreen to your exposed legs. To avoid that oily feeling, apply daily skincare products with SPF 15.

6.3.8 HAND PALMS, FOOT SOLES, AND NAIL BEDS

These don't appear to be high-risk places for skin cancer. They are not in Caucasians. However, if you have darkly colored skin, these are the places to look. Melanoma is uncommon in dark-skinned people. However, half of all melanomas in African Americans arise in the palms, soles, and nail beds.

6.3.9 MUCOSAL MEMBRANES

SCC and melanoma can both develop on the mucous membranes of the body. Lips, the interior of the mouth, nasal passageways, and genital tissues are all included. SCC appears as an open sore, a crusty area, or a raised, bleeding tumor. While anybody can develop melanoma in these regions, people with darker skin are more likely to develop it in their mucous membranes.

6.3.10 IN BETWEEN YOUR TOES

If you don't look between your toes regularly, you should. And not merely to keep them clean. To notice changes, you must first discover what is usual for you. In this area, which is normally free of skin problems, search for dark spots, unhealed wounds, or other lesions.

6.4 TREATMENT AVAILABLE NOWADAYS

6.4.1 SURGERIES

For non-melanocytic skin cancer surgery is the best option for treatment which is done via radical excision. Recurrence occurs in only 5% of instances when a tumor less than 2 mm in diameter is removed with a perimeter of 4 mm of healthy skin. A 2–3 mm boundary is suitable for superficial tumors. The excision has to go all the way down to the hypodermis (Orthaber et al., 2017). High-risk lesions, mainly those restricted to the head and neck, are treated using Mohs micrographic surgery. This approach eliminates the tumor in stages, reducing smaller margins of tissue while providing 100% visualization of the margins. The benefit is that the tumor cure rate is higher than it is with traditional excisional surgery, and the method is tissue sparing, resulting in smaller, more cosmetically acceptable scars (Craythorne et al., 2017; Garrubba et al., 2020). Radical excision of the skin tumor or biopsy site is used as a local therapy for Melanocytic Melanoma. It is comprised of a healthy skin border and a tumor. The border's size is determined by the tumor's thickness and goes up to the deep fascia (Orthaber et al., 2017).

6.4.2 RADIOTHERAPY

Radiation therapy is used when surgical treatment cannot be opted, like cancers in the craniofacial areas. It is seen that the recurrence rate for BCC was 5% when treated with radiotherapy. The diversity of radiotherapy makes it more approachable depending on various skin cancers. In radiation therapy, the dose is very important so that it remains confined to the affected area and does not harm the healthy tissues. Radionuclide brachytherapy, electronic brachytherapy, X-ray therapy, and electron beam therapy are various methods of radiation therapy. The side effects associated with this type of therapy are alopecia, acute skin toxicity, and change in skin pigment (Pashazadeh et al., 2019; Craythorne et al., 2017).

6.4.3 PHOTODYNAMIC

It is an FDA-approved light-based therapy. This therapy can be used to treat BCC, non-melanoma skin cancer, and actinic keratoses. It is a 2-step procedure that utilizes a photosensitizer, methyl aminolevulinate, or 5-aminolevulinic acid (ALA) and a light source for activation. The photosensitizer is applied to the skin which is absorbed by the keratinocytes and takes time to produce a sufficient amount of porphyrin IX. Once porphyrin is accumulated in the tissue a wavelength of specific requirement is introduced to the skin and this leads to the destruction of the tumor cells (Collins et al., 2019; Champeau et al., 2019).

6.4.4 CRYOSURGERY

Cryosurgery, also called cryotherapy utilizes sub-zero temperature which causes the destruction of the tumor cells. The freeze–slow thaw protocol is fast, and it reaches up to –50°C to –60°C. This causes the lesions to freeze in just 40–90 seconds. The time and temperature for the exposure of the affected skin depend upon the width and the depth of the tumor. It is seen that a decrease in the temperature causes improper eradiation of the tumor-affected skin. This method is effective to treat superficial BCC. The common reactions due to cryotherapy are pain, blistering, alopecia, delayed wound healing, etc. Also, due to a lack of knowledge in the histological margin, it is recommended to use this therapy for low-risk lesions. This method is very beneficial for superficial BCC (Collins et al., 2019; Zimmerman et al., 2012; Kauvar et al., 2015; Craythorne et al., 2017).

6.4.5 HEDGEHOG INHIBITORS

The Hedgehog (Hh) Inhibitors like Vismodegib (Erivedge, Genentech) or Sonidegib (Odomzo, Sun Pharma) are used for the treatment of BCC. Both of these drugs can be given orally. They have shown a response in decreasing the tumor size. This type of approach is mainly used to decrease the tumor size before any surgical intrusions or to be used as a long-term therapy by maintaining the size of the tumor. For patients undergoing this treatment method, a proper follow-up to manage the side effects is a must. The adverse effects of this treatment are muscle spasms, weight loss, dysgeusia, and alopecia. The studies have shown that alternative dosage regimes, such as one-to-three-week drug breaks, have been found to improve clinical outcomes and reduce toxicity (Collins et al., 2019; Villani et al., 2020).

6.4.6 HERBAL APPROACH

People nowadays prefer and use herbal skincare products since they have fewer negative effects and are more cost-effective. Herbal preparations are traditionally applied to a specific area or part of the skin to cure various skin disorders. Creams, gels, ointments, lotions, and foams are examples of topical formulations. Plant-derived natural compounds like alkaloids, phenols, essential oils, and isoflavones have been utilized for many dermatological problems. Several herbal remedies have been discovered for their ability to treat UV irradiation and are attracting a lot of attention (Sharma et al., 2022). Many spices show actions like anti-inflammatory, antioxidant, and anti-tumorigenic properties and the contribution of India is about 75% of global production in spices (Sreedhar et al., 2018). Some herbal medications are mentioned in subsections.

6.4.6.1 TURMERIC

It is the oldest known medication in Ayurveda. The main ingredient, curcumin is derived from the rhizome of turmeric (*Curcuma longa*). It possesses antiseptic, anti-inflammatory, antioxidant, and anti-tumorigenic properties (Gautam et al., 2020). A transcription factor NF-kB is upregulated in skin melanoma, and inhibition of this expression has shown a potential use of turmeric in skin cancer disorders (Sreedhar et al., 2018). Curcumin also has the property to stop or slow down the cell growth of cancerous cells (Trivedi et al., 2020). The problem of low bioavailability and low stability of turmeric via the oral route can be overcome by using a topical approach (Cullen et al., 2019).

6.4.6.2 GINGER

Ginger (*Zingiber officinale*) is a widely used spice as well as medication in Asian countries. It is considered to be a superfood since it has remarkable medicinal value (Sreedhar et al., 2018). The antioxidant and anti-inflammatory characteristics of ginger's active components help to prevent cancer from spreading (Trivedi et al., 2020). It also has the ability to suppress NF-kB activity by exerting anti-angiogenic and anti-inflammatory actions against it. Ginger extracts are being tried on cancer patients after multiple preclinical research revealed that ginger and its key components have anti-carcinogenic capabilities (Sreedhar et al., 2018). It was found that topical treatment of ginger (1 mg, 2 mg, or 4 mg/animal) was effective in preventing chemically induced carcinogenesis in mice for the first time (Katiyar et al., 1996).

6.4.6.3 GARLIC

Garlic (*Allium sativum*) is another typical flavoring component that has been used as an herbal treatment for generations. For its anti-inflammatory, antibacterial, and antioxidant characteristics, it is one of the most researched substances. Several studies have found an inverse relationship between daily garlic consumption and the risk of cancer. Garlic, both orally and topically applied, has demonstrated encouraging benefits in mice with chemically induced cutaneous pappilomagenesis. Ajoene was found to be efficacious when applied topically to patients with nodular or superficial base cell carcinoma (BCC) (Sreedhar et al., 2018). The bio-active allelic component is activated when the garlic bulb is chopped/crushed. Garlic is a well-known antibiotic that inhibits the growth of cancer-causing cells (Trivedi et al., 2020).

6.4.6.4 AMLA

In the Indian Ayurveda system, Indian gooseberry is a vital medicinal plant. Indian gooseberry is used for both medical and nutritional purposes. Because of its antioxidant qualities, it is utilized in cosmetics. Ascorbic acid is abundant in Amla. B-Glucogallin plays an important function in photoprotection effectiveness. It increases UV-B stress resistance by exhibiting a ROS inhibitory effect. It also prevents skin tanning caused by UV exposure by inhibiting UV-induced melanogenesis (Gautam et al., 2020). It's a superfood from the Ayurvedic tradition. Vitamin C is abundant in this fruit. It contains quercetin, phalambs compound, and gallic acid tannins, which boosts its rejuvenating power. Amla extract can kill tumor cells (Trivedi et al., 2020).

6.4.6.5 SANDALWOOD

Sandalwood (*Santalum album* L.) can prevent skin wrinkle and skin aging caused due to UV radiation. The main constituent, α- and β-santolol have been incorporated into herbal sunscreen (Trivedi et al., 2020). It shows therapeutic effects against eczema, atopic dermatitis (AD), and psoriasis (Sharma et al., 2022).

6.5 APPROACHES FOR TREATMENT OF SKIN CANCER

Nanotechnology is well acknowledged for being an essential method for therapeutic agent delivery in cancer therapy (Jarouliya et al., 2018). The systematic evolution of anticancer medication nanocarriers has resulted in improved systems that can target malignant tissues and cells (Marianecci et al., 2014). Given the quantity of events and obstacles involved in skin cancer, numerous types of NPs have been proposed and can be categorized firstly based on the main formulation component (Estanqueiro et al., 2015) Liposomes, transferosomes, niosomes, ETOs, solid lipid NPs, and liquid crystalline nanodispersions are examples of lipid-based nanoparticles; polymeric-based carriers include polymer NPs, polymeric micelles, and dendrimers (Pradhan et al., 2013). Combining nanostructured therapeutic ingredients in NPs with dose forms is a new and underutilized method of administering nanoparticles (Feitosa et al., 2019). These nanoparticles can be used in topical dosage forms such as creams (Hafeez et al., 2017; Abdulbaqi et al., 2016), hydrogels and ointments (Garg et al., 2016; Gabriel et al., 2016), patches (Abdulbaqi et al., 2016; Chen et al., 2015), and patches for topical penetration (Gabriel et al., 2016; Sun et al., 2017; Senyigit et al., 2012).

6.5.1 POLYMER-BASED NANOPARTICLES

Polymeric Nanoparticles have several appealing qualities as drug delivery vehicles, including ease of manipulation, functionalizing, and modifying capacity to functionalize and modify the surface with different ligands, control over behavior *in vivo*, biodegradability, and biocompatibility (Elzoghby et al., 2016; Ekladious et al., 2019). Though using such nanocarriers with various therapeutic compounds that can be transported across biological membranes is currently in development, polymeric NPs are most often supplied by systemic, intravenous injection (Ekladious et al., 2019). Protein NPs provide diverse interactions with drugs and three-dimensional networks to offer several reversible drug molecule assemblies (Elzoghby et al., 2012). Pluronics®, for example, is composed of poly(ethylene oxide)-poly(propylene oxide)-poly(ethylene oxide) (PEO-PPO-PEO). The PPO unit is a hydrophobic component that comprises 30% of the copolymer composition, as well as the PEO unit is the polymer's hydrophilic component. Pluronic F® (Bunjes et al., 2011) is a copolymer that has gained popularity due to its numerous therapeutic applications. Pluronic F® (Bunjes et al., 2011) is used to produce the hydrophobic core PPO, which provides the atmosphere for lipophilic drug inclusion. As a result, the PEO section prevents an integrated protein from adsorbing and aggregating (Muhammad et al., 2015). Drugs can be incorporated into polymeric micelles through physical, chemical, or electrostatic interactions (Park et al., 2008; Hamaguchi et al., 2007). Genexol-PM (PEG-poly(D,L-lactide)-paclitaxel, a polymeric micelle formulated paclitaxel, is an example of a polymeric micelle formulation (Senapati et al., 2018; Hamaguchi et al., 2007). Polymer-drug conjugates, on the other hand, are macromolecular agglomerates generated by one or more medicinal agents, such as small drug particles, proteins, and peptides, bound to a polymeric carrier structure via covalent bonds (Ekladious et al., 2019). Because proteins are natural polymers with such a wide range of molecular weights and sizes, uneven nanoparticle size distributions might vary from batch to batch (Malafaya et al., 2007). Animal proteins such as gelatin, collagen, albumin, silk proteins, and elastin are suitable raw materials since they are absorbable and their degradation products are less hazardous than synthetic polymers (Elzoghby et al., 2012). Furthermore, the availability of amino and carboxyl functional groups makes them more likely to bind, which is advantageous for targeting moieties and surface modifications (Senapati et al., 2018). Elastin-like polypeptide (ELP) nanoparticles are a promising medication delivery method for a variety of uses (Elzoghby et al., 2012; Oppen et al., 2019). Because of their amphiphilic nature, biodegradability, and immunogenicity in a unified system, these particles are great candidates. Because of their potential to penetrate deep into tumor sites after temperature-induced assembly with CPPs such as octa-arginine, ELP NPs were recently produced (Oppen et al., 2019), as well as the ability to reversibly self-assemble in micellar aggregates for photodynamic treatment (Pille et al., 2017). Furthermore, NPs derived from plant proteins like zein, and gliadin represent a novel approach for NP generation due to some advantages (Duclairoir et al., 1998). Due to the high hydrophobic nature of certain proteins, NPs made with them may require chemical or physical modification (Borgheti-Cardoso et al., 2020). Due to the structural diversity of such membranes, other polymer-based Nanoparticles, such as polymersomes, which are composed of liposomal membranes made of amphiphilic polymers, have received considerable interest (Schulz et al., 2012). A hybrid polymeric Nanoparticle system was developed and tested *in vitro* for benzocaine penetration and NP tracking in the artificial membrane (Grillo et al., 2019), as a method of medication delivery through the skin (Wakabayashi et al., 2018) created an appealing solid-in-oil (S/O) nanodispersion for transcutaneously administering hydrophilic molecules (Wakabayashi et al., 2018). Nanosized hydrogels in the submicrometer range are frequently referred to as nanogels, and they are created by chemical or physical cross-linking polymers. When swelled in water, this polymer network can expand to a few hundreds of nanometers in size (Li et al., 2015). Recently, it has been used for cancer imaging and medication delivery vehicles (Senapati et al., 2018).

6.5.2 LIPID-BASED NANOPARTICLES

Lipid nanoparticles are the most common nanocarriers, and they are mostly made up of lipid vesicles known as liposomes, which may transport both lipophilic and hydrophilic medicines (Grimaldi et al., 2016; Sala et al., 2018). The colloidal carriers are made up of lipids and phospholipids, which have the benefit of being physiologically equivalent (Pradhan et al., 2013). The majority of liposomes are phospholipid-based vesicles with a lipophilic chain and a hydrophilic head that can self-assemble (Sala et al., 2018). The absorption of hydrophilic compounds encapsulated within an aqueous core or hydrophobic compounds in the membrane bilayers is improved by these nanoparticles (Bellefroid et al., 2019). Furthermore, by utilizing appropriate preparation methods, amphiphilic compounds can be incorporated into a liposome core (Senapati et al., 2018). The content, elasticity, and deformability of these nanocarriers can be tailored to meet specific requirements (Sala et al., 2018). As a result, because big liposomes are restricted from the deeper skin layers, a microfluidic process can be used to create small and largely monodisperse liposomes with a width of roughly 30–40 nm to improve the ability of these lipid Nanoparticles to permeate the skin (Hood et al., 2014). Furthermore, *in vitro* experiments revealed that combining liposomes with biocompatible copolymers resulted in the creation of vesicles with improved potential to enter deep skin layers (Freitas et al., 2019). TRAs, which are deformable vesicles employed for medication administration to the skin, enter the SC pores by squeezing along an intracellular encapsulating lipid (Pradhan et al., 2013; Trotta et al., 2004). The production of niosomes is caused by hydrating synthetic non-ionic surfactants in the inclusion or exclusion of cholesterol as well as other lipids (Marianecci et al., 2014; Pradhan et al., 2013). ETOs are non-invasive nanocarriers composed mostly of phospholipids, ethanol, and water and are found in varying amounts in ethanol (Abdulbaqi et al., 2016). Touitou was the first to describe employing these NPs to improve medication penetration into deep epidermal layers (Touitou et al., 2000). Based on the influence of the matrix and nanoparticles components, small-sized vehicles in the lipid matrix release medicines (Bunjes et al., 2011). Solid lipid NPs, which range in size from 50 to 1,000 nm and are comprised of lipids that may organize and form a dispersion in water or surfactant solutions, are among these particles (Pradhan et al., 2013). Second-generation lipid NPs with a solid matrix containing liquid lipids in a ratio ranging from 70:30 to 99.9:0.1 are known as nanostructured lipid carriers (NLCs) (Sala et al., 2018; Qidwai et al., 2016). In addition to lipid-based delivery systems, liquid crystalline systems can integrate hydrophilic, lipophilic, and amphiphilic compounds, as well as modify their release depending on the phase in which NPs are formed. These lyotropic liquid crystalline NPs are made up of mesophases such as lamellar, hexagonal, and cubic phases. Each mesophase will produce nanosystems with distinct characteristics, such as different behaviors in molecule incorporation, varied sequences of molecule release, tissue penetration degree, and physically stable (Borgheti et al., 2017; Praca et al., 2017; Rossetti et al., 2016).

6.5.3 INORGANIC NANOPARTICLES

Because of their enormous surface area, better drug loading capacity, and less toxic side effects, inorganic nanocomposites have been studied for imaging and treatment (Senapati et al., 2018; Lu et al., 2010), excellent biocompatibility, and magnetic characteristics that are size-dependent 1 (Borgheti et al., 2017) Biomedical uses of gold nanorods (Au-NRs) have been investigated (Yang et al., 2015; Chen et al., 2016) due to their excellent photothermal conversion performance, and photothermic therapy (PTT) (Younis et al., 2019). Gold nanostructure-based plasmonic hybrids, on the other hand, have been developed to outperform PTT (Tan et al., 2017; Larsen et al., 2016). Due to its strong reactivity with endogenous hydrogen peroxide inside the tumor microenvironment, manganese dioxide (MnO_2) NPs have been employed to generate O_2, bypassing tumor photodynamic resistance by creating O_2 *in situ* (Zhu et al., 2016; Qian et al., 2016). Cancer cells proliferate rapidly and are also controlled by the cell cycle and DNA synthesis, and ruthenium-based anticancer medication candidates are utilized in one technique to treat DNA damage as one of many metallotherapeutics licensed by the US Food and Drug Administration (FDA) (Villemin et al., 2019; Komor et al., 2013). As a result, at a controlled rate, the metallopolymer prodrug generated by covalent attachment of the ruthenium complex to the polymer can be transformed into an active drug (Villemin et al., 2019), because of its minimally invasive nature, precise application, and localized scope of treatment, a combination of photodynamic therapy (PDT) and PTT is currently providing favorable applications in cancer treatment and is overcoming the inherent limitations of PDT, such that it has achieved attention for malignant tumor treatment, even surpassing conventional therapy technologies such as chemotherapy and radiotherapy (Younis et al., 2019). CNTs are artificial nanoparticles well known for their perfect near-infrared PDT potential, which allows them to raise the temperature within malignancies (Huang et al., 2010; Zhou et al., 2011). Because of its nontoxicity, ease of overcoming biological barriers, and capacity to transport compounds to the cytoplasm, water-soluble CNTs are all being studied for gene and medication delivery (Bianco et al., 2005). Furthermore, combining the effectiveness of different nanostructures in a hybrid construct demonstrates the increased physicochemical characteristics of both agents and demonstrates remarkable functioning by combining the impacts of two different nanostructures (Strelow et al., 2016; da Silva et al., 2016). Inorganic NPs' medication delivery potential and imaging capabilities have increased dramatically in recent years. These "nanotheranostic" NPs have been widely employed in breast and liver cancer treatment and diagnosis; however, few studies on skin cancer have been reported (Elzoghby et al., 2016; Lim et al., 2015). Although there are few studies on skin cancer, those that have been published have shown promising theranostic Nanoparticles for melanoma diagnosis and treatment, indicating that additional study is needed in this field. After irradiation with a NIR laser, gold nanoparticles (AuNPs) functionalized with anti-nucleolin aptamer (AS1) (Pille et al., 2017) and iron oxide nanoparticles functionalized with IR80 have been demonstrated to be effective magnetic resonance scanning probes that elicit selective toxicity in A375 melanoma cells (Grabowska-Jadach et al., 2019; Hou et al., 2017). Cobalt ferrite oxide nanotubes encapsulated in nanoemulsions demonstrated intense time-dependent aggregation in a mouse melanoma xenograft model, indicating that they could be used for MRI imaging. Li et al. studied a new strategy for tumor surveillance and therapy utilizing photoacoustic and ultrasonic technologies recently. They created a multifunctional polymeric NP containing Au-NRs and aqueous perfluorocarbon linked to a monoclonal antibody (MAGE-1 antibody). They discovered that theranostic NPs preferentially targeted melanoma tumor cells *in vivo*, and that they remained at the spot for a long time (Li et al., 2018). An ELP-conjugated gold NPs displayed photothermal properties in another investigation. Furthermore, a single intra-tumoral injection of ELP-gold NPs allowed for simultaneous photothermal, photoacoustic, and X-ray computerized tomographic imaging as well as PTT of the melanoma (Sun et al., 2017).

6.5.4 OTHER NANOPARTICLES

The conjugation of therapeutic drugs to polymeric carriers has other advantages as well. Polymer–drug conjugate therapeutics are constructs that include one or more therapeutic agents, including the first market-approved polymer–protein conjugate, and discuss advancements in various classes of polymer-drug conjugates, such as polymer-small-molecule and polymer–protein drug conjugates, dendrimers, and polymer nanoparticles (Ekladious et al., 2019). Furthermore, electrostatic interactions between cationic polymers and negative charge nucleic acids like plasmid DNA or small interfering RNA (siRNA) resulted in polyplexes (Novo et al., 2015; Lächelt et al., 2015). These structures are useful for the complex formation of genetic material since cationic lipids can also give negative charges. The form of these so-called lipoplexes is determined by the composition of cationic lipids, helper lipids, and the DNA or RNA (He et al., 2010; Schroeder et al., 2010). Lipopolyplexes are noncovalently linked constructions that combine cationic liposomes, cationic polymers, and RNA or DNA (Thomas et al., 2018; Heissig et al., 2016).

6.6 DRUGS AVAILABLE FOR TRANSDERMAL ADMINISTRATION (TABLE 6.1)

TABLE 6.1 Drugs Available for Transdermal Drug Delivery

Drug	Nano-Carrier	Target	Strategy for Drug Delivery	Outcome	References
Aluminum chloride phthalocyanine	Solid lipid nanoparticles	Cellular toxicity	Irradiation with lasers	Increased phototoxicity of NPs was observed when the laser light radiation was increased to 1.0 J/cm^{-2}. After being exposed to a free photosensitizer, cellular viability remains unchanged.	Goto et al. (2017)
Camptothecin	Magnetic nanoparticles	Controlled drug release	Size modification	Under the influence of a dynamic magnetic field, drug-loaded magnetic nanoparticles of 150 nm size form clusters by assembling or disassembling.	Kong et al. (2010); Soheilian et al. (2015)
Chlorine 6 and docetaxel	Polymeric nanoparticles	Cellular apoptosis	Ultrasound	When nanoparticles were combined with ultrasound exposure, the rate of apoptosis and cellular necrosis increased. Following sonodynamic therapy, elevated amounts of ROS were detected, which are responsible for cellular necrosis caused by mitochondrial damage.	Gaio et al. (2019)
Cisplatin	Dendrimer nano-bomb	Boost tumor penetration and treatment efficacy.	Modulation of the tumor microenvironment.	The drug-loaded dendrimer particles aggregate in the tumor's weakly acidic environment (at neutral pH, 80 nm, and at the tumor site, less than 10 nm).	Li et al. (2016)
Cisplatin	pH-responsive lipid nanoparticles.	Cytotoxicity	Microneedle	After treatments with microneedle and NP, a xenograft tumor model showed decreased tumor weight and volume. Apoptosis and tumor cell cytotoxicity were also markedly elevated.	Lan et al. (2018)
Curcumin and topotecan	Nano-capsule nanoconjugate and microbubble.	Growth rate of tumor and toxicity.	Ultrasound	Ultrasound causes moderate hyperthermia, which slows tumor development via a non-coagulative necrotic mechanism. Animals treated with ultrasonography survived at a rate of 93%, while untreated animals survived at a rate of 26%.	Prasad et al. (2019)

TABLE 6.1 *(Continued)*

Drug	Nano-Carrier	Target	Strategy for Drug Delivery	Outcome	References
Dasatinib	Micelle	Tumor tissue specification and improved circulation time with tumor accumulation.	Functionalization of ligand.	When compared to non-functionalized micelles, tumor targeting was improved.	Yao et al. (2017)
Docetaxel	Spiro pyran nanoparticles.	Tumor penetration.	Size modification.	When exposed to ultraviolet (UV), nanoparticles shrink to 49 nm from roughly 100 nm.	Tong et al. (2012, 2013)
Docetaxel	Micelle loaded nanocapsules.	Tumor penetration.	Size modification.	Pea-like nano-capsules for drug-loaded micelle transport can be aimed at tumor cells and activated by infrared (808 nm) radiation.	Lin et al. (2016)
Docetaxel	PEGylated gold nanorod and micelles.	Cellular necrosis.	Microneedle	When microneedle and photothermal treatment were combined the results were more effective than when the treatments were not combined.	Hao et al. (2017)
Doxorubicin	NO generating liposome	Controlled drug release	Size modification	Polyamidoamine dendrimers loaded with doxorubicin and NO-donating nitroso glutathione liposomes combined into a single big nanocarrier and targeted to tumors. Large nanocarriers were disrupted by ultra-sonic therapy, releasing dendrimers and liposomes.	Wang et al. (2017)
Ferrous chlorophyllin	Transethosomes	Tumor targeting	Irradiation with lasers	After *in vivo* photodynamic therapy treatment, 50% of mice demonstrated total tumor elimination after 2 months, and almost all animals reported a significant decrease in tumor volume over a 7-day period.	Rady et al. (2018)

TABLE 6.1 *(Continued)*

Drug	Nano-Carrier	Target	Strategy for Drug Delivery	Outcome	References
Metoxantrone	PEGylated gold NPs	–	Irradiation with lasers	The maximal photodynamic treatment efficacy of the nanoparticles was observed at a radiation intensity of 1.3 J/cm^2 and a drug concentration of 6 μm.	Keyal et al. (2019)
Paclitaxel	Transferosomes	R8H3 peptide as a cell-penetrating peptide.	–	Chemotherapeutic drugs penetrated the skin more effectively. The hydrogel of transfersomes improved its ability to permeate tumor stroma and transport through tumor cells.	Jang et al. (2017)
Phthalocyanine with dabrafenib and trametinib.	Mesoporous silica nanoparticles.	Controlled drug release and tissue penetration.	Microneedle	For the first 10 minutes, there was no noticeable difference in the number of nanoparticles in microneedle-treated versus untreated skin. However, the skin penetration rate of Nanoparticles increased in the microneedle-treated group to 63%, compared to 27.2% in the non-microneedle-treated group.	Tham et al. (2018)
Vertoporphyrin	Mesoporous silica nanoparticles	Cellular toxicity	Irradiation with lasers	Infrared irradiation for 120 and 180 seconds reduced cell growth by 50–70%.	Straten et al. (2017)
Vismodegib	Ultra-deformable liposomes.	Hyaluronic acid	Functionalization of ligand	Liposomes were modified to target specific binding sites on tumor-surface receptors.	Calienn et al. (2019)

6.7 PATENTED FORMULATION (TABLE 6.2)

TABLE 6.2 List of Patents

Patent Publication No.	Inventors	Year	Title	Description	References
US20120207840A1	Elisabet de losPinos	2012	Virion derived protein nanoparticles for delivering diagnostic or therapeutic agents for the treatment of non-melanoma skin cancer.	The invention provides a transdermal drug delivery system for the treatment of non-melanoma skin cancer that uses protein nanoparticles to deliver drugs to keratinocytes and basal membrane cells.	de LosPinos et al. (2012)
US8865772B2	Michael E. Silver	2017	Method for treating skin cancer.	The application of an isothiocyanate functional surfactant to a cancer-affected area on the skin for treating skin cancer.	Silver et al. (2017)
US5736154A	Richard C. Fuisz	1998	Transdermal delivery system.	The current invention drug delivery system and intra-lesioned injection of interferon to the individual in a controlled, sustained release way are used to treat individuals with nodulo-ulcerative carcinomas.	Fuisz et al. (1998)
US20040241249A1	Tina Sampalis	2004	Krill and/or marine extracts for prevention and/or treatment of cardiovascular diseases arthritis, skin cancer diabetes, premenstrual syndrome, and transdermal transport.	A medically effective amount of krill and/or marine oil is administered to a patient in this procedure. The study showed that krill oil when used transdermal showed an effect against the UVB radiation which is a cause of skin cancer.	Sampalis et al. (2004)

6.8 CONCLUSION

Skin cancer is a disease that can be prevented, mostly by lifestyle modifications, rather than an unavoidable cause of aging. The factors contributing to the proliferation of this disease are both manageable and non-manageable. The manageable factors are the ones that humans can work on. The newly developed non-invasive therapies help in increasing patient compliance in the treatment of skin cancer. Individuals not only opt for chemical therapy but also prefer herbal therapy as well. Herbal or Ayurvedic therapies seem to be less toxic and also have fewer side effects but may take a longer duration to show therapeutic effect than conventional therapies. Also, novel drug delivery treatment strategies should possess a number of characteristics. They should, for example, be more effective, less expensive, and pose no risk to the patient's life. Optimal treatment should be designed with increased overall treatment efficiency, very low possible toxicity, and a specific targeted site to achieve patient safety and compliance.

6.9 FUTURE PROSPECTIVES

Transdermal delivery methods were created as a way to avoid the issues that come with oral and injection dose forms. There are a variety of enhancement tactics that can be used to make transdermal delivery systems better. The emerging technology in the treatment of skin cancer has much potential in near future. The non-invasive treatment, as well as targeted treatment, will help in decreasing the side effects and toxic levels. To ensure the safety, effectiveness, and validity of clinical phase data, additional bioequivalence studies must be done. Furthermore, it is critical that manufacturing and industrial scale-up be adequately considered. Aseptic manufacturing and large-scale production procedures are frequently linked to this topic. Furthermore, it is unsurprising that modern technology and high-tech equipment will be required for the required quality assurance methods. As a result, the final product's pricing will be influenced by this high-cost process. Furthermore, before a product can be considered for use in clinical settings, the necessary regulatory authorities must provide guidelines on acceptable production conditions so that systems can be manufactured efficiently.

KEYWORDS

- **cryosurgery**
- **drugs**
- **inorganic nanoparticles**
- **mucosal membranes**
- **radiotherapy**
- **skin cancer**
- **transdermal drug delivery**

REFERENCES

Abdulbaqi, I. M., Darwis, Y., Khan, N. A. K., Assi, R. A., & Khan, A. A., (2016). Ethosomal nanocarriers: The impact of constituents and formulation techniques on ethosomal properties, *in vivo* studies, and clinical trials. *Int. J. Nanomedicine, 11*, 2279–2304. https://doi.org/10.2147/IJN.S105016.

Akash, M. S. H., & Rehman, K., (2015). Recent progress in biomedical applications of Pluronic (PF127): Pharmaceutical perspectives. *J. Control. Release, 209*, 120–138. https://doi.org/10.1016/J.JCONREL.2015.04.032.

Akhtar, N., Singh, V., Yusuf, M., & Khan, R. A., (2020). Non-invasive drug delivery technology: Development and current status of transdermal drug delivery devices, techniques and biomedical applications. *Biomedical Engineering/Biomedizinische Technik, 65*(3), 243–272. https://doi.org/10.1515/bmt-2019-0019.

Apalla, Z., Nashan, D., Weller, R. B., & Castellsagué, X., (2017). Skin cancer: Epidemiology, Disease burden, pathophysiology, diagnosis, and therapeutic approaches. *Dermatol. Ther. (Heidelb.), 7* (Suppl 1), 5–19. https://doi.org/10.1007/s13555-016-0165-y.

Ascha, M., Ascha, M. S., Tanenbaum, J., & Bordeaux, J. S., (2017). Risk factors for melanoma in renal transplant recipients. *JAMA Dermatol., 153*(11), 1130. https://doi.org/10.1001/jamadermatol.2017.2291.

Bala, P., Jathar, S., Kale, S. N., & Pal, K., (2014). Transdermal drug delivery system (TDDS) – a multifaceted approach for drug delivery. *Journal of Pharmacy Research*, 1805–1835.

Bellefroid, C., Lechanteur, A., Evrard, B., & Piel, G., (2019). Lipid gene nanocarriers for the treatment of skin diseases: Current state-of-the-art. *Eur. J. Pharm. Biopharm., 137*, 95–111. https://doi.org/10.1016/j.ejpb.2019.02.012.

Bianco, Kostarelos, K., & Prato, M., (2005). Applications of carbon nanotubes in drug delivery. *Curr. Opin. Chem. Biol., 9*, 674–679. https://doi.org/10.1016/j.cbpa.2005.10.005.

Borgheti-Cardoso, L. N., Kooijmans, S. A. A., Fens, M. H. A. M., Van, D. M. R., Vicentini, F. T. M. C., Fantini, M. C. A., Bentley, M. V. L. B., & Schiffelers, R. M., (2017). In situ gelling liquid crystalline system as local siRNA delivery system. *Mol. Pharm., 14*, 1681–1690. https://doi.org/10.1021/acs.molpharmaceut.6b01141.

Bunjes, H., (2011). Structural properties of solid lipid based colloidal drug delivery systems. *Curr. Opin. Colloid Interface Sci., 16,* 405–411. https://doi.org/10.1016/j.cocis.2011.06.007.

Calienni, M. N., Febres-Molina, C., Llovera, R. E., Zevallos-Delgado, C., Tuttolomondo, M. E., Paolino, D., Fresta, M., et al., (2019). Nanoformulation for potential topical delivery of vismodegib in skin cancer treatment. I*nternational Journal of Pharmaceutics, 565,* 108–122. https://doi.org/10.1016/j.ijpharm.2019.05.002.

Carr, S., Smith, C., & Wernberg, J., (2020). Epidemiology and risk factors of melanoma. *Surg. Clin. North Am., 100*(1), 1–12. https://doi.org/10.1016/j.suc.2019.09.005.

Carter, P., Narasimhan, B., & Wang, Q., (2019). Biocompatible nanoparticles and vesicular systems in transdermal drug delivery for various skin diseases. *International Journal of Pharmaceutics, 555,* 49–62. https://doi.org/10.1016/j.ijpharm.2018.11.032.

Champeau, M., Vignoud, S., Mortier, L., & Mordon, S., (2019). Photodynamic therapy for skin cancer: How to enhance drug penetration? *J. Photochem. Photobiol. B, 197*(111544), 111544. https://doi.org/10.1016/j.jphotobiol.2019.111544.

Chen, G., Hao, B., Ju, D., Liu, M., Zhao, H., Du, Z., & Xia, J., (2015). Pharmacokinetic and pharmacodynamic study of triptolide-loaded liposome hydrogel patch under microneedleson rats with collagen-induced arthritis. *Acta Pharm. Sin. B., 5,* 569–576. https://doi.org/10.1016/j.apsb.2015.09.006.

Chen, W., Zhang, S., Yu, Y., Zhang, H., & He, Q., (2016). Structural-engineering rationales of gold nanoparticles for cancer theranostics. *Adv. Mater., 28,* 8567–8585. https://doi.org/10.1002/adma.201602080.

Chen, X., (2018). Current and future technological advances in transdermal gene delivery. *Adv. Drug Deliv. Rev., 127,* 85–105. https://doi.org/10.1016/j.addr.2017.12.014.

Collins, A., Savas, J., & Doerfler, L., (2019). Nonsurgical treatments for nonmelanoma skin cancer. *Dermatol. Clin., 37*(4), 435–441. https://doi.org/10.1016/j.det.2019.05.003.

Craythorne, E., & Al-Niami, F., (2017). Skin cancer. *Medicine (Abingdon), 45*(7), 431–434. https://doi.org/10.1016/j.mpmed.2017.04.003.

Cullen, J. K., Simmons, J. L., Parsons, P. G., & Boyle, G. M., (2020). Topical treatments for skin cancer. *Adv. Drug Deliv. Rev., 153,* 54–64. https://doi.org/10.1016/j.addr.2019.11.002.

Da Silva, A. G. M., Rodrigues, T. S., Correia, V. G., Alves, T. V., Alves, R. S., Ando, R. A., Ornellas, F. R., et al., (2016). Plasmonic nanorattles as nextgeneration catalysts for surface plasmon resonance-mediated oxidations promoted by activated oxygen. *Angew. Chem. Int. Ed., 55,* 7111–7115. https://doi.org/10.1002/anie.201601740.

Das, P., Colombo, M., & Prosperi, D., (2019). Recent advances in magnetic fluid hyperthermia for cancer therapy. *Colloids Surf. B: Biointerfaces, 174,* 42–55. https://doi.org/10.1016/j.colsurfb.2018.10.051.

De Freitas, C. F., Calori, I. R., Da Silva, A. C. P., De Castro, L. V., Sato, F., Silva, P. D., Tessaro, A. L., et al., (2019). PEG-coated vesicles from Pluronic/lipid mixtures for the carrying of photoactive erythrosine derivatives. *Colloids Surf. B: Biointerfaces, 175,* 530–544. https://doi.org/10.1016/j.colsurfb.2018.12.031.

De Los Pinos, E., (2012). *Virion Derived Protein Nanoparticles for Delivering Diagnostic or Therapeutic Agents for the Treatment of Non-Melanoma Skin Cancer.* 20120207840, A1.

Dehdashtian, A., Stringer, T. P., Warren, A. J., Mu, E. W., Amirlak, B., & Shahabi, L., (2018). Anatomy and physiology of the skin. In: *Melanoma* (pp. 15–26). Springer International Publishing: Cham.

Duclairoir, C., Nakache, E., Marchais, H., & Orecchioni, A. M., (1998). Formation of gliadin nanoparticles: Influence of the solubility parameter of the protein solvent. *Colloid Polym. Sci., 276*, 321–327. https://doi.org/10.1007/s003960050246.

Eckhart, L., Lippens, S., Tschachler, E., & Declercq, W., (2013). Cell death by cornification. *Biochimica et Biophysica Acta (BBA) – Molecular Cell Research, 1833*(12), 3471–3480. https://doi.org/10.1016/j.bbamcr.2013.06.010.

Ekladious, Colson, Y. L., & Grinstaff, M. W., (2019). Polymer–drug conjugate therapeutics: Advances, insights and prospects. *Nat. Rev. Drug Discov., 18*, 273–294. https://doi.org/10.1038/s41573-018-0005-0.

Elzoghby, A. O., Hemasa, A. L., & Freag, M. S., (2016). Hybrid protein-inorganic nanoparticles: From tumor-targeted drug delivery to cancer imaging. *J. Control. Release, 243*, 303–322. https://doi.org/10.1016/j.jconrel.2016.10.023.

Elzoghby, A. O., Samy, W. M., & Elgindy, N. A., (2012). Protein-based nanocarriers as promising drug and gene delivery systems. *J. Control. Release, 161*, 38–49. https://doi.org/10.1016/j.jconrel.2012.04.036.

Estanqueiro, M., Amaral, M. H., Conceição, J., & Sousa, L. J. M., (2015). Nanotechnological carriers for cancer chemotherapy: The state of the art. *Colloids Surf. B: Biointerfaces, 126*, 631–648. https://doi.org/10.1016/j.colsurfb.2014.12.041.

Feitosa, R. C., Geraldes, D. C., Beraldo-de-Araújo, V. L., Costa, J. S. R., & Oliveira, N. L., (2019). Pharmacokinetic aspects of nanoparticle-in-matrix drug delivery systems for oral/buccal delivery. *Front. Pharmacol., 10*. https://doi.org/10.3389/fphar.2019.01057.

Fuisz, R. C., (1998). *Transdermal Delivery System*. 5736154.

Gabriel, D., Mugnier, T., Courthion, H., Kranidioti, K., Karagianni, N., Denis, M. C., Lapteva, M., et al., (2016). Improved topical delivery of tacrolimus: A novel composite hydrogel formulation for the treatment of psoriasis. *J. Control. Release, 242*, 16–24. https://doi.org/10.1016/j.jconrel.2016.09.007.

Garg, B. J., Garg, N. K., Beg, S., Singh, B., & Katare, O. P., (2016). Nanosized ethosomes-based hydrogel formulations of methoxsalen for enhanced topical delivery against vitiligo: Formulation optimization, *in vitro* evaluation and preclinical assessment. *J. Drug Target., 24*, 233–246. https://doi.org/10.3109/1061186X.2015.1070855.

Garrubba, C., & Donkers, K., (2020). Skin cancer. *JAAPA, 33*(2), 49–50. https://doi.org/10.1097/01.jaa.0000651756.15106.3e.

Gautam, K., Pandit, V., & Ashawat, M. S., (2020). Herbs used in skin protection from ultraviolet sun radiation. *Res. J. Top. Cosmet. Sci., 11*(2), 95–97. https://doi.org/10.5958/2321-5844.2020.00017.5.

Gautam, S. P., Keservani, R. K., Gautam, T., Gupta, A. K., & Sharma, A. K., (2015). An alternative approach for acetylation of amine terminated polyamidoamine (PAMAM) dendrimer. *ARS Pharmaceutica, 56*(3), 155–159.

Grabowska-Jadach, Kalinowska, D., Drozd, M., & Pietrzak, M., (2019). Synthesis, characterization, and application of plasmonic hollow gold nanoshells in a photothermal therapy—New particles for theranostics. *Biomed. Pharmacother., 111*, 1147–1155. https://doi.org/10.1016/j.biopha.2019.01.037.

Grillo, R., Dias, F. V., Querobino, S. M., Alberto-Silva, C., Fraceto, L. F., De Paula, E., & De Araujo, D. R., (2019). Influence of hybrid polymeric nanoparticle/thermosensitive hydrogels systems on formulation tracking and *in vitro* artificial membrane permeation: A promising system for skin drug-delivery. *Colloids Surf. B: Biointerfaces, 174*, 56–62. https://doi.org/10.1016/j.colsurfb.2018.10.063.

Grimaldi, N., Andrade, F., Segovia, N., Ferrer-Tasies, L., Sala, S., Veciana, J., & Ventosa, N., (2016). Lipid-based nanovesicles for nanomedicine. *Chem. Soc. Rev., 45*, 6520–6545. https://doi.org/10.1039/C6CS00409A.

Hafeez, & Kazmi, I., (2017). Dacarbazine nanoparticle topical delivery system for the treatment of melanoma. *Sci. Rep., 7*, 16517. https://doi.org/10.1038/s41598-017-16878-1.

Hamaguchi, T., Kato, K., Yasui, H., Morizane, C., Ikeda, M., Ueno, H., Muro, K., et al., (2007). A phase I and pharmacokinetic study of NK105, a paclitaxel-incorporating micellar nanoparticle formulation. *British Journal of Cancer, 97*(2), 170–176. https://doi.org/10.1038/sj.bjc.6603855.

Hao, Y., Dong, M., Zhang, T., Peng, J., Jia, Y., Cao, Y., & Qian, Z., (2017). Novel approach of using near-infrared responsive PEGylated gold nanorod coated poly(L-lactide) microneedles to enhance the antitumor efficiency of docetaxel-loaded MPEG-PDLLA micelles for treating an A431 tumor. *ACS Applied Materials & Interfaces, 9*(18), 15317–15327. https://doi.org/10.1021/acsami.7b03604.

He, C. X., Tabata, Y., & Gao, J. Q., (2010). Non-viral gene delivery carrier and its three-dimensional transfection system. *Int. J. Pharm., 386*, 232–242. https://doi.org/10.1016/j.ijpharm.2009.11.006.

Heissig, P., Klein, P. M., Hadwiger, P., & Wagner, E., (2016). DNA as tunable adaptor for siRNA polyplex stabilization and functionalization. *Mol. Ther. Nucleic Acids, 5*, e288. https://doi.org/10.1038/mtna.2016.6.

Hood, R. R., Kendall, E. L., Junqueira, M., Vreeland, W. N., Quezado, Z., Finkel, J. C., & DeVoe, D. L., (2014). Microfluidic-enabled liposomes elucidate size-dependent transdermal transport. *PLoS One, 9*, e92978. https://doi.org/10.1371/journal.pone.0092978.

Hou, X., Zhou, H., Wang, L., Tang, J., Chen, C., Jiang, G., & Liu, Y., (2017). Multifunctional near infrared dye-magnetic nanoparticles for bioimaging and cancer therapy. *Cancer Lett., 390*, 168–175. https://doi.org/10.1016/j.canlet.2016.12.026.

Huang, N., Wang, H., Zhao, J., Lui, H., Korbelik, M., & Zeng, H., (2010). Single-wall carbon nanotubes assisted photothermal cancer therapy: Animal study with a murine model of squamous cell carcinoma. *Lasers Surg. Med., 42*, 798–808. https://doi.org/10.1002/lsm.20968.

India Sees High Number of Skin Cancer Cases in North, Northeast Regions, ICMR Study Finds. https://theprint.in/health/india-sees-high-number-of-skin-cancer-cases-in-north-northeast-regions-icmr-study-finds/741687/ (accessed on 1 November 2023).

Jang, E. J., Choi, W. R., Kim, S. Y., Hong, S. S., Rhee, I., Lee, S. J., Choi, S. W., et al., (2017). 2-hydroxyoleic acid-inserted liposomes as a multifunctional carrier of anticancer drugs. *Drug Delivery, 24*(1), 1587–1597. https://doi.org/10.1080/10717544.2017.1388452.

Jarouliya, U., Kesharwani, R. K., & Kesharwani, R. K., (2018). Advances of nanotechnology in cancer therapy. In: *Nanobiomaterials* (pp. 291–328). Apple Academic Press. ISBN: 9781771885911.

Jiang, T., Xu, G., Chen, G., Zheng, Y., He, B., & Gu, Z., (2020). Progress in transdermal drug delivery systems for cancer therapy. *Nano Res., 13*(7), 1810–1824. https://doi.org/10.1007/s12274-020-2664-5.

Jijie, R., Barras, A., Boukherroub, R., & Szunerits, S., (2017). Nanomaterials for transdermal drug delivery: Beyond the state of the art of liposomal structures. *Journal of Materials Chemistry B, 5*(44), 8653–8675. https://doi.org/10.1039/c7tb02529g.

Jordan, A. H., Sandler, G., & Aldrink, J. H., (2022). Melanoma and skin cancer(s). In: *Pediatric Surgical Oncology* (pp. 256–271). CRC Press: Boca Raton.

Karimi, K., Lindgren, T. H., Koch, C. A., & Brodell, R. T., (2016). Obesity as a risk factor for malignant melanoma and non-melanoma skin cancer. *Rev. Endocr. Metab. Disord.*, *17*(3), 389–403. https://doi.org/10.1007/s11154-016-9393-9.

Katiyar, S. K., Agarwal, R., & Mukhtar, H., (1996). Inhibition of tumor promotion in SENCAR mouse skin by ethanol extract of zingiber officinale rhizome. *Cancer Res.*, *56*(5), 1023–1030.

Kauvar, A. N. B., Arpey, C. J., Hruza, G., Olbricht, S. M., & Bennett, R., (2015). Consensus for nonmelanoma skin cancer treatment, part II: Squamous cell carcinoma, including a cost analysis of treatment methods. *Dermatol. Surg.*, *41*(11), 1214–1240. https://doi.org/10.1097/dss.0000000000000478.

Keservani, R. K., & Gautam, S. P., (2020). Formulation and evaluation of baclofen liposome vesicles using lecithin. *ARS Pharmaceutica, 61*(3), 175–180.

Keservani, R. K., & Gautam, S. P., (2022). Skeletal muscle relaxant activity of different formulation of span 60 niosome. *ARS Pharmaceutica, 63*(91), 32–44.

Keservani, R. K., Bandopadhyay, S., Bandyopadhyay, N., & Sharma, A. K., (2020a). Design and fabrication of transdermal/skin drug-delivery system. In: *Drug Delivery Systems* (pp. 131–178). Academic Press.

Keservani, R. K., Sharma, A. K., & Ramteke, S., (2010). Novel vesicular approach for topical delivery of baclofen via niosomes. *Lat. Am. J. Pharm., 29*, 1364–1370.

Keyal, U., Bhatta, A. K., Zhang, G., & Wang, X. L., (2019). Present and future perspectives of photodynamic therapy for cutaneous squamous cell carcinoma. *Journal of the American Academy of Dermatology, 80*(3), 765–773. https://doi.org/10.1016/j.jaad.2018.10.042.

Khan, N. H., Mir, M., Qian, L., Baloch, M., Ali Khan, M. F., Rehman, A. U., Ngowi, E. E., et al., (2022). Skin cancer biology and barriers to treatment: Recent applications of polymeric micro/nanostructures. *J. Adv. Res.*, *36*, 223–247. https://doi.org/10.1016/j.jare.2021.06.014.

Komor, A. C., & Barton, J. K., (2013). The path for metal complexes to a DNA target. *Chem. Commun., 49*, 3617–3630. https://doi.org/10.1039/c3cc00177f.

Kriplani, P., & Guarve, K., (2021). Transdermal drug delivery: A step towards treatment of cancer. *Recent Patents on Anti-Cancer Drug Discovery, 16*. https://doi.org/10.2174/15748 92816666211202154000.

Kuttan, R., Sudheeran, P. C., & Josph, C. D., (1987). Turmeric and curcumin as topical agents in cancer therapy. *Tumori*, *73*(1), 29–31. https://doi.org/10.1177/030089168707300105.

Lächelt, U., & Wagner, E., (2015). Nucleic acid therapeutics using polyplexes: A journey of 50 years (and beyond). *Chem. Rev., 115*, 11043–11078. https://doi.org/10.1021/cr5006793.

Lai, V., Cranwell, W., & Sinclair, R., (2018). Epidemiology of skin cancer in the mature patient. *Clin. Dermatol.*, *36*(2), 167–176. https://doi.org/10.1016/j.clindermatol.2017.10.008.

Lan, X., She, J., Lin, D., Xu, Y., Li, X., Yang, W., Lui, V. W. Y., et al., (2018). Microneedle-mediated delivery of lipid-coated cisplatin nanoparticles for efficient and safe cancer therapy. *ACS Applied Materials & Interfaces, 10*(39), 33060–33069. https://doi.org/10.1021/acsami.8b12926.

Larsen, G. K., Farr, W., & Hunyadi, M. S. E., (2016). Multifunctional Fe_2O_3-Au nanoparticles with different shapes: Enhanced catalysis, photothermal effects, and magnetic recyclability. *J. Phys. Chem. C., 120*, 15162–15172. https://doi.org/10.1021/acs.jpcc.6b03733.

Li, H. J., Du, J. Z., Liu, J., Du, X. J., Shen, S., Zhu, Y. H., Wang, X., et al., (2016). Smart superstructures with ultrahigh ph-sensitivity for targeting acidic tumor microenvironment: Instantaneous size switching and improved tumor penetration. *ACS Nano, 10*(7), 6753–6761. https://doi.org/10.1021/acsnano.6b02326.

Li, X., Wang, D., Ran, H., Hao, L., Cao, Y., Ao, M., Zhang, N., et al., (2018). A preliminary study of photoacoustic/ultrasound dual-mode imaging in melanoma using MAGE-targeted gold nanoparticles. *Biochem. Biophys. Res. Commun., 502*, 255–261. https://doi.org/10.1016/j.bbrc.2018.05.155.

Li, Y., Maciel, D., Rodrigues, J., Shi, X., & Tomás, H., (2015). Biodegradable polymer nanogels for drug/nucleic acid delivery. *Chem. Rev., 115*, 8564–8608. https://doi.org/10.1021/cr500131f.

Lim, E. K., Kim, T., Paik, S., Haam, S., Huh, Y. M., & Lee, K., (2015). Nanomaterials for theranostics: Recent advances and future challenges. *Chem. Rev., 115*, 327–394. https://doi.org/10.1021/cr300213b.

Lin, C. T., Chieh, I. L., Sung, S. Y., Su, Y. L., Huang, Y. F., Chiang, C. S., & Hu, S. H., (2016). Dual-targeted photopenetrative delivery of multiple micelles/hydrophobic drugs by a nanopea for enhanced tumor therapy. *Advanced Functional Materials, 26*(23), 4169–4179. https://doi.org/10.1002/adfm.201600498.

Linares, M. A., Zakaria, A., & Nizran, P., (2015). Skin cancer. *Primary Care: Clinics in Office Practice, 42*(4), 645–659. https://doi.org/10.1016/j.pop.2015.07.006.

Lu, W., Senapati, D., Wang, S., Tovmachenko, O., Singh, A. K., Yu, H., & Ray, P. C., (2010). Effect of surface coating on the toxicity of silver nanomaterials on human skin keratinocytes. *Chem. Phys. Lett., 487*, 92–96. https://doi.org/10.1016/j.cplett.2010.01.027.

Malafaya, P. B., Silva, G. A., & Reis, R. L., (2007). Natural-origin polymers as carriers and scaffolds for biomolecules and cell delivery in tissue engineering applications. *Adv. Drug Deliv. Rev., 59*, 207–233. https://doi.org/10.1016/j.addr.2007.03.012.

Marianecci, C., Di Marzio, L., Rinaldi, F., Celia, C., Paolino, D., Alhaique, F., Esposito, S., & Carafa, M., (2014). Niosomes from 80s to present: The state of the art. *Adv. Colloid Interf. Sci., 205*, 187–206. https://doi.org/10.1016/j.cis.2013.11.018.

Marks, R., (1995). An overview of skin cancers. Incidence and causation. *Cancer, 75*(2 Suppl), 607–612. https://doi.org/10.1002/1097-0142(19950115)75:2+<607::aid-cncr2820751402>3.0.co;2-8.

Melanoma of the Skin – Cancer Stat Facts. https://seer.cancer.gov/statfacts/html/melan.html (accessed on 1 November 2023).

Novo, L., Mastrobattista, E., Van, N. C. F., Lammers, T., & Hennink, W. E., (2015). Decationized polyplexes for gene delivery. *Expert Opin. Drug Deliv., 12*, 507–512. https://doi.org/10.1517/17425247.2015.988136.

Orthaber, K., Pristovnik, M., Skok, K., Perić, B., & Maver, U., (2017). Skin cancer and its treatment: Novel treatment approaches with emphasis on nanotechnology. *J. Nanomater., 2017*, 1–20. https://doi.org/10.1155/2017/2606271.

Park, J. H., Lee, S., Kim, J. H., Park, K., Kim, K., & Kwon, I. C., (2008). Polymeric nanomedicine for cancer therapy. *Prog. Polym. Sci., 33*, 113–137. https://doi.org/10.1016/j.progpolymsci.2007.09.003.

Pashazadeh, A., Boese, A., & Friebe, M., (2019). Radiation therapy techniques in the treatment of skin cancer: An overview of the current status and outlook. *J. Dermatolog. Treat., 30*(8), 831–839. https://doi.org/10.1080/09546634.2019.1573310.

Pille, J., Van, L. S. A. M., Van, H. J. C. M., & Leenders, W. P. J., (2017). Self-assembling VHH-elastin-like peptides for photodynamic nanomedicine. *Biomacromolecules, 18*, 1302–1310. https://doi.org/10.1021/acs.biomac.7b00064.

Praca, F. G., Petrilli, R., Eloy, J. O., Lee, R. J., & Lopes, B. B. M. V., (2017). Liquid-crystalline nanodispersions containing monoolein for photodynamic therapy of skin diseases: A mini-review. *Curr. Nanosci., 13*, 1–8. https://doi.org/10.2174/1573413713666170529115831.

Pradhan, M., Singh, D., & Singh, M. R., (2013). Novel colloidal carriers for psoriasis: Current issues, mechanistic insight and novel delivery approaches. *J. Control. Release, 170*, 380–395. https://doi.org/10.1016/j.jconrel.2013.05.020.

Prasad, C., & Banerjee, R., (2019). Ultrasound-triggered spatiotemporal delivery of topotecan and curcumin as combination therapy for cancer. *Journal of Pharmacology and Experimental Therapeutics, 370*(3), 876–893. https://doi.org/10.1124/jpet.119.256487.

Prausnitz, M. R., & Langer, R., (2008). Transdermal drug delivery. *Nature Biotechnology, 26*(11), 1261–1268. https://doi.org/10.1038/nbt.1504.

Qian, C., Yu, J., Chen, Y., Hu, Q., Xiao, X., Sun, W., Wang, C., et al., (2016). Light-activated hypoxia-responsive nanocarriers for enhanced anticancer therapy. *Adv. Mater., 28*, 3313–3320. https://doi.org/10.1002/adma.201505869.

Qidwai, Khan, S., Md, S., Fazil, M., Baboota, S., Narang, J. K., & Ali, J., (2016). Nanostructured lipid carrier in photodynamic therapy for the treatment of basal-cell carcinoma. *Drug Deliv., 23*, 1476–1485. https://doi.org/10.3109/10717544.2016.1165310.

Rady, M., Gomaa, I., Afifi, N., & Abdel-Kader, M., (2018). Dermal delivery of Fe-chlorophyllin via ultradeformable nanovesicles for photodynamic therapy in melanoma animal model. *International Journal of Pharmaceutics, 548*(1), 480–490. https://doi.org/10.1016/j.ijpharm.2018.06.057.

Ramadon, D., McCrudden, M. T. C., Courtenay, A. J., & Donnelly, R. F., (2021). Enhancement strategies for transdermal drug delivery systems: Current trends and applications. *Drug Deliv. Transl. Res., 12*(4), 758–791. https://doi.org/10.1007/s13346-021-00909-6.

Rizvi, S. M. H., Aagnes, B., Holdaas, H., Gude, E., Boberg, K. M., Bjørtuft, Ø., Helsing, P., et al., (2017). Long-term change in the risk of skin cancer after organ transplantation: A population-based nationwide cohort study. *JAMA Dermatol., 153*(12), 1270. https://doi.org/10.1001/jamadermatol.2017.2984.

Roohnikan, M., Laszlo, E., Babity, S., & Brambilla, D., (2019). A snapshot of transdermal and topical drug delivery research in Canada. *Pharmaceutics, 11*(6), 256. https://doi.org/10.3390/pharmaceutics11060256.

Rossetti, F. C., Depieri, L. V., Praça, F. G., Del, C. J. O., Fantini, M. C. A., Pierre, M. B. R., Tedesco, A. C., & Bentley, M. V. L. B., (2016). Optimization of protoporphyrin IX skin delivery for topical photodynamic therapy: Nanodispersions of liquid-crystalline phase as nanocarriers. *Eur. J. Pharm. Sci., 83*, 99–108. https://doi.org/10.1016/j.ejps.2015.12.003.

Sala, M., Diab, R., Elaissari, A., & Fessi, H., (2018). Lipid nanocarriers as skin drug delivery systems: Properties, mechanisms of skin interactions and medical applications. *Int. J. Pharm., 535*, 1–17. https://doi.org/10.1016/j.ijpharm.2017.10.046.

Sampalis, T., (2004). *Krill and/or Marine Extracts for Prevention and/or Treatment of Cardiovascular Diseases Arthritis, Skin Cancer Diabetes, Premenstrual Syndrome and Transdermal Transport*. 20040241249:A1.

Schroeder, Levins, C. G., Cortez, C., Langer, R., & Anderson, D. G., (2010). Lipid-based nanotherapeutics for siRNA delivery. *J. Intern. Med., 267*, 9–21. https://doi.org/10.1111/j.1365-2796.2009.02189.x.

Schulz, M., Olubummo, A., & Binder, W. H., (2012). Beyond the lipid-bilayer: Interaction of polymers and nanoparticles with membranes. *Soft Matter, 8*, 4849–4864. https://doi.org/10.1039/c2sm06999g.

Senapati, S., Mahanta, A. K., Kumar, S., & Maiti, P., (2018). Controlled drug delivery vehicles for cancer treatment and their performance. *Signal Transduct. Target. Ther., 3*, 7. https://doi.org/10.1038/s41392-017-0004-3.

Senyigit, T., Ozcan, I., & Ozer, O., (2012). Innovative topical formulations for treatment of dermatitis. *Recent Patents Inflamm. Allergy Drug Discov., 6*, 186–201. https://doi.org/10.2174/187221312802652785.

Sharma, R. R., Deep, A., & Abdullah, S. T., (2022). Herbal products as skincare therapeutic agents against ultraviolet radiation-induced skin disorders. *J. Ayurveda Integr. Med., 13*(1), 100500. https://doi.org/10.1016/j.jaim.2021.07.016.

Silver, M. E., (2017). *Method for Treating Skin Cancer*. 9642827.

Skin Cancer Statistics, https://www.wcrf.org/dietandcancer/skin-cancer-statistics/ (accessed on 1 November 2023).

Strelow, Theuerholz, T. S., Schmidtke, C., Richter, M., Merkl, J. P., Kloust, H., Ye, Z., et al., (2016). Metal–semiconductor nanoparticle hybrids formed by self-organization: A platform to address exciton–plasmon coupling, *Nano Lett., 16*, 4811–4818. https://doi.org/10.1021/acs.nanolett.6b00982.

Sun, L., Liu, Z., Wang, L., Cun, D., Tong, H. H. Y., Yan, R., Chen, X., et al., (2017). Enhanced topical penetration, system exposure and anti-psoriasis activity of two particle-sized, curcumin-loaded PLGA nanoparticles in hydrogel. *J. Control. Release, 254*, 44–54. https://doi.org/10.1016/j.jconrel.2017.03.385.

Sun, M., Peng, D., Hao, H., Hu, J., Wang, D., Wang, K., Liu, J., et al., (2017). Thermally triggered in situ assembly of gold nanoparticles for cancer multimodal imaging and photothermal therapy. *ACS Appl. Mater. Interfaces, 9*, 10453–10460. https://doi.org/10.1021/acsami.6b16408.

Tan, C., Cao, X., Wu, X. J., He, Q., Yang, J., Zhang, X., Chen, J., et al., (2017). Recent advances in ultrathin two-dimensional nanomaterials. *Chem. Rev., 117*, 6225–6331. https://doi.org/10.1021/acs.chemrev.6b00558.

Tham, H. P., Xu, K., Lim, W. Q., Chen, H., Zheng, M., Thng, T. G. S., Venkatraman, S. S., et al., (2018). Microneedle-assisted topical delivery of photodynamically active mesoporous formulation for combination therapy of deep-seated melanoma. *ACS Nano, 12*(12), 11936–11948. https://doi.org/10.1021/acsnano.8b03007.

Thomas, T. J., & Thomas, T., (2018). Collapse of DNA in packaging and cellular transport. *Int. J. Biol. Macromol., 109*, 36–48. https://doi.org/10.1016/j.ijbiomac.2017.12.076.

Tong, R., Chiang, H. H., & Kohane, D. S., (2013). Photoswitchable nanoparticles for *in vivo* cancer chemotherapy. *Proceedings of the National Academy of Sciences, 110*(47), 19048–19053. https://doi.org/10.1073/pnas.1315336110.

Tong, R., Hemmati, H. D., Langer, R., & Kohane, D. S., (2012). Photoswitchable nanoparticles for triggered tissue penetration and drug delivery. *Journal of the American Chemical Society, 134*(21), 8848–8855. https://doi.org/10.1021/ja211888a.

Touitou, E., Dayan, N., Bergelson, L., Godin, B., & Eliaz, M., (2000). Ethosomes – novel vesicular carriers for enhanced delivery: Characterization and skin penetration properties. *J. Control. Release, 65*, 403–418. http://www.ncbi.nlm.nih.gov/pubmed/10699298.

Trivedi, D., Gupta, R., Scholar, M. S., & Radhakrishnan, S., (2020). Cancer in ayurveda and its preventive measure. *World J. Pharm. Res.* https://doi.org/10.20959/wjpr202010-18474.

Trotta, M., Peira, E., Carlotti, M. E., & Gallarate, M., (2004). Deformable liposomes for dermal administration of methotrexate. *Int. J. Pharm., 270*, 119–125. https://doi.org/10.1016/j.ijpharm.2003.10.006.

Van, O. L. M. P. E., Pille, J., Stuut, C., Van, S. M., Van, D. V. L. N., Smeitink, J. A. M., Koopman, W. J. H., et al., (2019). Octaarginine boosts the penetration of elastin-like polypeptide nanoparticles in 3D cancer models. *Eur. J. Pharm. Biopharm., 137*, 175–184. https://doi.org/10.1016/j.ejpb.2019.02.010.

Van, S. D., Mashayekhi, V., De Bruijn, H., Oliveira, S., & Robinson, D., (2017). Oncologic photodynamic therapy: Basic principles, current clinical status, and future directions. *Cancers, 9*(12), 19. https://doi.org/10.3390/cancers9020019.

Villani, A., Cinelli, E., Fabbrocini, G., Lallas, A., & Scalvenzi, M., (2020). Hedgehog inhibitors in the treatment of advanced basal cell carcinoma: Risks and benefits. *Expert Opin. Drug Saf., 19*(12), 1585–1594. https://doi.org/10.1080/14740338.2020.1837773.

Villemin, E., Ong, Y. C., Thomas, C. M., & Gasser, G., (2019). Polymer encapsulation of ruthenium complexes for biological and medicinal applications. *Nat. Rev. Chem., 3*, 261–282. https://doi.org/10.1038/s41570-019-0088-0.

Wakabayashi, R., Sakuragi, M., Kozaka, S., Tahara, Y., Kamiya, N., & Goto, M., (2018). Solid-in-oil peptide nanocarriers for transcutaneous cancer vaccine delivery against melanoma. *Mol. Pharm., 15*, 955–961. https://doi.org/10.1021/acs.molpharmaceut.7b00894.

Wakabayashi, R., Sakuragi, M., Kozaka, S., Tahara, Y., Kamiya, N., & Goto, M., (2018). Solid-in-oilpeptide nanocarriers for transcutaneous cancer vaccine delivery against melanoma. *Mol. Pharm., 15*, 955–961. https://doi.org/10.1021/acs.molpharmaceut.7b00894.

Wang, B., Zhai, Y., Shi, J., Zhuang, L., Liu, W., Zhang, H., Zhang, H., & Zhang, Z., (2017). Simultaneously overcome tumor vascular endothelium and extracellular matrix barriers via a non-destructive size-controlled nanomedicine. *Journal of Controlled Release, 268*, 225–236. https://doi.org/10.1016/j.jconrel.2017.10.029.

Worldwide Cancer Data, https://www.wcrf.org/dietandcancer/worldwide-cancer-data/ (accessed on 1 November 2023).

Yang, X., Yang, M., Pang, B., Vara, M., & Xia, Y., (2015). Gold nanomaterials at work in biomedicine. *Chem. Rev., 115*, 10410–10488. https://doi.org/10.1021/acs.chemrev.5b00193.

Yao, Q., Choi, J. H., Dai, Z., Wang, J., Kim, D., Tang, X., & Zhu, L., (2017). Improving tumor specificity and anticancer activity of dasatinib by dual-targeted polymeric micelles. *ACS Applied Materials & Interfaces, 9*(42), 36642–36654. https://doi.org/10.1021/acsami.7b12233.

Younis, M. R., Wang, C., An, R., Wang, S., Younis, M. A., Li, Z. Q., Wang, Y., et al., (2019). Low power single laser activated synergistic cancer phototherapy using photosensitizer functionalized dual plasmonic photothermal nanoagents. *ACS Nano, 13*, 2544–2557. https://doi.org/10.1021/acsnano.8b09552.

Zhou, F., Wu, S., Wu, B., Chen, W. R., & Xing, D., (2011). Mitochondria-targeting single-walled carbon nanotubes for cancer photothermal therapy. *Small, 7*, 2727–2735. https://doi.org/10.1002/smll.201100669.

Zhu, W., Dong, Z., Fu, T., Liu, J., Chen, Q., Li, Y., Zhu, R., et al., (2016). Modulation of hypoxia in solid tumor microenvironment with MnO_2 nanoparticles to enhance photodynamic therapy. *Adv. Funct. Mater., 26*, 5490–5498. https://doi.org/10.1002/adfm.201600676.

Zimmerman, E. E., & Crawford, P., (2012). Cutaneous cryosurgery. *Am. Fam. Physician, 86*(12), 1118–1124.

CHAPTER 7

Follicular Delivery of Nanocarriers to Improve Skin Disease Treatment

BHUSHAN R. RANE,[1] AKASH J. AMKAR,[1] SHIVANI S. PAWAR,[1] PUNAM S. GADEKAR,[1] RAJ K. KESERVANI,[2] and ASHISH S. JAIN[1]

[1]Shri D.D. Vispute College of Pharmacy and Research Center, Devad-Vichumbe, Panvel, Navi Mumbai, Maharashtra, India

[2]Faculty of B. Pharmacy, CSM Group of Institutions, Prayagraj, Uttar Pradesh, India

ABSTRACT

Skin-related diseases surround a vast array of situations ranging in severity from benign to life threatening. Skin diseases were believed to have insignificant impact on patient's quality of life. The fourth most common source of non-lethal disease was skin and cutaneous abnormalities. In the past few generations, topical implementations of nanocarrier-assisted drug delivery technologies have gained great attention. Selective follicular targeting is possible by modifying the nanocarrier size meaning that specific nanocarrier sizes show deeper follicular penetration than others. According to the findings of the studies, that nanocarrier between 300 and 650 nm penetrated significantly deeper than smaller or larger particles. The novel deliveries towards skin disorders are emulgels, micellar microparticles, and Small interfering ribonucleic acid (siRNA) delivery through nanocarriers. Polymeric nanoparticle, lipid nanoparticles, metallic nanoparticle, ethosomes (ETOs), niosomes are the carriers that shows proofs of follicular pathway to give a specific therapeutic effect. Some of the traditional treatments are found to be very effective in treatment of skin problems are Ayurveda from India, Chinese traditional medicines and Kampo medicines from Japan. Some of

Novel Nanocarriers forSkin Diseases: Advances and Applications.
Raj K. Keservani and Júlia Scherer Santos (Eds.)

the patented formulations are available for the treatment of skin disease through follicular pathway in which drugs like 5-alpha Reductase inhibitors like Finasteride, Minoxidil are found to be very effective for alopecia.

7.1 INTRODUCTION

Today, skin diseases and skin troubles are emerging aspects and afflict millions of people every day. Throughout history, skin diseases have mainly been caused by numerous infection pathogens or inflammatory situation. Skin-related diseases surround a vast array of situations ranging in severity from benign to life threatening (Sigmundsdottir et al., 2010). Scientific data reveal that dermatologic diseases are very acute and commonly influence populations in many developing countries. While these problems have not gained much attention from an international audience, there seems to be a high demand by healthcare workers for more consideration to be given to skin diseases (Gupta et al., 2012).

Despite the great progress in dermatological treatment, many skin problems are related to infectious skin disease and remain difficult to treat. These problems depend on the types of pathogens involved, the integrity of skin layer and their structure (Fleischer et al., 2000). Dermatitis (atopic and contact) and Psoriasis are examples of chronic skin infections that originate from the inflammatory T lymphocytes and enhance cytokine production in that region (Dawson et al., 2012). These diseases are significant cause of morbidity and mortality.

The term "nanomaterial" refers to substances with one or more dimension under 100 nm. According to the 2011 definition provided by the European Council, a nanomaterial is any natural, manufactured material that contains molecules in an unbound form, as an agglomeration, as an aggregate, and where at least 50% of the particles in the number size distribution have at least one exterior dimension that falls within the size range less than 100 nm (Ozkan et al., 2019).

Nanomaterials are the material which affects the nanomedicine through drug delivery, biosensors, microfluidics, and synthetic biology, can be simply characterized as materials with diameters ranging from 1 to 100 nm (Patra et al., 2018). Numerous new studies and patents on nanomedicine in the field of health sciences have been published throughout the past century (Brower et al., 2006). The goal of nanomedicine is to identify and maintain health while causing any negative side effects through non-invasive procedures. Among the properties that nonmaterials can improve in a drug delivery method are solubility, surface area growth, site-targeted delivery, and control release (Escobar et al., 2012).

New surgical instruments, improved diagnostics chips, novel body structural replacement materials, and medication delivery systems are all example of how nanosystem is being applied in the biomedical sciences to treat a diverse range of disorders. These nanostructures can be created from a wide range of materials, and they vary significantly in terms of both their chemical characteristics and structural makeup. These nanostructures collectively referred to as nanocarriers, and they can all be administered to organisms topically or transdermally. As they are too minute for the immune response to recognize them and can carry the drug to the specific receptor, nanocarriers are a potent tool against many diseases. As a result, negative impacts using nanocarriers are greatly reduced (Keservani et al., 2018; Escobar et al., 2012).

Drug targeting and Controlled drug delivery to a specific organ, cell, or tissue are the two major applications of drug nanocarriers or nanosystem. The foundation of drug delivery is comprised of targeting molecules and nontoxic nanoparticles. Target specific compounds are usually antibody or biotin/avidin that target particular a cells, tissue, or organ. The drug release properties of the nanocarrier system are provided by the environmentally sensitive nature of the carrier (Ozkan et al., 2019).

Lane and Hadgraft provide a clear overview of the development of permeation studies (Hadgraft & Lane, 2005). When a topical, systemic, or regional effect is needed, the skin has proven to be a significant pathway for drug administration (Escobar et al., 2012). Skin is a great barrier and creating challenges for the transdermal delivery of therapeutic substances, but several medications have the properties to permeate across the stratum corneum (SC) in enough proportions to achieve therapeutic concentrations within the blood (Rizwan et al., 2009).

Several recent innovations have been made in the field of skin disease treatment as likewise with other fields. Intensive research proposes that the effective treatment of skin disorders requires timely identification, estimation, and management of the causative agent and adoptability of efficient treatment, as well as drug administration via the optimal route with an optimized dosing schedule. To this end, there are a host of new treatment options available to combat skin disorders. In addition, the understanding of skin morphology, the barrier nature of SC, transport route in skin as well as barrier properties of diseased skin have expanded rapidly over the past few decades. This new knowledge has provided the recognition of molecular targets and the rapid progress for development of new, specific, targeted therapies for treating skin diseases (Gupta et al., 2012).

7.2 DEFINITION OF NANOCARRIERS

Nanomaterials employed as a transport module for another chemical, such as a medicine, are known as nanocarriers. Recently topical applications of nanocarrier aided drug delivery techniques have attracted growing attention. Numerous models of nanocarriers are now being designed in order to satisfy specific criteria because various clinical needed different kinds of drug delivery systems (DDSs) (Su & Kang, 2020). Nanocarriers used to deliver therapeutic agents have to be biocompatible and nontoxic (Farah et al., 2019). Drug release nanocarriers are available in the shape of polymeric nanoparticle, solid lipid nanoparticles (SLNs), as well as inorganic nanoparticles, micelles, liposomes, and microemulsion (Behera et al., 2010; Gupta et al., 2013). Because of their benefits over traditional formulations, nanostructured carriers are becoming a popular medication delivery method. Colloidal particulate systems comprising size between 10 and 1,000 nm provide targeted therapies, prolonged releases, minimal toxicities, and prevention of unstable moieties from deterioration and it also gives drug adhesiveness to the skin (Gupta et al., 2013). Nanocarriers have been shown to improve drug absorption, penetration, half-life, bioavailability, and stability, among other things. Nanocarriers are so small that they are undetectable by the immune system, and they can carry drugs to the target organ with lower medication doses, reducing adverse effects. Nanocarriers can be injected into organisms via a variety of methods, one of which is the dermal route (Escobar-Chávez et al., 2012).

It is anticipated that the usage of nanocarriers in delivery of drugs will increase therapeutic selectivity and hence minimize negative impact while also reducing dosages of drug. Polymeric nanoparticles are promising for topical application due to the controlled delivery of enclosed active ingredients that must permeate through the polymeric network to enter into the skin. Because of their hard matrix, they are structurally stable and may keep their structure for lengthy periods of time when applied topically. Nanocarriers composed of different substances are expected to penetrate differently into the hair follicle. However, a particle's physical properties such as particle size, shape, and stiffness appear to have greater impact than nanocarrier composition (Friedman et al., 2021).

Nanocarrier-assisted DDSs have gained increasing recognition in recent years for topical applications. As different clinical needs require different types of DDSs, various designs of nanocarriers are being developed in order to meet specific requirements.

7.2.1 POLYMERIC NANOCAPSULES

Polymeric nanocapsules are vesicular particles with a polymeric wall maintained by steric agents or surfactants, surrounded by an oily core of diameter which is less than one meter (Bronaugh & Stewart, 1985). The properties of the polymeric wall affect the diffusion of the active substance from the oily center (Gupta et al., 2013). PLGA-based nanoparticles, Chitosan-modified PLGA nanoparticles may be useful in skin delivery as they propose a number of advantages including non-toxicity and biodegradability and entrapment of various therapeutic moieties (Deng et al., 2020).

7.2.2 LIPIDIC NANOPARTICLES

The effect of skin barrier damage on the penetration profile of various bioactives applied as SLNs or nanostructured lipid nanoparticles (NLCs) (Baig et al., 2018) composed of different lipids, varying in polarity, was studied. It is appreciated that the topical delivery of drugs in skin diseases by lipidic nanoparticles serves as an excellent tool in the dermatological field (Jensen et al., 2011).

7.2.3 INORGANIC NANOPARTICLES

Inorganic nanoparticles cover a broad range of substances including elemental metals, metal oxides, and metal salts (Ángela & Miguel, 2014). A titanium dioxide (TiO_2) and zinc oxide (ZnO) used in sunscreens are prime examples. They are not only translucent, but also attractive. TiO_2 is more effective in the UVB range and ZnO is more efficient in the UVA region, and the mixture of these particles gives extensive UV protection (Schneider et al., 2018). Because of their antibacterial properties, Silver-containing nanoparticles are used.

7.2.4 GOLD NANOPARTICLES (AUNPS)

These are aggregated particles with a core of gold and a coat of gold that range in size less than 100 nanometers. A gold nanoparticle's essential properties are determined by its gold core. AuNPs are particular an excellent intracellular targeting vector because:

i. From 0.8 to 200 nanometers, they could be quickly adjusted to a desired size;
ii. A range of functionalities and biocompatibility can be provided by altering their surfaces;
iii. They have observable light extinction behavior, allowing nanoparticle paths in cells to be tracked.

7.2.5 CARBON NANOTUBES (CNTS)

Carbon nanotubes (CNTs) are long, persistent carbon nanoparticles having antioxidant and cytoprotective properties. Their mean sizes are exceedingly tiny (less than 100 nanometers). Their enormous interior volume allows small biomolecules to be loaded, while their outside surface can be chemically changed to create a variety of unique characteristics that can be utilized for the loading of genes and proteins successful for drug delivery (Xu et al., 2006). CNTs conductivity can be used to create a highly sensitive sub-organellar biomarker sensor, allowing for early detection of chronic skin infections and cancers (Gupta et al., 2013).

7.2.6 FULLERENES

Fullerenes are carbon spheres with 60 carbon atoms that are 1 nm in size. Despite their hydrophobic nature, fullerenes can be chemically functionalized by attaching a hydrophilic moiety, making them water soluble and capable of transporting DNA, proteins, and other biomolecules for delivery (Xu et al., 2006). Because of their small size, spherical form, and hollow interior, they can be used for medicinal purposes. These have been advocated as rejuvenating cosmetics such as sunscreens, moisturizer sand long-lasting makeup, among other things. Slow-release kinetics are significant in scents since they might last all day (Nasir et al., 2010). Fullerenes, C_{60}, which include fewer than 300 carbons, are examples of endohedral fullerenes and buckyball cluster, respectively (Mahor et al., 2021).

7.2.7 DENDRIMERS

Dendrimers are monodispersing populations that are structurally and chemically uniform. They allow conjugation with numerous functional groups due to the nature of their branches. The amount of branches increases exponentially, and dendrimers growth is typically about 1 nm per generation (Svenson & Tomalia, 2005). Dendrimers have a high surface-charge density due to ionizable groups that help them to attach drugs by electrostatic forces, regardless of the stoichiometry. This dendrimer drug association provides drugs with better solubility, increasing their transport through biological membranes and sometimes increasing drug stability (Escobar-Chávez et al., 2012). Dendrimers are composed of monomers associated radially from a central core (Caminade et al., 2016).

7.2.8 ETHOSOMES (ETOS)

Ethosomes (ETOs) the only difference between conventional liposomes and ETOs is that ethanol, instead of cholesterol, is used as constituent in ETOs. An ethanol content of up to 45% may be present in ETOs, which is responsible for skin penetration resulting in drug delivery into deep layers of the skin (Liu & Hu, 2007). In the process of exploration of new approaches for enhanced cutaneous delivery, ETOs were studied and explored as potential carriers in dermatologic area (Touitou et al., 2000). Antibiotics could be effectively delivered via ETOs to microbes located in the deep layers of skin in order to prevent staphylococcal infection.

7.2.9 TRANSFERSOMES (TRAS)

Deformable liposomes are a critical advancement in topical vesicular drug delivery and have the potential to dramatically improve drug delivery (Cevc et al., 1996). These first generations of elastic vesicles are reported to penetrate intact skin carrying the drugs. They consist mainly of phospholipids with an edge activator that destabilizes lipid bilayers of the vesicles and contribute to the deformability of the bilayers (Honeywell & Bouwstra,

2005). Nanocarriers as TRAs having ability to pass through skin barrier's restrictions because they can modify their shape (Opatha et al., 2020).

7.2.10 NIOSOMES

Niosome are non-ionic surfactant vesicles obtained by hydrating mixture of cholesterol and nonionic surfactants. It can be used as carriers of amphiphilic drug (Kumavat et al., 2021). In niosomes DDS, the medication is encapsulated in a vesicle. Niosomes (Keservani et al., 2010, 2020, 2022) are biodegradable, biocompatible, and non-immunogenic, and their structural characterization is flexible (Sharma et al., 2018).

7.2.11 CERAMIC NANOSTRUCTURES

Ceramic nanostructures or nanocarrier are made of nontoxic inorganic components like alumina, silica, calcium phosphate, and Titania and also, they are porous in nature. Ceramic nanostructures are thought to be effective transporters for medications, DNA, and proteins in the biomedical industry (Lu et al., 2016).

7.3 NOVEL APPROACHES FOR SKIN DISEASE TREATMENT

The NDDS with their unique aspects provide suitable skin interactions as desired in the diseased conditions. Scrutinize the benefits; there have been several recent attempts are used in NDDS approach to improve the existing topical drug formulations in Skin disorders. Novel carriers such as liposome, niosomes, ETOs, silver nanoparticles (AgNPs), SLNs have been utilizing through almost all the routes of administration because of less painful effects as given by injections (Chenthamara et al., 2019). However, the topical route has been used as one of the most appropriate substances to treat dermatological disorders more effectively. In spite of the conventional formulations based on creams & ointments, these novel dermatological systems are different in their composition & concentration. Several pharmaceutical and dermatological variables influence the choice of the system as per the need of the drug and disease. The applications of such novel nanovehicle systems are able to deliver potent drugs to the preferred site in a very accurate manner. The composition of Nanomedicines based on Nanosystems apparently control the release of a therapeutic moiety to the affected region at the skin site with localized effect by creating skin reservoirs. Such a fact that skin acts even as negatively charged membrane; the existence of charge on the surfaces of Nanocarriers influences their drug diffusion through the skin. A positively charged delivery system would strongly interact with cells & has shown better permeability and prolonged pharmacological activity (Tamanna & Harmeet, 2021). The novel deliveries towards skin disorders are emulgels and micellar microparticles.

7.3.1 EMULGEL

Emulgel are dosage formulations made up of gels and emulsions that have been mixed. These are either water-in-oil emulsions or oil-in-water emulsions that have been gelled by adding a gelling agent. Hydrophobic medications include the use of emulgels as a topical drug delivery device. The primary goal of this formulation is to introduce hydrophobic drugs into the systemic circulation via the skin. Emulgel is a new topical drug formulation that is gaining popularity as a result of its benefits over traditional topical preparations. Drugs may be used to achieve local or systemic effects. Emulgels have turned out to become one of the most innovative topical delivery methods due to dual release control system, which combines both gel and emulsion (Bhosale et al., 2007). Emulgels are greaseless, thixotropic, spreadable, and easy to remove, stain-free, emollient, water-soluble, and have a long shelf life. They can be used in a variety of cosmetics preparations as well (Patel et al., 2018).

7.3.1.1 METHOD OF PREPARATION OF EMULGEL

There are various methods of formulation of Emulgel, employing different kinds of ingredient.

- Chemical enhancement;
- Physical enhancement;
- Biochemical enhancement;
- Super saturation enhancement.

Emulgel are prepared by incorporating gel and emulsion. The emulsion and gel are prepared separately and mixed together.

- **Step 1:** Create an emulsion that is either O/W or W/O.
- **Step 2:** Build the gel foundation.
- **Step 3:** Continuous emulsion incorporation into gel base agitation (Abhijeet et al., 2017).

7.3.2 MICELLAR MICROPARTICLES

Microparticle entrapped micelles is a delivery system in which the particles of the micellar range are ensemble for drug and gene delivery in specific parts of the body. Micelle-containing microparticles may be used to deliver micelle encapsulated hydrophobic drug on targeted site. Micelles have been used as drug carriers for administration and exhibit many advantages including their ease of production, long circulation times and having surfaces that are readily modified with targeting ligands. Hydrophobic agents could be successfully incorporated into micelles. The major goals in designing colloidal microparticles topical formulation are to improve topical dose formulations that locally distribute the API. Micellar delivery systems that are smaller than 100 nm can be readily prepared.

Micellar DDSs are used because they improve bioavailability, reduce drug degrading, and minimize negative side effects. Drugs that are poorly soluble can be made more bioavailable by being solubilized using micellar systems. The ability to manufacture a variety of slightly soluble to practically insoluble molecules in the solution state through solubilization in aqueous surfactant solutions at surfactant concentrations surpassing the critical micelle concentration is well known. The solubility of medicines is increased through micellar solubilization. Micelle entrapped into microparticle is a sensible approach of converting an aqueous micellar solution into solid for ease of administration and patient compliance (Bansal et al., 2018).

7.3.3 SIRNA FOR TOPICAL DRUG DELIVERY SYSTEMS (DDSS)

Small interfering ribonucleic acid, i.e., siRNA administration can be used to suppress the abnormal gene expression that results in the synthesis of proteins associated to the progression of the disease. For the administration of siRNA, the skin comes to be the most vulnerable organ. Some skin conditions, including psoriasis, wounds, melanoma, alopecia areata (AA), pachyonychia congenita (PC), and rheumatoid arthritis (RA), are brought on by gene abnormalities. By administering the suitable siRNA to the intended site in the skin, various gene abnormalities are rectified.

7.3.3.1 PSORIASIS

Psoriasis is the most prominent skin conditions impacting people worldwide. It demonstrates a notable increase in keratinocytes, which produce plaque with chronic inflammatory responses. Psoriasis can be genetically cured by targeting a particular gene that involved in the elevation of the inflammatory cytokines. An important target for the therapy of psoriasis is TNF-α.

7.3.3.2 ALLERGIC CONTACT DERMATITIS (ACD)

Allergic contact dermatitis (ACD) consists of important immunized component. Atopic and contact dermatitis are the two most prevalent types of ACD. It is found that CD86 expressed in allergic skin. Hence, decreased in CD86 expression suppressed the Inflammation and immune response of the system. Using small interfering ribonucleic acid that targets CD86 can lower the expression of CD86.

7.3.3.3 PACHYONYCHIA CONGENITA (PC)

Pachyonychia congenita (PC) is rare genetic condition occurs due to alterations within one of the keratin genes. Depending upon the type of the mutant gene, it is divided into two subsets. A variation in the K6a gene induced PC-1, whereas a variation in the K6b gene triggered PC-2. These modifications result from the substitution of one nucleotide in the keratin gene, which is in charge of producing keratin fiber. Therefore, by using silencing effect of siRNA to target the mutant gene that leads to the development of PC is beneficial for its treatment (Aldawsari et al., 2015).

7.3.3.4 ALOPECIA AREATA (AA)

Alopecia areata (AA) is a disease occurred due to autoimmune response initiated by gene abnormality in which hair loss. According to research, patients with AA had T lymphocytes, CD4 and CD8 leaking surrounding their hair follicles. Th1 is a potential target for siRNA therapy to suppress abnormal gene expression in this skin disorder (Vicentini et al., 2013).

7.3.3.5 MELANOMA

Melanoma develops prominently between the junctions of epidermis and dermis layer. In that junction's pigment is buildup that defines as a melanoma. It is discovered that melanoma is caused by a mutation of particular proteins are BRAF V600E and Protein kinase B (Aldawsari et al., 2015; Vicentini et al., 2013). By using siRNA to target the mutated gene, the development of melanoma is prevented (Vicentini et al., 2013).

Administration approaches to deliver small interfering ribonucleic acid topically include liposomes, polymeric nanoparticles, polymer-drug conjugates, dendrimers, oil nanoemulsions, nanoparticles containing silica, and iron oxide nanoparticles (Aldawsari et al., 2015).

7.4 WHAT IS SKIN DISEASE?

Teenagers and adults alike are affected by the widespread problem of skin conditions. The consequence of skin conditions on patient's quality of life was once thought to be minimal but now it was concluded that it is getting worsen (Kassab et al., 2019). Skin and subcutaneous disorders were the 4th leading cause of non-fatal disease burden, directly following iron-deficiency anemia, tuberculosis, and sense organ diseases (Seth et al., 2017).

7.4.1 MOSTLY CONSIDERED SKIN DISORDERS

7.4.1.1 BACTERIAL SKIN DISEASES

Cellulitis usually shows as a swelled, red spot on the surface of skin, when touch, is sensitive and burning. The most frequent causes are Streptococcus and Staphylococcus (Sullivan & Debarra, 2018).

Hair follicle infections called folliculitis are quite prevalent (Lugović-Mihić et al., 2011). A hair follicle gets infected painfully by a furuncle, often described as a boil. It is an infection of the entire of pilosebaceous unit.

The upper part of skin's epidermis becomes infected with microbes in impetigo (Sukumaran & Senanayake, 2016).

7.4.1.2 FUNGAL SKIN DISEASE

Specifically, dermatophytosis and superficial mycoses were separated into two categories of skin fungal diseases. Dermatophytes like Microsporum, Epidermophyton, and Trichophyton, are the principal causes behind skin fungal diseases (White et al., 2014). Tinea infections are a common name for dermatophytoses (Kim et al., 2015).

7.4.1.3 INFLAMMATORY SKIN DISEASE

The body folds, scalp, and face, and are locations with a high concentration of sebaceous glands where seborrheic dermatitis frequently manifests as an inflamed skin condition with a papulosquamous shape (Tucker & Masood, 2022).

Atopic dermatitis (AD) is chronic inflammatory skin disorders that is characterized by intense itching and recurrent eczematous lesions (Bieber et al., 2021).

Psoriasis is an inflammatory response which is a chronic skin disorder with significant hereditary susceptibility and having auto-immune pathogenic features (Rendon & Schäkel, 2019).

7.4.1.4 VIRAL SKIN DISEASES

The exanthem (skin rashes) and enanthem (Abrasions in mucus membrane) of viral skin infections are the primary symptoms. The several viral skin conditions are examined, such as skin rashes like measles, erythema infectiosum, roseola, and rubella that affect children (Biesbroeck & Sidbury, 2013). Herpes viral skin conditions, as well as a number of other viral skin conditions, Gianotti-Crosti syndrome, and human papilloma virus (HPV) are found to be hazardous (Ramdass et al., 2015).

7.4.1.5 PSORIASIS

Psoriasis is a T-cell mediated autoimmune inflammatory disorder (Jarouliya et al., 2018; Barker et al., 1998). It is considered as skin surface inflammation, epidermal proliferation, which sometimes leads to hyperkeratosis, angiogenesis, and anomalous keratinization (Tamanna & Singh, 2021).

It appears in a variety of manifestations such as plaque psoriasis, inverse psoriasis, pustular, and erythrodermic psoriasis (Rahman et al., 2015). Lymphocyte activation is the cause of psoriasis (Lowes et al., 2014). Other cause is the risk factors in psoriasis which include abnormal alterations in eicosanoid metabolism, polyunsaturated fatty acids metabolic abnormalities, and gene expression (Tamanna & Singh, 2021).

7.4.1.6 ATOPIC DERMATITIS (AD)

AD is also known as Atopic eczema (Nutten et al., 2015). It is a type of inflammatory skin disorder characterized by severe itching and repetitive eczematous lesions (Eckhart et al., 2013). The pathophysiology of this disease is not fully understood. It seems to be the outcome of the complex interactions between the defects in skin barrier functions, environmental factors, infectious agents, and immune abnormalities (Thomsen et al., 2014).

7.4.1.7 IMPAIRED WOUND HEALING

Non-healing wounds are the results in inhibition of the normal sequence of cellular and biochemical events towards the fixing of the skin's integrity (Saini et al., 2016). Wounds that do not heal within 3 months are called or considered as chronic wounds (Frykberg & Banks, 2015). In acute wounds, production & degradation of molecules such as collagen is lost & as in chronic wounds balance is lost and degradation plays a large role in healing (Tamanna & Singh, 2021).

7.4.1.8 ACNE VULGARIS

Acne Vulgaris exists as a chronic disorder of the pilosebaceous follicles of the skin (Aydemir et al., 2014). The root cause of acne Vulgaris is the comedo and is initiated by hyperkeratosis of the lining of the pilosebaceous follicles with recognition of keratin and sebum. The comedo is a non-inflamed lesion and it usually relapses automatically. Certain diseases which block passage through the follicular pores for example hidadenitis, suppurativa and necrotizing cellulites of the scalp, perhaps related to acne (Tamanna & Singh, 2021).

7.4.1.9 MELANOMA

Skin cancers are of different types based on cells that become malignant. Melanocyte exists as a melanin-producing cell located inside basal layer of the epidermis, these cells can give birth to melanoma (Wang et al., 2016). Melanoma is more susceptible to occur and proliferate to different regions. Cancerous cells spread when they separate from the origin and entered into lymphatic or blood vessels. Thus, neighboring lymphatic nodules may contain cancerous cells (Ji et al., 2016).

7.4.1.10 SCABIES

Scabies is a severe skin disorder brought on by a mite's infestation (Gilson & Crane, 2021). The *Sarcoptes scabiei* mite penetrates the skin and produces painful irritation (Chandler & Fuller, 2019). Scabies is found to be highly infectious among the members who are in contact with infectious person because it could be transmits through skin-to-skin contact.

7.5 FOLLICULAR DELIVERY APPROACHES OF NANOCARRIERS

In 2007, the relationship between massage which induces movement of the hairs and the follicular penetration depths was detected by applying 320 nm polymer particles (Patzelt & Lademann, 2020). In 2011, it was shown that selective follicular targeting is possible by modifying the nanocarrier size meaning that specific nanocarrier sizes show deeper follicular penetration than others. In this study, it was found that nanocarriers between 300 and 650 nm penetrated significantly deeper than smaller or larger particles (Patzelt et al., 2011). It was hypothesized that this size dependency might be related to the thickness of the cuticula size, which was determined to be around 530 nm in human terminal hairs and 320 nm in porcine ear skin and therefore within the same size range (Lademann et al., 2009).

To target specific structures within the hair follicle without increasing the systemic or skin bioavailability of the corresponding drug (intrafollicular application) or it can be utilized to promote transfollicular delivery of the transported drug and consecutively the drugs bioavailability (transfollicular application) depending on the clinical and pharmaceutical requirements.

If intrafollicular drug deposition is desired, it is important to define the target structure of interest within the hair follicle, which might be the sebaceous gland or the bulge region, which is hosting the stem cells. It has also been shown that nanoencapsulation can improve the therapeutic outcome of hair loss and that poly(lactide-co-glycolide) nanoparticles, polymeric micelle nanocarriers and chitosan nanoparticles can provide an enhanced drug delivery within the hair follicles (Patzelt & Lademann, 2020).

For transfollicular delivery, it is important that the active is released from the carrier system at the right time point and at the right location as the likelihood of a transfollicular penetration of the nanocarrier itself is very low, especially in intact skin. The follicular penetration of polymer particles and found them to be located in the infundibulum without any translocation into viable cells of the external root sheath (Desai et al., 2010). So, in diseased skin, the barrier function can be changed in many different ways such as altered differentiation of keratinocytes, lipid composition or microbial colonization (Vogt et al., 2016), which can lead to increased nanocarriers penetration in disrupted skin (Schneider et al., 2009).

The encapsulated active substances are shielded from degradation in the particles because of which there is an obvious advantage of particulate substances is the possibility of sustained release (Singh et al., 2010), resulting in extended activity or enhanced uptake and the possible reduction of adverse effects.

There are now three main approaches to taking advantage of selective follicular penetration of particle drugs:

i. By selecting precise particle sizes, particles can be used to deliver therapeutic compounds into hair follicles, more specifically to predetermined target areas within the follicle.
ii. Particles can be used to transport therapeutic chemicals to viable skin after skin barrier disruption.
iii. A more elegant way to deliver therapeutic substances deep into the hair follicles, where they are actively released and then translocated independently to the viable skin particles having a particular releasing mechanism.

- **The First Approach:** Selection of suitable particle sizes, pharmacological active compounds that can be delivered into the hair follicles or to predestined targeted areas of hair follicle without translocating to the viable tissue. Recently, it was demonstrated that a nanoparticle-emulsion containing polyhexanide was able to achieve a better and long-lasting antisepsis for the human skin. The nanoparticle emulsion containing polyhexanide was demonstrated to block the endogenous recontamination pathway, i.e., through follicles (Ulmer et al., 2013). PLGA particles were shown to increase their permeation into the hair follicles (Jeong et al., 2019).

- **The Second Approach:** It is to translocate therapeutic substances to the viable skin is to disrupt the skin barrier prior to topical application of substances (Gorzelanny et al., 2020). Therefore, various techniques such as cyanoacrylate skin surface stripping, chemical enhancers, microneedles, electroporation, and ultrasound have been developed.
- **The Third Approach:** It is to equip particles with specific release mechanism. In this case, the particles are only responsible to deliver the therapeutic substances deeply into the hair follicles where they are released actively and subsequently translocated independently to the viable skin (Patzelt & Lademann, 2013).

7.5.1 POLYMERIC NANOPARTICLES

Polymeric nanoparticle might follow follicular and has been reported as the primary penetration route for nanoparticles (Wu et al., 2009). Hence, they accumulate preferentially in skin furrows and hair follicles and create high local concentrations of loaded drugs that can subsequently diffuse into the skin layers. It is believed that it is a size-dependent phenomenon where smaller nanoparticles show highest penetration. Hence, they may target the drug to the follicles followed by their accumulation, depot formation, and subsequent release of a drug may be used to provide more effective, sustained release (Gupta et al., 2012). Polymeric nanoparticles are either composed of natural polymers (Zielińska et al., 2020; Keservani et al., 2017a). A Demonstration that shows an increased percutaneous absorption and follicular penetration of retinal by topical application of chitosan-based nanoparticles (Limacharoen et al., 2019). PLA and PLGA copolymers are applied as synthetic polymers with the aim of drug delivery into the hair follicles has been demonstrated (Lademann et al., 2007).

7.5.2 LIPID NANOPARTICLES

Lipid nanoparticles an increased follicular uptake was observed such as for nanostructured lipid carriers (NLCs), Solid lipid nanocarrier, nanoemulsion, and liposomes. Suggested mechanism of liposomes through follicular route is that upon dehydration of liposomal bilayer can partition at pack into the follicular or hair ducts. This partitioning is favorable since the follicular ducts contain lipids (Picardo et al., 2009). The filling of the follicular opening with the liposomal bilayer not only results in entrapped drugs being carried into the follicles but also allows partitioning of unentrapped drugs into the bilayer matrix within the follicles (Prajapati et al., 2012). The use of nano-liposomal formulations in topical drug delivery has been found to improve the penetration of several entrapped agents into the skin and have been proven to be a valuable module for follicular drug targeting (Gupta et al., 2012).

7.5.3 METALLIC NANOPARTICLE

Demonstrate in the study states that quantum dots of 40 nm penetrate into the outer root sheath of the follicles (Zhang et al., 2008). Iron sulfate nanoparticles of only 10 nm in the hair follicles and around the hair follicles, which could indicate that they were able to penetrate transfollicularly (Baroli et al., 2007).

7.5.4 ETHOSOMES (ETOs)

Ethosomes (ETOs) are ideally suitable to serve as carrier for certain medications through the skin for the conditions relates with sebaceous gland and hair follicle, because they remain in the dermis and skin appendages for a longer time period than other types of skin cells (Yang et al., 2017). Targeting of minoxidil through ETOs to pilosebaceous units, the results showed localization of minoxidil in the pilosebaceous units that indicate higher delivery of minoxidil using ethosomal carriers (Nainwal et al., 2018).

7.5.5 NIOSOMES

Niosomes have been shown to be efficient in delivering bioactive substances to specific cells (Akbarzadeh et al., 2020). Proniosomes are formed of cholesterol and nonionic surfactants, consumes less time to prepare, and are more stable during storage (Sammour et al., 2019). Proniosomes can be converted into niosomes. It can be prepared by mixing the drug's aqueous phase with proniosomes with constant stirring or agitation at a temperature higher than transition phase temperature of surfactant (Wichayapreechar et al., 2019; Varsha & Savitha, 2019). Proniosmes are proven to be effective for skin problems through follicular route in mice (Rungseevijitprapa et al., 2021).

7.6 TRADITIONAL TREATMENT FOR SKIN DISEASES

7.6.1 TRADITIONAL HERBS USE FOR SKIN DISORDERS

Plants include phytochemical compounds that are used to treat skin disorders. Plant constituents, also known as phytoconstituents, are classified as primary or secondary metabolites (Mendoza & Silva, 2018). Secondary metabolites have been shown to have a wide range of biological effects, providing scientific support for the use of herbs in traditional medicine by many ancient civilizations (Hussein et al., 2018).

Tannins are naturally astringent substances that are applied topically to cure acne. The bark extract of witch hazel also called *Hamamelis virginiana* is frequently used as a home medicine and is thought to be quite safe to apply topically (McGuffin et al., 1997). In China, topical duckweed, scientifically known as Lemna minor, is commonly used to cure acne (Fleming et al., 2000). Dabao for the treatment of androgenic alopecia (Kessel et al., 1991). For the topical application of fungal and bacterial diseases, tea tree oil is used (Carson et al., 2006). Thus, the symptomatic treatment of onychomycosis, tinea pedis, and wounds may benefit from the use of tea tree oil (Faoagali et al., 1997). Antibacterial and anticandidal agents have been applied topically with thyme oil from *Thymus vulgaris* (Vanwyk et al., 2004). Carrot oil is considered a powerhouse of richly available vitamins A and E that are highly beneficial for hair and skin (Shebaby et al., 2013). The vitamin present in carrot oil helps in preventing hair loss and nourishes the hair shafts. The hair and skin benefit greatly from the moisturizing properties of carrot oil. The oil extracted from the seeds of *Daudus carota* has unique antiseptic and calming effects (Alves-Silva et al., 2016). It detoxifies the bodies which help to treat eczema and skin rashes (Ahuja et al., 2021). The leaves of aloe vera give a juice and gel or latex (Surjushe et al., 2008). The gel is derived from the leaf's inner core and has been applied topically for generations (Pierce et al., 1999). Aloe vera improved wound healing by lowering inflammatory cell infiltration, boosting CD^{4+}/CD^{8+} lymphocytes, and improving epidermal thickness and collagen deposition (Sánchez et al., 2020). Aloe sterols are involved in this UV protection (Misawa et al., 2017).

7.6.2 AYURVEDIC TREATMENTS FOR SKIN DISORDERS

Panchkarma treatment is a very renowned tool to cure many big problems. For skin related issues, *Panchkarma* has many therapies for skin protection and treatment like (Kour et al., 2016):

- *Virechana* (very effective for skin);
- *Vaman*;
- Swedan;
- Basti;
- *Udvartan* (scrub);
- Herbal face pack; and
- *Potli* massage.

Virechana is the best measure for *Kushta* (dermatological disorders). Most of the *Kushta* come under the heading of Raktapradshajavyadhi. The mala of Rakta is Pitta. As a result, *Pitta* and *Rakta* have inseparable connections. Pitta overproduction contributes to *Rakta* purification and the healing of *Rakta Pradoshaja Vikaras* like *kushta* as it leaves the human body. Rasa, *Rakta*, *Lasika*, *Udaka*, *Vata*, *Pitta*, and *Kapha*, are the primary causes of skin problems according to ayurveda, are specifically targeted by *virechana karma*. *Virechana* is hence the most effective shodhana karma in pitta pradhana kushta and to stop recurrences (Chaganti & Prasad, 2015). Similarly, in *Raktadushti* conditions *malaroopapitta* gets increased in the body, which is located in the liver and gall bladder. To eliminate such *malrropapita*, *Virechanakarma* is the only line of treatment.

7.6.3 OTHER TRADITIONAL TREATMENTS

Over 1,500 years ago, Chinese traders brought kampo therapy to the West. There is significant difference between Chinese traditional medicine and kampo medicine which is uniquely developed in Japan and Kampo prescriptions have been prescribed to treat a variety of diseases in Japan. AD can be effectively treated with kampo therapy. The indications of AD can be treated with standard Kampo preparations (Shimizu et al., 2013).

7.7 PATENTED FORMULATION

Following topical application to both human and animal skin, some investigations have demonstrated that nanocarriers or nanosystems can invade deeper into hair follicles. Some researchers have hypothesized that follicular delivery is more effective with nanocarriers with diameters around 300 nm as compared to larger nanocarriers (Silvia et al., 2022).

From patent WO2017046728A1 the purpose of the current concept is to create a nanocarrier that can transfer therapeutically active chemicals transfollicularly while also allowing for targeted distribution and release of substances in the vicinity of the pilosebaceous unit.

The present invention WO2006095778A1 relates to a hair-growth component-containing nanoparticle in which herbal medicine is encapsulated as a hair-growth component in the nanoparticle.

Acne treatments by reduce the accumulation of sebum and microorganisms within follicles and the sebaceous gland from patent US20140371656A1.

From patent JP2015526484A the drug's absorption and retention at the intended target area in treatment of androgenic alopecia needs to be through follicular route that provides to be cure for it using active components finasteride and minoxidil with the help of nanocarriers (Table 7.1).

TABLE 7.1 Various Patented Formulations for the Treatment of Skin Cancer

Application Number	Title	Results	Year
WO2017046728A1	Nanocarrier for transfollicular delivery of active substances and associated formation process.	A polymeric and phospholipidic derived aqueous product, and also a process for forming the nanocarrier, is used in a nanoparticle system for direct percutaneous release of therapeutic compounds.	2017
US20140371656A1	Hair removal with coated metal nanoparticle.	Photoactive substances and UV light, which including nanoparticles and formulations, are used to cure various skin tissue in animals such as humans for cosmetic, diagnosis, and clinical purposes.	2014
WO2006095778A1	Nanoparticles contain ingredients that stimulate hair development, methods for their production, and hair growth stimulants using the same.	Nanoparticles containing a hair-growth-stimulating component that are made by encapsulating a crude medicinal ingredient in a biocompatible polymer to produce nano-sized particles. These nanoparticles reach the deepest area of the scalp through pores and the scalp surface. As a result, the crude pharmaceutical substance can be transmitted to the deep area of the scalp, where it will be gradually released from nanoparticles.	2006
JP2015526484A	Finasteride and minoxidil polymer nanoparticles, methods for their preparation, aqueous suspensions containing them, pharmaceutical compositions, and uses thereof.	This present invention is a topical pharmacological formulation for alopecia therapy, consisting of polymer nanoparticles, particularly nanocapsules, having two active substances finasteride and minoxidil.	2015

7.8 CONCLUSION

Due to undesirable physicochemical properties and high toxicity profiles, therapeutic efficacy is restricted. Due to its distinctive features such as excellent biocompatibility, ease of surface modification, and tiny size, vesicular nanocarriers have the potential to reduce the downsides of specific medications that will be useful for skin disorders. The expanding use of nanocarriers or nanosystems for topical medication delivery systems has the potential to provide an opportunity for the deployment of highly capable and secure therapies with a high benefit-risk ratio. Nanocarriers can successfully preserve APIs on the layers of the skin from degradation, raise their concentration gradient in the top skin layers, and allow for progressive release. The utilization of particulate compounds that have been found to penetrate preferentially into the hair follicles or of controlled drug release systems are current areas of optimization. In this case, the particles are only used as transporters to a specific depth within the hair follicle, where the active medicine is then released and can translocate to the deeper viable skin layers around the hair follicles on its own. In terms of follicular penetration, the hair follicle is a complex three-dimensional dynamic structure with numerous roles, the reservoir and barrier functions being of particular significance. Follicular medication delivery using smart nanocarrier-based DDSs is a promising way to boost the percutaneous absorption and epidermal and systemic bioavailability of topically applied drugs. To get effective penetration into the hair follicles and to reach the depth of the hair bulb for pharmacological activity purposes, one should aim for the size range of carriers that suits the target region inside the hair follicle.

7.9 FUTURE PROSPECTIVES

The technique that shows promise for boosting the absorption of topically administered drugs is follicular drug delivery using innovative nanocarrier-based DDSs. The uses of internal or external stimuli for controlled drug release from the particulates are interesting concepts to optimize drug delivery to hair follicles and to advantageously utilize particulate substances for effective follicular drug delivery. Lipid nanocarriers are an efficient means of preventing the API from deteriorating on the skin's surface, enhancing their gradient of concentration in the top skin layers, and facilitating controlled release. Lipid nanoparticles for topical application may be produced with high lipid matrix content or may be dispersed in various bases. Topical administration of the API is safe, efficacious, and biocompatible because it doesn't harm cells or modify the way the skin looks. Nanoparticles are important for keeping the medicine at the point of action and changing the release profile for treating skin pathologies such as highly proliferative skin disorders. In addition to being compatible and capable of forming a protective lipid layer, using lipids similar to those found in skin structures in the creation of lipid nanocarriers has further benefits. The ability to design novel, more potent treatments for psoriasis and skin chemotherapy is made possible by the enhanced retention of antiproliferative medicines in the skin without causing major and irreversible alterations to its barrier function. Since androgenetic alopecia only affects pilosebaceous units, enhancing drug delivery at the site of action within hair follicles may be able to improve the success of alopecia treatment. Drug dose reduction and systemic drug absorption will both benefit from follicular drug targeting. The most promising method for topical delivery is nanostructured drug delivery technologies, which may enhance drug distribution or absorption in the hair follicle region while minimizing adverse effects and lowering dosage requirements. Additionally, by overcoming the skin's barriers to penetration, the use of nanotechnologies could enhance medication solubility while concurrently increasing the concentration of the drug at the target region.

KEYWORDS

- **ayurvedic treatments**
- **ethosomes**
- **follicular delivery**
- **lipid nanoparticles**
- **nanoparticles**
- **niosomes**
- **skin disease**

REFERENCES

Ahuja, A., Gupta, J., & Gupta, R., (2021). Miracles of herbal phytomedicines in treatment of skin disorders: Natural healthcare perspective. *Infect. Disord. Drug Targets, 21*(3), 228–338.

Akbarzadeh, I., Fatemizadeh, M., Heidari, F., & Mousavi-Niri, N., (2020). Niosomal formulation for co-administration of hydrophobic anticancer drugs into MCF-7 cancer cells. *Arch. Adv. Biosci., 11*, 1–9.

Aldawsari, M., Chougule, M. B., & Babu, R. J., (2015). Progress in topical siRNA delivery approaches for skin disorders. *Curr. Pharm. Des.*, *21*(31), 2594–4605.

Alves-Silva, J. M., Zuzarte, M., & Gonçalves, M. J., (2016). New claims for wild carrot (*Daucus carota* subsp. carota) essential oil. *Evid Based Complement Alternat Med.*, 2045196.

Aydemir, E. H., (2014). Acne vulgaris. *Turk Pediatri Ars.*, *49*(1), 23–16.

Baig, M. S., Keservani, R. K., Ahmad, M. F., & Baig, M. E., (2018). Smart delivery of nanobiomaterials in drug delivery. In: *Nanobiomaterials* (pp. 241–287).

Bansal, M. & Jamil, S., (2018). Micellar microparticles: A novel approach to topical drug delivery system. *International Journal of Applied Pharmaceutics, 10*(5), 1.

Barker, J. N., (1998). Psoriasis as a T cell-mediated autoimmune disease. *Hosp Med.*, *59*(7), 230–533.

Baroli, B., Ennas, M. G., Loffredo, F., et al., (2007). Penetration of metallic nanoparticles in human full-thickness skin. *J. Invest. Dermatol., 127*, 2701–1712.

Behera, J., Keservani, R. K., Yadav, A., Tripathi, M., & Chadoker, A., (2010). Methoxsalen loaded chitosan coated microemulsion for effective treatment of psoriasis. *International Journal of Drug Delivery, 2*(2).

Bieber, T., (2021). Atopic dermatitis: An expanding therapeutic pipeline for a complex disease. *Nat. Rev. Drug Discov*., 21–40.

Biesbroeck, L., & Sidbury, R., (2013). Viral exanthems: An update. *Dermatol Ther*., *26*(6), 233–438.

Caminade, A. M., (2016). Inorganic dendrimers: Recent advances for catalysis, nanomaterials, and nanomedicine. *Chemical Society Reviews, 45*(19), 5174–5186.

Carson, C. F., Hammer, K. A., & Riley, T. V., (2006). Melaleuca alternifolia (tea tree) oil: A review of antimicrobial and other medicinal properties. *Clin. Microbiol Rev*., *19*(1), 20–62.

Chaganti, S., & Prasad, B. S., (2015). Analysis of virechana karma with Danti avaleha: A retrospective study. *J. Ayurveda Integr. Med*., *6*(4), 200–304.

Chandler, D. J, & Fuller, L. C., (2019). A review of scabies: An infestation more than skin deep. *Dermatology, 235*, 29–90.

Chenthamara, D., Subramaniam, S., & Ramakrishnan, S. G., (2019). Therapeutic efficacy of nanoparticles and routes of administration. *Biomater Res*., *23*, 20.

Choudhury, B., (2021). Scopes of skin disease management through ayurveda. *IJATM, 3*, 5–7.

Deng, S., Gigliobianco, M. R., Censi, R., Di Martino, P., (2020). Polymeric nanocapsules as nanotechnological alternative for drug delivery system: Current status, challenges and opportunities. *Nanomaterials (Basel)*, *10*(5), 247.

Desai, P., Patlolla, R. R., & Singh, M., (2010). Interaction of nanoparticles and cell-penetrating peptides with skin for transdermal drug delivery. *Mol Membr Biol*., *27*(7), 247–259.

Eckhart, L., Lippens, S., & Tschachler, E., (2013). Cell death by cornification. *Biochimica et Biophysica Acta (BBA)-Molecular Cell Research, 1833*(12), 2471–2480.

Faoagali, J., George, N., & Leditschke, J. F., (1997). Does tea tree oil have a place in the topical treatment of burns? *Burns, 23*, 249–251.

Farah, F., & Farah, F. H., & Farah, F., (2019). Nanocarriers as delivery systems for therapeutics agents. *International Journal of Pharmaceutical Sciences and Research, 10*, 1000–1022.

Filisa, C., Annamaria, C., Donatella, P., Massimo, F., Angelo, M., & Giuseppe, O., (2017). *Nanocarrier for Transfollicular Delivery of Active Substances and Associated Formation Process.* WO2017046728A1.

Fleming, T., (2000). Medical economics Co.. *PDR for Herbal Medicines* (2nd edn.). Montvale, NJ.

Frykberg, R. G., & Banks, J., (2015). Challenges in the treatment of chronic wounds. *Adv Wound Care (New Rochelle)*, *4*(9), 260–582.

Gautam, S. P., Keservani, R. K., Gautam, T., Gupta, A. K., & Sharma, A. K., (2015). An alternative approach for acetylation of amine terminated polyamidoamine (PAMAM) dendrimer. *ARS Pharmaceutica, 56*(3), 155–159.

Gilson, R. L., & Crane, J. S., (2021). Scabies. In: *StatPearls*. Treasure Island (FL): StatPearls Publishing.

Gorzelanny, C., Mess, C., Schneider, S. W., Huck, V., & Brandner, J. M., (2020). Skin Barriers in dermal drug delivery: Which barriers have to be overcome and how can we measure them? *Pharmaceutics, 12*(7), 284.

Gupta, M., Agrawal, U., & Vyas, S. P., (2012). Nanocarrier-based topical drug delivery for the treatment of skin diseases. *Expert. Opin. Drug Deliv.*, *9*(7), 283–804.

Hiroyuki, T., Kaori, H., & Yusuke, T., (2006). *Nanoparticles Containing Hair Growth-Stimulating Ingredient, Method of Producing the Same and Hair Growth Stimulant Using the Same.* WO2006095778A1.

Hussein, R. A., & El-Anssary, A. A., (2018). Plants Secondary metabolites: The key drivers of the pharmacological actions of medicinal plants. In: *Herbal Medicine*. IntechOpen.

Jarouliya, U., & Keservani, R. K., (2018). Nutraceutical components in the treatment of psoriasis and psoriatic arthritis. In: Siba, P. R., Smriti, R., & Debasis, B., (eds.), *Psoriasis and Psoriatic Arthritis Pathophysiology, Therapeutic Intervention, and Complementary Medicine*. CRC Press,Taylor & Francis Group.

Jeong, W. Y., Kim, S., & Lee, S. Y., (2019). Transdermal delivery of minoxidil using HA-PLGA nanoparticles for the treatment in alopecia. *Biomater Res.*, *23*, 16.

Ji, R. C., (2016). Lymph Nodes and cancer metastasis: New perspectives on the role of intranodal lymphatic sinuses. *Int. J. Mol Sci.*, *18*(1), 21.

Kassab, Y. W., Muhamad, S. A., Aldahoul, H. K., Mohammed, I. K., Paneerselvam, G. S., et al., (2019). The impact of skin disorders on patients' quality of life in Malaysia. *J. Clin. Intensive Care Med., 4*, 001–009.

Keservani, R. K., & Gautam, S. P., (2020). Formulation and evaluation of baclofen liposome vesicles using lecithin. *ARS Pharmaceutica, 61*(3), 175–180.

Keservani, R. K., & Gautam, S. P., (2022). Skeletal muscle relaxant activity of different formulation of span 60 niosome. *ARS Pharmaceutica, 63*(91), 32–44.

Keservani, R. K., Kesharwani, R. K., & Sharma, A. K., (2017a). Introduction to nanotechnology in drug delivery. In: *Drug Delivery Approaches and Nanosystems* (pp. 1–19).

Keservani, R. K., Sharma, A. K., & Kesharwani, R. K., (2018). Nanoparticulate nanocarriers in drug delivery. In: *Nanobiomaterials* (pp. 3–22).

Keservani, R. K., Sharma, A. K., & Ramteke, S., (2010). Novel vesicular approach for topical delivery of baclofen via niosomes. *Lat. Am. J. Pharm., 29,* 1364–1370.

Kessels, A. G. H., Cardynaals, R. L. L. M., & Borger, R. L. L., (1991). The effectiveness of the hair restorer "Dabao" in males with alopecia androgenetica: A clinical experiment. *J. Clin. Epidemiol., 44*, 239–247.

Khan, H. A., Sakharkar, M. K., Nayak, A., Kishore, U., & Khan, A., (2018). 14-nanoparticles for biomedical applications: An overview. In: Narayan, R., (ed.), *Nanobiomaterials* (pp. 357–384). Cambridge: Woodhead Publishing.

Kim, S. H., Cho, S. H., Youn, S. K., et al., (2015). Epidemiological characterization of skin fungal infections between the years 2006 and 2010 in Korea. *Osong. Public Health Res. Perspect.*, *6*(6), 241–345.

Knorr, F., Patzelt, A., Darvin, M. E., et al., (2016). Penetration of topically applied nanocarriers into the hair follicles of dog and rat dorsal skin and porcine ear skin. *Vet. Dermatol.*, *27*(4), 256–e60.

Kour, B., (2016). Beauty Care & skin diseases treatment in ayurveda. *Int. J. Complement. Alt Med.*, *2*(3), 00052.

Kumavat, S., Sharma, P. K., Koka, S. S., Sharma, R., Gupta, A., & Darwhekar, G. N., (2021). A Review on niosomes: Potential vesicular drug delivery system. *Journal of Drug Delivery and Therapeutics*, *11*(5), 208–212.

Lademann, J., Patzelt, A., & Richter, H., (2009). Determination of the cuticula thickness of human and porcine hairs and their potential influence on the penetration of nanoparticles into the hair follicles. *J. Biomed. Opt.*, *14*, 221014.

Lademann, J., Richter, H., & Teichmann, A., (2007). Nanoparticles–an efficient carrier for drug delivery into the hair follicles. *Eur. J. Pharm. Biopharm.*, *66*, 259–164.

Limcharoen, B., Toprangkobsin, P., & Banlunara, W., (2019). Increasing the percutaneous absorption and follicular penetration of retinal by topical application of proretinal nanoparticles. *Eur. J. Pharm. Biopharm.*, *139*, 23–100.

Lowes, M. A., Suárez-Fariñas, M., & Krueger, J. G., (2014). Immunology of psoriasis. *Annu Rev Immunol.*, *32*, 227–255.

Lu, H., Wang, J., Wang, T., Zhong, J., Bao, Y., & Hao, H., (2016). Recent progress on nanostructures for drug delivery applications. *Journal of Nanomaterials*, 1–12.

Lugović-Mihić, L., Barisić, F., & Bulat, V., (2011). Differential diagnosis of the scalp hair folliculitis. *Acta Clin. Croat.*, *50*(3), 295–402.

Mahor, A., Singh, P. P., Bharadwaj, P., Sharma, N., Yadav, S., Rosenholm, J. M., & Bansal, K. K., (2021). *Carbon-Based Nanomaterials for Delivery of Biologicals and Therapeutics: A Cutting-Edge Technology. C*, *7*, 19.

McGuffin, M., Hobbs, C., Upton, R., & Goldberg, A., (1997). *Botanical Safety Handbook.* Boca Raton, FL: CRC Press.

Meenakshi, D. (2013). Emulgel A novel approach to topical drug delivery. *Int J Pharma Bio Sci*, *4*, 847–856.

Mendoza, N., & Silva, E. M. E., (2018). Introduction to phytochemicals: Secondary metabolites from plants with active principles for pharmacological importance. In: Asao, T., & Asaduzzaman, M., (eds.), *Phytochemicals – Source of Antioxidants and Role in Disease Prevention.* IntechOpen.

Misawa, E., Tanaka, M., Saito, M., Nabeshima, K., Yao, R., Yamauchi, K., Abe, F., et al., (2017). Protective effects of aloesterols against UVB-induced photoaging in hairless mice. *Photodermatology, Photoimmunology & Photomedicine*, *33*(2), 101–111.

Nethanel, F., Arie, D., Jhonathan, E., Sharon, M., & Ofra, B., (2021). Physical properties of gold nanoparticles affect skin penetration via hair follicles. *Nanomedicine: Nanotechnology, Biology and Medicine*, *36*, 102414.

Nidhi, N., Sunil, J., Singh, R., & Saharan, V. A., (2018). Transdermal applications of ethosomes – A detailed review. *Journal of Liposome Research*, *29*, 1–32.

Nutten, S., (2015). Atopic Dermatitis: Global epidemiology and risk factors. *Ann. Nutr. Metab.*, *66*, 8–16.

Ojha, A., Ojha, M., & Madhav, N. S., (2017). Recent Advancement in emulgel: A novel approach for topical drug delivery. *Int. J. Adv. Pharm.*, *6*, 17–23.

Opatha, S. A. T., Titapiwatanakun, V., & Chutoprapat, R., (2020). Transfersomes: A promising nanoencapsulation technique for transdermal drug delivery. *Pharmaceutics*, *12*(9), 255.

Patra, J. K., Das, G., Fraceto, L. F., et al., (2018). Nano based drug delivery systems: Recent developments and future prospects. *J. Nanobiotechnol.*, *16*, 71.

Patzelt, A., & Lademann, J., (2013). Drug delivery to hair follicles. *Expert Opin. Drug Deliv.*, *10*(6), 287–797.

Patzelt, A., & Lademann, J., (2020). Recent advances in follicular drug delivery of nanoparticles. *Expert Opin. Drug Deliv.*, *17*(1), 29–60.

Patzelt, A., Richter, H., Knorr, F., et al., (2011). Selective follicular targeting by modification of the particle sizes. *J. Control Release, 150*, 25–48.

Paulman, Adriana, R. G., Dennis, S. D., Ludmila, P. D., & Silvia, S., (2015). *Finasteride and Minoxidil Polymer Nanoparticles, Methods for their Preparation, Aqueous Suspensions Containing Them, Pharmaceutical Compositions, and Uses Thereof.* JP2015526484A.

Peirce, A., Fargis, P., & Scordato, E., (1999). *The American Pharmaceutical Association Practical Guide to Natural Medicines.* New York: Stonesong Press Inc.

Picardo, M., Ottaviani, M., Camera, E., & Mastrofrancesco, A., (2009). Sebaceous gland lipids. *Dermatoendocrinol.*, *1*(2), 28–71.

Prajapati, B., (2012). Topical liposomes in drug delivery: A review. *IJPRT*.

Rahman, M., Akhter, S., & Ahmad, J., (2015). Nanomedicine-based drug targeting for psoriasis: Potentials and emerging trends. *Expert Opinion on Drug Delivery, 12*(4), 235–252.

Ramdass, P., Mullick, S., & Farber, H. F., (2015). Viral skin diseases. *Prim Care*, *42*(4), 217–567.

Rendon, A., & Schäkel, K., (2019). Psoriasis pathogenesis and treatment. *Int. J. Mol. Sci.*, *20*(6), 2475.

Rungseevijitprapa, W., Yingngam, B., & Chaiyasut, C., (2021). Improvement of biophysical skin parameters of topically applied fermented soybean extract-loaded niosomes with no systemic toxicity in ovariectomized rats. *Pharmaceutics, 13*, 1068.

Saini, S., Dhiman, A., & Nanda, S., (2016). Traditional Indian medicinal plants with potential wound healing activity: A review. *International Journal of Pharmaceutical Sciences and Research, 7*(5), 2809.

Saising, J., Maneenoon, K., Sakulkeo, O., Limsuwan, S., Götz, F., & Voravuthikunchai, S. P., (2022). Ethnomedicinal plants in herbal remedies used for treatment of skin diseases by traditional healers in Songkhla province, Thailand. *Plants*, *11*, 880.

Sammour, R. M. F., Taher, M., Chatterjee, B., Shahiwala, A., & Mahmood, S., (2019). Optimization of aceclofenac proniosomes by using different carriers, part 1: Development and characterization. *Pharmaceutics, 11*, 350.

Sánchez, M., González-Burgos, E., Iglesias, I., & Gómez-Serranillos, M. P., (2020). Pharmacological update properties of aloe vera and its major active constituents. *Molecules, 25*(6), 1324.

Sankar, V., Ramesh, S., & Siram, K., (2018). Ethosomes: An exciting and promising alcoholic carrier system for treating androgenic alopecia. In: *Alopecia*. IntechOpen.

Schneider, M., Stracke, F., Hansen, S., & Schaefer, U. F., (2009). Nanoparticles and their interactions with the dermal barrier. *Dermatoendocrinol.*, *1*(4), 297–206.

Seth, D., Cheldize, K., Brown, D., & Freeman, E. F., (2017). Global burden of skin disease: Inequities and innovations. *Curr. Dermatol. Rep.*, *6*(3), 204–210.

Sharma, D., Ali, A. A. E., & Aate, J. R., (2018). Niosomes as novel drug delivery system: Review article. *Pharmatutor, 6*(3), 58.

Shebaby, W. N., El-Sibai, M., Smith, K. B., Karam, M. C., Mroueh, M., & Daher, C. F., (2013). The antioxidant and anticancer effects of wild carrot oil extract. *Phytother Res.*, *27*(5), 237–744.

Shimizu, T., (2013). Efficacy of kampo medicine in treating atopic dermatitis: An overview. *Evid. Based Complement Alternat Med.*, 260235.

Singh, M. N., Hemant, K. S., Ram, M., & Shivakumar, H. G., (2010). Microencapsulation: A promising technique for controlled drug delivery. *Res. Pharm. Sci.*, *5*(2), 25–77.

Souto, E. B., De Souza, A. L. R., Dos Santos, F. K., Sanchez-Lopez, E., Cano, A., Zielińska, A., Staszewski, R., et al., (2021). Lipid nanocarriers for hyperproliferative skin diseases. *Cancers*, *13*, 5619.

Stefanov, S. R., & Andonova, V. Y., (2021). Lipid nanoparticulate drug delivery systems: Recent advances in the treatment of skin disorders. *Pharmaceuticals.*, *14*,1083.

Sukumaran, V., & Senanayake, S., (2016). Bacterial skin and soft tissue infections. *Aust. Prescr.*, *39*(5), 259–163.

Sullivan, T., de Barra, E., (2018). Diagnosis and management of cellulitis. *Clin Med (Lond).*, *18*(2), 260–163.

Surjushe, A., Vasani, R., & Saple, D. G., (2008). Aloe vera: A short review. *Indian J. Dermatol.*, *53*(4), 263–166.

Tamanna, & Singh, H., (2021). Nanotechnology: A novel approach for treatment of skin disorder. *Journal of Drug Delivery and Therapeutics.*, *11*(4-S), 271–277.

Thomsen, S. F., (2014). *Atopic Dermatitis: Natural History, Diagnosis, and Treatment*. ISRN allergy.

Todd, J. H., & Alice, A. C. K., (2014). *Hair Removal with Coated Metal Nanoparticles*. US20140371656A1.

Tucker, D., & Masood, S., (2022). *Seborrheic Dermatitis.* In: StatPearls [Internet]. Treasure Island (FL): StatPearls Publishing.

Ulmer, M., Patzelt, A., Vergou, T., et al., (2013). *In vivo* investigation of the efficiency of a nanoparticle-emulsion containing polihexanide on the human skin. *Eur. J. Pharm. Biopharm.*, *84*(2), 225–329.

Van, W. B., & Wink, M., (2004). *Medicinal Plants of the World*. Portland, OR: Timber Press.

Varsha, V. R., & Savitha, S. K., (2019). Proniosomes: As a potential drug delivery system. *Curr. Drug Deliv.*, *11*, 2594–2597.

Vicentini, F. T., Borgheti-Cardoso, L. N., Depieri, L. V., et al., (2013). Delivery systems and local administration routes for therapeutic siRNA. *Pharm. Res.*, *30*, 915–931.

Vogt, A., Wischke, C., & Neffe, A. T., (2016). Nanocarriers for drug delivery into and through the skin – do existing technologies match clinical challenges? *J. Control Release*, *242*, 2–15.

Wang, J. X., Fukunaga-Kalabis, M., & Herlyn, M., (2016). Crosstalk in skin: Melanocytes, keratinocytes, stem cells, and melanoma. *J. Cell Commun Signal*, *10*(3), 191–196.

White, T. C., Findley, K., & Dawson, T. L. Jr., (2014). Fungi on the skin: Dermatophytes and Malassezia. *Cold Spring Harb. Perspect. Med.*, *4*(8), a019802.

Wichayapreechar, P., Anuchapreeda, S., Rungseevijitprapa, W., & Ampasavate, C., (2019). Dermal targeting of *Centella asiatica* extract using hyaluronic acid surface modified niosomes modified niosomes. *J. Liposome Res.*, *30*, 197–207.

Wu, X., Price, G., & Guy, R., (2009). Disposition of nanoparticles and an associated lipophilic permeant following topical application to the skin. *Molecularpharmaceutics*, *6*. 1441-1448.

Yang, L., Wu, L., Wu, D., Shi, D., Wang, T., & Zhu, X., (2017). Mechanism of transdermal permeation promotion of lipophilic drugs by ethosomes. *Int. J. Nanomedicine*, *12*, 2357-3364.

Zhang, L. W., Yu, W. W., Colvin, V. L., et al., (2008). Biological interactions of quantum dot nanoparticles in skin and in human epidermal keratinocytes. *Toxicol. Appl. Pharmacol.*, *228*, 200–211.

Zielińska, A., Carreiró, F., Oliveira, A. M., et al., (2020). Polymeric nanoparticles: Production, characterization, toxicology and ecotoxicology. *Molecules*, *25*(16), 2731.

CHAPTER 8

Nanocarriers for Atopic Dermatitis Treatment

MAILINE GEHRCKE and LETÍCIA CRUZ

Laboratory of Pharmaceutical Technology, Graduate Program in Pharmaceutical Sciences, Center of Health Sciences, Federal University of Santa Maria, Santa Maria, Brazil

ABSTRACT

Atopic dermatitis (AD) is a chronic and immune-inflammatory skin disease that has a complex pathophysiology initiated by skin barrier impairment. Although it is incurable, the treatment of this eczema is based on the control of its clinical signs (itching, dehydration, papules, and wound formation, and edema). However, in addition to the lack of a single treatment, pharmacological therapy for atopic skin is associated with limited efficacy and many adverse effects. The drawbacks of current therapies lead to the development of novel therapeutic strategies such as nanotechnology-based formulations. Different types of nanocarriers can be designed to transport active substances, enhancing their therapeutic efficacy and reducing their adverse effects. This chapter first introduces what pathophysiology of AD involves and the current treatments available on the market. Then, with numerous findings reported, it dwells on nanocarriers and their advancements in AD. Similarly, nano-based dosage forms are highlighted shedding light on both nanocarriers skin penetration and animal models for screening potential nanoformulations. But it is important to mention that although there is progress in nanotechnology-based approaches to treat AD, more confirmatory *in vivo* studies about their effectiveness and toxicity are encouraged.

Novel Nanocarriers forSkin Diseases: Advances and Applications.
Raj K. Keservani and Júlia Scherer Santos (Eds.)

8.1 ATOPIC DERMATITIS (AD)

Atopic dermatitis (AD) or atopic eczema is a chronic and non-contagious inflammatory cutaneous disease, characterized by intense itching. In addition, this eczema is associated with clinical features that include papules and plaques, along with xerosis and keratosis, involving the face, scalp, and extremity areas. Thus, the patients skin presents redness with or without wounds and exudation (Malik & Heitmiller, 2017; Rerknimitr et al., 2017). This eczema is part of the atopic triad (asthma, allergic rhinitis and dermatitis) and affects up to 20% of children and 1–3% of adults globally (Misery et al., 2019).

The pathophysiology of AD is a complex interrelationship among genetic, environmental, immunological, pharmacological, and psychological factors, as well as skin barrier dysfunction (Malik & Heitmiller, 2017). Besides, this pathology can present heterogeneous manifestations with severity ranges from mild, moderate to severe. The diagnosis can be assessed using eczema area severity index (EASI) which defines the lesions extent in each body region and then a lesion in each of these areas is evaluated for formation of the erythema, edema or papules, excoriation, and lichenification. Another severity score used is the scoring AD (SCORAD) which is based on the extent and severity of the lesion and the presence of subjective symptoms, such as pruritus and sleeplessness (Rullo et al., 2008).

The skin has a complex structure, playing an important role in protection, thermoregulation, and immune response and is constantly subject to stimuli, such as pathogens and mechanical, chemical, and physical agents. The main physical barrier to the entry of chemicals and pathogens is the *stratum corneum* (SC), the outermost epidermis layer formed by corneocytes, dead cells, and keratin, which are immersed in a lipid matrix composed mainly by ceramides, cholesterol, and fatty acids (Wickett & Visscher, 2006). This lipid organization prevents excessive water loss through the skin. The skin barrier disruption in the AD may be related to changes in the corneocytes structural proteins expression and the lipids composition present in the SC (Yang et al., 2020).

Corneocytes are composed of densely cross-linked proteins such as filaggrin (FLG), loricrin, and involucrin. FLG is crucial for keratin alignment and its metabolites integrate the natural moisturizing factor which is essential for appropriate SC hydration (Wickett & Visscher, 2006). FLG genes mutations are highly associated with AD development (Yang et al., 2020). Regarding lipid disorders, studies show that individuals with AD have a long chains reduction of lipids, an increase of unsaturated free fatty acids and a decrease in the ceramide levels. The ceramides reduction is due to an increased pH and high epidermal serine protease activity (Smeden & Bouwstra, 2016).

The allergens penetration through the skin leads to loss of tissue homeostasis. Dendritic cells induce the differentiation of naive CD4(+) T cells into T helper 2 (Th2) cells which secret Th2 cytokines (IL-4, IL-5, and IL-13). These cytokines stimulate the differentiation of B cells to IgE-producing plasma cells and the eosinophils activation. In addition to eosinophils activation, AD is also characterized by the infiltration of other inflammatory cells, such as lymphocytes, macrophages, and mast cells (Malik & Heitmiller, 2017; Rerknimitr et al., 2017; Yang et al., 2020). Some authors categorize the AD into extrinsic and intrinsic types. Extrinsic or allergic type has high serum levels of total IgE with presence of specific IgE for environmental and food allergens. On the other hand, the intrinsic type has lower expression of specific IgE and Th2 cytokines but presents higher expression of interferon-γ (IFN-γ) (Bieber, 2017; Tokura, 2010) (Figure 8.1).

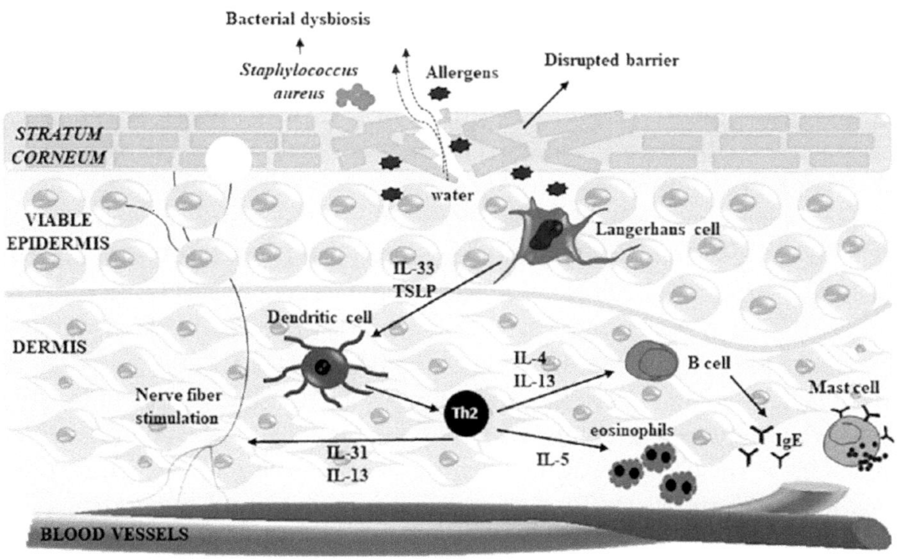

FIGURE 8.1 Barrier impairment and immunological contributing to the pathogenesis of atopic dermatitis (skin structure not drawn to scale).

Pruritus in AD may be related to the release of mediators, such as thymic stromal lymphopoietin (TSLP), IL-13, and IL-31, which stimulate nerve fibers (Rerknimitr et al., 2017). During scratching the skin barrier is frequently removed and a constant release of cytokines occurs. This process is known as the vicious cycle of AD. The itch-scratch cycle is crucial to progression and inflicts a substantial psychosocial burden on patients (Malik & Heitmiller, 2017; Rerknimitr et al., 2017; Sibbald & Drucker, 2017). Moreover, in atopic skin is observed an abnormal microbial colonization with pathogenic organisms, mainly *Staphylococcus aureus*, which exacerbates the immune response. It is estimated that more than 90% of AD lesions are colonized with this pathogen (Malik & Heitmiller, 2017).

In addition to inflammatory/immunological modulation, reactive oxygen species (ROS) have been reported as important contributors to the pathogenesis of AD (Bertino et al., 2020). ROS damage epidermal keratinocytes through alterations in cellular DNA and/or through lipid peroxidation of cellular structures. Furthermore, enzymatic antioxidants such as superoxide dismutase, superoxide reductase, catalase, and the entire glutathione system may be reduced, while malondialdehyde levels may be increased. Thus, the oxidative stress contributes to exacerbation of cutaneous inflammation and disruption of skin barrier function, as well as enables infections by pathogens (Ji & Li, 2016).

8.2 CURRENT TREATMENTS

AD is not yet curable and presents a great individual clinical variability making its management difficult. The severity ranges of the AD generally determine the choice of therapy and its treatment is based on pruritus minimization and achieve long-term disease control. Prevention of skin dryness and contact with irritating agents are the primary approach that is achieved (Ghosalkar et al., 2022; Singh et al., 2022). The use of products composed by emollients, humectants, and occlusive substances is necessary to preserve skin hydration and restore the integrity of the skin barrier (Mancuso et al., 2021).

The anti-inflammatory topical therapy is the first-line treatment for AD. Topical corticosteroids are the main options for acute flares, and they differ in potency. The choice of which one to use depends on the disease severity and the application site. Topical calcineurin inhibitors are used as second-line treatment in patients with inadequate response to topical corticosteroids (Tier et al., 2021). Patients with severe AD refractory to the habitual topical treatment can be medicated with systemic drugs, such as oral immunosuppressive drugs and biological therapy (Simpson et al., 2017). Topical and systemic approaches most frequently used in AD and their respective mechanisms of action are shown in Table 8.1.

Other therapies may be beneficial for the treatment of AD. Ultraviolet (UV) based phototherapy (UVB, narrow-band UVB or UVA) reduces

TABLE 8.1 Current Drugs for AD Treatment

Treatment type	Class	Drug	Mechanism of action	Reference
Topical	Calcineurin Inhibitors	Tacrolimus, Pimecrolimus	It inhibits calcineurin-dependent T-cell activation, blocking the production of proinflammatory cytokines and mediators	(Carroll and Fleischer, 2015; Huang and Xu, 2015)
	Corticosteroids	Clobetasol propionate, Halobetasol propionate, Betamethasone dipropionate, Mometasone furoate, Hydrocortisone valerate, Triamcinolone acetonide	It suppresses inflammatory cytokines and immune cells	(Ghosalkar et al., 2022)
Systemic	Immunosuppressants	Cyclosporin	It inhibits calcineurin blocking transcription of IL-2 and decreases activation of T cells	(Schmitt et al. 2007)
		Azathioprine	It is a 6-mercaptopurine analog. It inhibits purine synthesis, hindering cellular metabolism and preventing mitosis mainly in leukocytes	(Meggitt and Reynolds, 2001)
		Mycophenolate mofetil	It inhibits lymphocyte activation by monophosphate dehydrogenase reversible inhibition	(Neuber et al., 2000)
		Methotrexate	It is a folic acid antagonist. It inhibits dihydrofolate reductase, blocking division and lymphocyte proliferation	(Deo et al., 2014)
	Biologic	Dupilumab	It is human monoclonal antibody that inhibits IL-4 receptor α, a common part of IL-4 and IL-13 receptors, blocking IL-4 and IL-13 signaling	(Ferreira and Torres, 2018)

inflammation and induces apoptosis in pathogenic cells. First-generation oral antihistamines can be used to control the pruritus associated sleep disturbances. Antibiotics are used for the treatment of infected lesions associated with AD (Berger et al., 2014; Singh et al., 2022).

However, conventional topical and systemic treatments present drawbacks. Topical corticosteroids can cause rashes, rosacea-like eruptions and systemic effects (Ghosalkar et al., 2022), while topical calcineurin inhibitors are associated to burning, pain, and greater incidence of viral infection (Huang & Xu, 2015). Oral immunosuppressive drugs suffer from poor target-specific effect, low bioavailability, and pronounced side effects (Hemrajani et al., 2022). In consequence, patient satisfaction and compliance to therapy are often poor among the individuals affected by AD. Thus, novel drug delivery systems (DDSs) have been studied in the last years to alter the landscape of therapeutic options for AD management.

8.3 DRUG DELIVERY NANOCARRIERS

Nanocarriers development have been offered new opportunities in designing of drug delivery strategies for cutaneous disorders management, including AD (Ramanunny et al., 2021). Over the past few decades there has been extensive research demonstrating the effectiveness of classical drug-loaded nanocarriers (corticosteroids, immunosuppressants, and antihistamines) to treat AD. The main benefits provided by the nanoencapsulation of traditional drugs are in terms of increased bioavailability and improved skin permeability, which enables dose reduction and consequently, diminishes side effects (Alam et al., 2013; Badihi et al., 2020; Hussain et al., 2014; Li et al., 2012; Wang et al., 2019). However, research involving the nanoencapsulation of non-traditional drugs (drug repositioning) and novel therapeutic molecules to treat AD have increased (Cervi et al., 2021; Espinoza et al., 2020; Lin et al., 2021; Weber et al., 2018).

Most studies focus on the development of novel nanocarriers for topical application, including micro- and nano-emulsions (NEs) (Behera et al., 2020), liposomes, ethosomes (ETOs), transfersomes (TRAs), solid lipid nanoparticles (SLNs), nanostructured lipid carriers (NLCs), polymeric micelles, nanofibers, polymeric nanoparticles and inorganic nanoparticles (Figure 8.2). In fact, in addition to being the first-line treatment for AD, topical therapy is more advantageous than systemic administration because of the direct contact with the site of action. Moreover, specifically for AD, the formulation components can contribute to restore the skin barrier

(Paiva-Santos et al., 2022). The choice of the ideal nanocarrier and its components should be based on the encapsulated drug characteristics and the objective to be achieved. In topical treatment, the type and the composition of the nanocarrier may influence the drug skin permeation (Figure 8.3) (Roberts et al., 2017). In the following sections of this chapter is approached an overview of the several nanocarriers along with their applications for AD treatment.

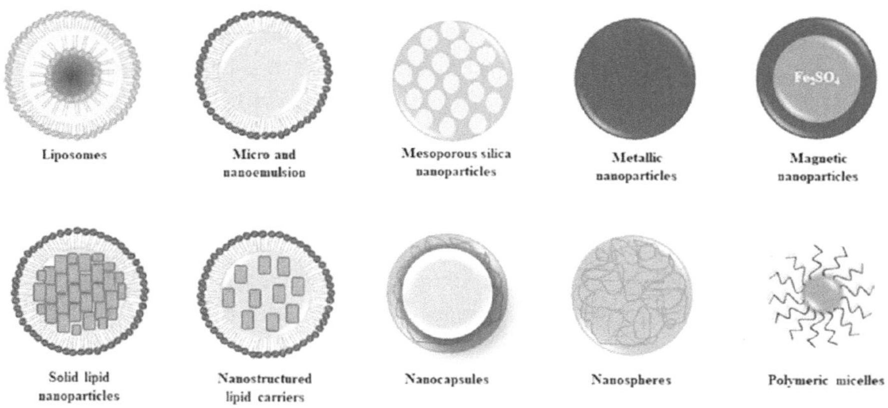

FIGURE 8.2 Representative figures of nanocarriers investigated for drug delivery in atopic dermatitis treatment.

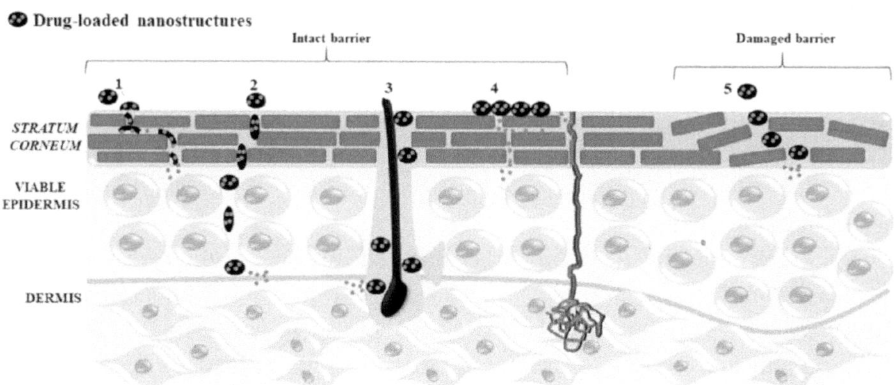

FIGURE 8.3 Main penetration routes of nanocarrier-based formulations on skin (skin structure not drawn to scale). (1) Nanocarrier fusion with lipid structure of stratum corneum (e.g., liposomes, nanoemulsions); (2) nanocarrier intact penetration across skin (flexible nanocarriers, e.g., ethosomes, transferomes); (3) increased penetration by nanocarrier accumulation in hair follicles (e.g., polymeric nanoparticles); (4) skin nanoparticles deposition with improved occlusion and penetration (e.g., lipid nanoparticles); and (5) increased penetration across inflamed skin.

8.3.1 LIPID-BASED NANOSTRUCTURES

8.3.1.1 VESICULAR SYSTEMS

Lipid-based vesicular carriers have been extensively studied for AD treatment due to their advantageous characteristics as low toxicity, biodegradability, and low cost. The amphiphilic structure of nanovesicles enables encapsulation of both hydrophobic and hydrophilic drugs. In addition, the vesicles composition influences in their physicochemical properties, stability, and efficacy (Kushwaha et al., 2021; Paiva-santos et al., 2021; Souto et al., 2021). Different vesicular systems have been studied for AD treatment such as liposomes, ETOs, niosomes (Keservani et al., 2010; Keservani & Gautam, 2022); and transferosomes.

Conventional liposomes are hollow vesicles composed of phospholipids bilayer surrounding an aqueous core with similar composition of the biological membranes. Besides, liposomes may include other lipids, such as cardiolipin, cholesterol or sphingomyelin which may affect stability, membrane fluidity or degree of hydration (Kushwaha et al., 2021). Liposomes were developed to reduce the side effects of betamethasone valerate and diflucortolone valerate, medium, and high potency topical corticosteroids, respectively. The vesicles were prepared by thin-film hydration method using Phospholipon® 90G and cholesterol for lipid bilayer formation and with only 10% of corticosteroid concentrations used in commercial creams. Despite the lower drug concentration, the *in vitro* skin permeation and *in vivo* therapeutic efficacy studies (2,4-dinitrofluorobenzene-induced AD of rats) showed that the liposomal formulations had amounts of drug retained in the skin and values of skin hydration similar to conventional formulations for both corticosteroids used, suggesting a possible side effects minimization (Eroğlu et al., 2016).

X_L-DNA-loaded liposomes composed of 1,2-dioleoyl-sn-glycero-3-phosphocholine (DOPC), 1,2-dioleoyl-sn-glycero-3-phospho-(1′-rac-glycerol) (DOPG) and cholesterol were produced by emulsion transfer method and presented a mean diameter of 115 nm, a narrow size range and a negative zeta potential. Transdermal delivery was assessed in rat back skin fragments mounted in a Franz cell system using fluorescein-labeled X_L-DNA. Skin samples observed under confocal microscopy revealed that non-nanoencapsulated X_L-DNA remained only on the skin surface while X_L-DNA-loaded liposomes were distributed in the epidermal and dermal layers. Besides, the efficacy of liposomes was evaluated using a NC/Nga mouse model stimulated with house dust mite plus 2,4-dinitrochlorobenzene (DNBC). The results clearly showed that X_L-DNA encapsulated into liposomes allows a Th1/Th2 balance, reducing the levels of GATA3, IL-4 and IL-5 (cell transcription factor and Th2 cytokines, respectively) and increasing the expression of T-bet (Th1 cell transcription factor) and IFN-γ, being an effective immunomodulatory formulation for the treatment of AD (Yang et al., 2018).

In both studies, an increase in permeation of active substances was found when associated with liposomes, which may have increased therapeutic efficacy. Liposomes can be fused with the stratum corneum (SC) releasing the drug in deeper layers of the skin. However, liposomes do not cross the SC intact (Kushwaha et al., 2021). To improve drug penetration, liposomes were modified by adding edge activators or single chain surfactant, being designated flexible or elastic or highly deformable liposomes (TRAs). This unilamellar vesicle is more effective because its flexibility permits the vesicles to squeeze themselves penetrating through the SC in their intact form, reaching deeper skin layers (Souto et al., 2021).

Increasing liposome flexibility may be beneficial in the treatment of AD. Cetirizine dihydrochloride-loaded transferosomes composed of Phospholipon® 90G phospholipid, stearylamine, and edge activator (sodium deoxycholate, Tween® 80 or Span® 80) were prepared by the thin film hydration method. Among tested edge activators, 10% Span® 80 was selected for the elastic vesicles development because presented maximum drug entrapment efficiency. This optimized formulation was compared to conventional liposomes prepared using 10% cholesterol. It was showed that conventional liposomes are reduced in size by half when subjected to extrusion to assess their degree of deformability, while elastic vesicles maintained their size close to their initial value, proving their flexibility. Notably, the TRAs increased skin permeation rates of cetirizine by almost two-fold. Besides, the developed formulation reduced the itch score and the dermal eosinophil count compared to conventional cetirizine cream in AD model induced by topical treatment with oxazolone on female BALB/c mice (Goindi et al., 2013).

Skin permeation and consequently the therapeutic effect of elastic liposomes may be improved by the permeation enhancers addition (Keservani & Gautam, 2020; Keservani et al., 2020a). Kang and colleagues developed conventional and elastic liposomes associated with the TAT peptide (transactivator of transcription) as a permeation enhancer for oregonin delivery, a natural and hydrophilic substance. The addition of the peptide did not change the initial physicochemical characteristics of the vesicles (average diameter of 130–140 nm, negative zeta potential and loading efficiency of around 50%), as well as maintained the flexibility of the elastic liposomes. However, TAT peptide increased the permeation flux of about 20% and showed a greater reduction in the lesion scores and inducible nitric oxide synthase (iNOS) and cyclooxygenase (COX)-2 levels (Kang et al., 2010). The same research group in another study developed elastic liposomes for the taxifolin glycoside skin delivery conjugated with Pep-1 peptide, a type of penetrating peptide. This formulation presented enhanced drug skin permeation (*in vitro*), as well as improved skin hydration and reduced IL-4 and IgE blood levels in AD-induced by 2,4,6-trinitro-1-chrolobenzene on NC/Nga mice (Kang et al., 2010).

ETOs also emerged in the investigation of novel techniques to improve cutaneous delivery. ETOs display a phospholipid bilayer and a high ethanol concentration (20–45%) as an alternative to cholesterol. The ethanol presence makes these vesicles smaller and with higher entrapment efficiency, deformability, fluidity, and stability than liposomes. In addition, it improves the extension and efficiency of skin penetration (Paiva-santos et al., 2021). Studies have shown promising performances of ethosomal formulations designed for dermal delivery of drugs in AD treatment. In one of these works, ETOs containing the immunosuppressant tacrolimus were prepared from Lipoid® S100 and 30% ethanol versus traditional liposomes containing only Lipoid® S100. In addition to reducing the nanovesicles size, the presence of ethanol increased the drug encapsulation efficiency. Moreover, ETOs showed increased tacrolimus permeation through SC, reaching the target of AD (Li et al., 2012). In another study involving an immunosuppressant drug, Carreras and co-workers compared the skin permeation of four novel lipid vesicles containing cyclosporine A: liposomes (formulated with Phospholipon® 90G and cholesterol), TRAs 1 (prepared with Phospholipon® 90G and Tween® 80), TRAs 2 (containing Phospholipon® 90G and Tween® 20 and D-limonene) and ETOs (formulated with Phospholipon® 90G and ethanol). ETOs were the most flexibles among the produced nanovesicles, reducing only a 14% of their initial size after extrusion. The cyclosporine A permeation using human heat-separated epidermis (HHSE) was ordered as follows: ETOs > TRAs 1 > TRAs 2. No cyclosporine A diffusion was detected from conventional liposomes (Carreras et al., 2020).

In recent studies conducted by Kumar and team, ETOs were formulated for the AD management varying the concentrations of phosphatidylcholine and ethanol, for skin delivery of piperine or tea tree oil. In both studies, the entrapment efficiency was increased with the increase in phosphatidylcholine and ethanol concentrations, while the size was increased with the increase in phosphatidylcholine concentration and reduced with the increase in ethanol concentration. The optimized piperine-loaded ethosomal dispersion was formulated with 3% phosphatidylcholine and 40% ethanol, which presented size of 318.1 nm and entrapment efficiency of 74.30%. The optimized tea tree oil-loaded ETOs were produced with 3% phosphatidylcholine and 30% ethanol and presented size and entrapment efficiency of 333.6 nm and 76.19%, respectively. These ethosomal formulations were incorporated into creams and showed higher deposition in the epidermis and dermis in comparison to their respective conventional creams. Moreover, the drug-loaded ethosomal creams were more effective than their conventional creams, reducing the inflammatory response in DNBC-induced female BALB/c mice model (Kumar et al., 2021a, b).

Binary ETOs has also been developed for topical drug delivery in AD treatment. The vesicle dispersion was produced by adding another alcohol type to the classical ethosome dispersion, such as propylene glycol and isopropyl alcohol (Abdulbaqi et al., 2016). Akhtar and colleagues developed binary ETOs with ethanol plus propylene glycol aiming to improve the penetration of topical corticosteroids into deeper epidermis to treat atopic skin. In the first study, the authors explored the role of binary solvents in topical drug delivery of triamcinolone acetonide. A reduction in vesicle size was observed with the increase in both propylene glycol and ethanol concentrations, suggesting an improved bilayer flexibility (Akhtar et al., 2017). Besides, binary ETOs presented higher entrapment efficiency and permeated amount of triamcinolone acetonide through the skin than conventional ETOs. In the second study, the use of β-cycloamylose as penetration enhancer in binary ETOs (β-cycloethosomes) was investigated in comparison to reference ETOs (without β-cycloamylose) for fluocinolone acetonide topical delivery. β-cycloethosomes showed maximum *in vitro* permeability and presented a deeper uniform penetration of fluorescent dye deep into the epidermis, suggesting a synergistic effect exerted by binary ETOs and β-cycloamylose (Akhtar et al., 2018).

The drug systemic absorption may be reduced and its residence time in the upper skin layers (stratum corneum and epidermis) may be improved by niosomes development. This vesicular carrier is composed by cholesterol and non-ionic surfactants, as alternatives to phospholipids (Limongi et al., 2021). In addition to skin retention, niosomes may prevent water loss from the skin and replenish lost cutaneous lipids, improving the skin barrier. Considering this, a comparative study between levocetirizine loaded polymeric nanoparticles and niosomal formulation was conducted by Pal and co-workers. Niosomes were prepared by thin film hydration method with Span® 20, Tween® 40 and cholesterol, while chitosan nanoparticles were prepared by ionic gelation method. Both nanocarriers exhibited particle size around 380 nm, but niosomes presented higher entrapment efficiency than nanoparticles. Besides, it was observed higher skin retention percentage of levocetirizine provided by niosomes. In the *in vivo* test, levocetirizine niosomes reduced the erythema score and scratching frequency in DNBC-induced AD animal model (Pal et al., 2021).

Phytosomes have been developed to improve the effectiveness of natural actives, including for AD treatment. Phytosomes are formed by bound between phospholipids of the lipid membrane and phytomolecules (Limongi et al., 2021). The effects of *Centella asiatica* phytosome were examined by using phthalic anhydride-induced AD mouse model. This phytosome inhibited infiltration of inflammatory cells and decreased the hyperkeratosis and proinflammatory cytokines release such as IL-1β and IgE (Ho et al., 2018). In a registry study, Togni and co-workers evaluated the effects of curcumin phytosome (Meriva®) as supplementary management of patients affected by AD. After 90 days, it was observed a better response in the group that received standard management (commercially available moisturizers and ceramide creams) plus phytosomes, with reduction of clinical manifestations such as itch, eczema, dryness, loss of sensitivity, and edema, as well as reduction in oxidative stress and improvement in skin oxygenation and hydration (Togni et al., 2019).

8.3.1.2 LIPID NANOPARTICLES

As well as vesicular nanocarriers, lipid nanoparticles present low toxicity and improved drug skin permeability, being widely studied for the topical treatment of AD. These nanoparticles adhere to the skin forming a lipid film, presenting occlusive properties, as well as being able to provide drug slow release. However, these carriers are restricted to the encapsulation of lipophilic substances (Sengar et al., 2018). Lipid nanoparticles comprise SLNs and NLCs (Keservani et al., 2018).

SLNs are composed by solid lipids at room temperature which are involved by surfactants in aqueous environment (Roberts et al., 2017). Hydroxyzine SLNs were developed to enhance drug skin permeation and to improve its antidermatitis effect. Different formulations were prepared by the double emulsification method varying the lipid type (cholesterol or glyceryl dibehenate), soybean lecithin amount and Tween® 80 concentration. The optimized formulation presented negative zeta potential, average diameter of 111 nm and encapsulation efficiency of 75%. Besides, it presented higher values of rate transdermal flux and permeability coefficient, reaching a cumulative percent of permeating drug of 75% after 12 h. Moreover, DNBC-induced AD mice model showed the potential of gels containing hydroxyzine SLNs to reduce scratching behavior, IL-4 and substance P levels, as well as to improve hypertrophy of epidermis (El-Telbany et al., 2021).

Aiming to develop cyclosporine A-loaded SLNs for topical AD treatment, the formulations were prepared using the hot ultrasonication method and were composed of Softisan® 649 and Tween® 80. After preparation, the nanoparticles presented sizes of around 200 nm, negative zeta potential and encapsulation efficiency of 88%. Then, lipid nanoparticles were freeze-dried, resulting in an oleogel formation. This oleogel presented *in vitro* drug-controlled permeation profile in comparison to lipid nanoparticles in aqueous dispersion, indicating its potentiality for topical administration (Silva et al., 2020).

In another study approaching the nanoencapsulation of an immunosuppressant drug in SLNs, Pople & Singh (2010) optimized a formulation containing glyceryl trimyristate, polysorbate 80 and sorbitan monooleate for tacrolimus dermal targeting with reduced adverse effects. This formulation presented superior drug release profile, skin penetration and accumulation in comparison to the marketed product. Skin visualization by confocal laser scanning microscopy confirmed that lipid nanoparticles targeted into deeper cutaneous layers. Moreover, no skin irritations were observed in the Draize test, while the reference ointment presented irritation signs (Pople & Singh, 2010). In a subsequent study, the same investigators evaluated the dermato pharmacokinetics, biodistribution, efficacy, and safety of tacrolimus-loaded lipid nanoparticles. The results showed that lipid nanoparticles presented a bioavailability 3.02-fold higher than reference tacrolimus. Biodistribution evaluation showed the nanoparticles localization at the target-skin-area without spreading to other body organs. The *in vivo* efficacy and toxicity studies showed that tacrolimus-loaded lipid nanoparticles reduced inflammatory atopic-like skin lesions and presented no evident toxicity, representing an efficient alternative for AD management (Pople & Singh, 2012).

The therapeutic effectiveness of tetrahydrocurcumin-loaded SLNs-based gels was investigated by Saini et al. in atopic skin treatment. These particles were prepared by microemulsification method using Tween® 80,

Phospholipon® 90G and Compritol® 888 ATO and presented mean size of 109 nm. *Ex vivo* and *in vivo* hydration tests showed that SLNs enhanced skin hydration and achieved C_{max} greater and T_{max} earlier than non-nanoencapsulated tetrahydrocurcumin gel in both epidermis and dermis. Confocal laser scanning microscopy proved an improved drug penetration through the skin reaching cutaneous deeper layers. In addition, tetrahydrocurcumin-loaded solid lipid nanoparticle reduced the levels of inflammatory cytokines and presented a complete healing in DNBC-induced AD mice model (Saini et al., 2022).

NLCs are the second generation of lipid nanoparticles and are composed by a mixture of solid and liquid lipids (Roberts et al., 2017). Usually, this lipid nanocarrier has higher encapsulation efficiency and greater stability than SLNs due to the presence of liquid lipids in the particles core making it less ordered and with lower melting point, preventing recrystallization of solid lipids (Man et al., 2007).

A skin care formulation containing microsilver complexed with NLCs was developed. The nanocarriers were composed by cetylpalmitate, Inutec® SP1, hemp seed oil and TegoCare® 450 and presented a size of about 200 nm. The final formulation was applied to the skin of volunteers with AD for 3 weeks, twice daily. *In vivo* studies revealed the potential of microsilver-NLCs to minimize the symptoms of AD (Keck & Schwabe, 2009). In a further study, these microsilver-NLCs showed a pronounced antimicrobial activity against *Staphylococcus aureus* strain. Moreover, erythema and edema induced by 2,4-dinitro-1-fluorobenzene was attenuated in an AD mice model (Keck et al., 2014).

For topical treatments, a high skin retention with low drug penetration is desired. For this, an ointment-based NLC for betamethasone dipropionate topical application was produced with Precirol® ATO5, oleic oil and Tween® 80 by melt emulsification method. It was observed that drug permeation and skin retention increase with enhancing Tween® 80 and oleic acid concentrations in the formulation. The optimized formulation presented tissue distribution as follows: skin > muscle > blood and no skin irritation (Kong et al., 2016).

8.3.1.3 MICRO- AND NANO-EMULSIONS

Micro- and nano-emulsions are colloidal dispersions composed by an oily phase (oil blend or single oil plus lipophilic surfactants) and an aqueous phase (surfactants, co-surfactant, and other components). Generally, these colloidal dispersions are non-irritating and have high drug skin permeation and drug-loading capacity (Dinshaw et al., 2021; Nastiti et al., 2017). Although micro- and nano-emulsions (NEs) present many similarities, they also have differences that allow their identification and classification. Microemulsions are formed spontaneously when the precise amounts of immiscible liquids are mixed with surfactants at the specific conditions of pressure and temperature. These nanosystems present thermodynamic stability with droplet size usually below 100 nm and are visually transparent or translucent (Mariyate & Bera, 2022). On the other hand, nanoemulsions are kinetically stable with droplet in the size range 100–600 nm, presenting milky appearance (Bouchemal et al., 2004).

The oily components of nanoemulsions may offer benefits for the treatment of AD. Negatively and positively charged nanoemulsions were formulated for topical administration of SC lipids (ceramide 3B, ceramide 3, palmitic acid, cholesterol, and vitamin E). Negative nanoemulsion was prepared with myristic acid and positive nanoemulsion with phytosphingosine. Both nanoemulsions presented size of about 200 nm. A clinical study carried out on healthy female volunteers showed that positively charged nanoemulsion significantly increased skin hydration and elasticity than negatively charged nanoemulsion (Yilmaz & Borchert, 2006). Another study reported the evaluation of the skin hydration capacity of nanoemulsions composed of rice bran oil, castor oil and surfactants sorbitan oleate/PEG-30 on volunteers with normal and diseased skin types. Nanoemulsions were classified as non-irritating in the HET-CAM assay. The topical nanoemulsion application on skin of volunteers increased the hydration, oiliness, and maintained the skin pH values (Bernardi et al., 2011). Moreover, nanoemulsions containing linseed oil were prepared by ultrasonic emulsification method using isopropyl myristate, DL-alpha tocopherol acetate, isodecyl neopentanoate, undecyl alcohol, Labrafil® M1944, Transcutol® HP and capric/caprylic triglyceride. Linseed oil nanoemulsion presented a mean droplet size of about 99 nm and negative zeta potential and no mutagenic effect was observed on strains of *Salmonella typhimurium*. *In silico* evaluations showed that this nanoemulsion may be an effective strategy to treat AD because ω-3 fatty acids in linseed oil did not show allergen properties and presented appropriate skin permeability values (Kildaci et al., 2021).

Considering drug association, clobetasol propionate-loaded nanoemulsions were prepared by aqueous phase titration method, using eucalyptus oil, ethyl alcohol and Tween® 20. The efficacy of this formulation was evaluated against nickel-induced dermatitis. The results showed an increased NTPDase activity in lymphocytes by clobetasol nanoemulsions, which is responsible for the adenosine triphosphate hydrolysis, reducing the inflammatory processes (Alam et al., 2013).

In a recent study, nanoemulsion-based gels of cetirizine, a second-generation antihistamine, were developed to avoid the drug side effects and to enhance skin permeation. The formulations were prepared by water titration method and their optimized composition consisted of palm oil and Cremophor® RH40/ethanol. Cetirizine-loaded nanoemulsion presented higher permeability parameters through skin than free cetirizine. Moreover, in a clinical study, it was observed a significant decrease in the degree of wheals and itching in urticarial patients treated with cetirizine-loaded nanoemulsion compared with free cetirizine after 4 weeks of treatment (Wang et al., 2019).

Moreover, the effectiveness of an optimized pioglitazone-loaded nanoemulsion composed by Capryol® 90, Labrasol®, and Transcutol® P was evaluated on AD model using oxazolone-sensitized mice. A high retention of pioglitazone was found in the skin without achieve receptor compartment. Pioglitazone nanoemulsions reduced oxazolone-induced skin lesions, prevented transepidermal water loss (TEWL) and suppressed pro-inflammatory cytokines (TNF-α, IL-6, and IL-17). Moreover, atomic force microscopy demonstrated a reversal of skin rigidification caused by treatment with nanoemulsions (Espinoza et al., 2020).

Similarly, like nanoemulsions, microemulsions also stand out as an interesting strategy for topical drug delivery. Due to their reduced droplet size, microemulsions were developed to increase the penetration and to reduce the local side effects (burning sensation and irritation) of tacrolimus. Menthol/camphor eutectic oil solution was chosen as the oily phase because both compounds provide a cool sensation, reducing pruritus and pain, as well as presenting skin penetration enhancing effects. Besides, Cremophor® EL and Transcutol® P were used as the surfactant and co-surfactant, respectively. Tacrolimus-loaded microemulsions presented an average droplet size of 26.59 nm enhanced 2-fold the percutaneous delivery of drug in comparison to the commercial ointment. In addition, microemulsions potentiated the therapeutic effect of tacrolimus, reducing the ear thickness, the scratch frequency and the IgE levels, as well as restoring the skin barrier (Wang et al., 2019).

8.3.2 POLYMER-BASED NANOSTRUCTURES

8.3.2.1 POLYMERIC NANOPARTICLES

Polymeric nanoparticles have gained considerable attention in the last few years for AD treatment. These polymeric nanocarriers generally are obtained with size smaller than 500 nm and include both nanospheres and nanocapsules. Nanocapsules are reservoir-type nanoparticles presenting an aqueous or oily core surrounded by a polymeric layer. In this nanosystem, the drug may be adsorbed onto the polymeric shell and/or dissolved in the core. In turn, nanospheres are matrix-type nanoparticles where drugs can be entrapped or adsorbed onto their surface (Mora-Huertas et al., 2010; Pohlmann et al., 2016; Quintanar-Guerrero et al., 1998). Several biodegradable polymers, with natural or synthetic origin, such as chitosan, poly(lactide-co-glycolide) (PLGA), poly-?-caprolactone (PCL) can be applied in the formulation of nanoparticles (Abdel-Mottaleb & Lamprecht, 2016). However, polymers of class of copolymers of poly(ethylacrylate, methyl-methacrylate, and chlorotrimethyl-ammonioethyl methacrylate), such as Eudragit® RS100 has aroused interest for topical formulations due to their bioadhesive potential (Cervi et al., 2021; Prado et al., 2021).

The most accepted cutaneous permeation mechanism for polymeric nanoparticles is their deposition on SC surface and accumulation in the furrows and cavities of hair follicles after skin application. This accumulation generates a depot effect with high drug concentrations into skin tissue and subsequent release in a sustained manner into deep skin layers (Abdel-Mottaleb & Lamprecht, 2016; Pohlmann et al., 2016). Polymeric nanoparticles have a negligible penetration across the SC in intact form. However, in diseased skin, the nanoparticle absorption into epidermal and dermal layers can be significantly enhanced (Kahraman et al., 2017). Try and co-workers evaluated the size influence of polymeric nanoparticles on their penetration through atopic skin. PLGA nanoparticles linked to fluoresceinamine were produced with two sizes (70 nm and 300 nm) and their cutaneous distributions in both mice and pig skins with oxazolone-induced AD were compared to healthy skin. Regardless of size, nanoparticles remained on SC after topical application on both pig and mouse healthy skins. On the other hand, in excised biopsies of atopic skins, the lower-sized nanoparticles presented greater penetration depth with fluorescence intensity 5-fold higher than nanoparticles with 300 nm. The diffusion of smaller nanoparticles through the inflamed skin can be due to the alteration of the skin barrier, with accumulation of interstitial fluid in cutaneous tissue and spatial rearrangement of viable epidermis cells (Try et al., 2016).

The sustained skin release of drugs from polymeric nanoparticles favors a localized effect with reduced blood absorption and systemic side effects (Kahraman et al., 2017). To reduce the transcutaneous absorption of hydrocortisone, a low-potency corticosteroid, chitosan nanoparticles were produced via ionic gelation. Hydrocortisone-loaded nanoparticles showed a reduction in flux and permeability coefficient across the full-thickness skin, as well as an increase in the drug accumulation in the epidermis and dermis. Besides, *in vivo* studies using a model similar to AD induced by 2,4 dinitro-fluorobenzene revealed that the treatment with hydrocortisone-containing chitosan nanoparticles prevented TEWL and reduced the dermatitis index and erythema formation, showing anti-inflammatory and antifibrotic activities (Hussain et al., 2013). In another study, these same authors explored the immunomodulatory effects of 214 nm-sized chitosan nanoparticles containing hydrocortisone. It was possible to observe a release suppression of cytokines involved in the dermatitis pathology such as IL-4, IL-5, IL-6, IL-13, IL-12, IFN-γ, and TNF-α in both serum and skin homogenates. Furthermore, histological findings indicated that hydrocortisone-loaded nanoparticles maintained the integrity of elastic connective tissues by inhibiting fibroblast infiltration and fragmentation of elastic fibers (Hussain et al., 2014).

To obtain additional benefits for AD treatment, co-encapsulation of hydrocortisone and hydroxytyrosol into chitosan nanoparticles has been the focus of several studies involving their development and both pre-clinical and clinical evaluations. Hydroxytyrosol is a potent antimicrobial and antioxidant and was added to the formulation to improve the efficacy against AD. Co-loaded nanoparticles were prepared by ionic cross-linking, and the optimized formulation showed about 235 nm and positive zeta potential. Notably, nanoparticles reduced the permeability and increased the skin retention (epidermis and dermis) for both hydroxytyrosol and hydrocortisone. This greater cutaneous retention may have favored the better performance observed for the nanoformulation in an animal model of AD (controlled TEWL, decreased erythema, dermatitis index reduction) (Hussain et al., 2013). Further, *in vivo* studies showed that chitosan nanoparticles penetrated 2.46-fold deeper into the skin than the commercial formulation without spreading to the surrounding tissues. Besides, dermal pharmacokinetic showed a higher C_{max} for nanoparticles than the commercial formulation. This nanoformulation also inhibited the *in vitro* growth of *Staphylococcus aureus* and *Escherichia coli* strains and presented no evidence of toxicity in repeated dermal application (Siddique et al., 2016). Also, co-loaded nanoparticles presented LD_{50} 100-fold higher than the normal human dose of hydrocortisone and did not cause skin irritation and adverse effects after repeated dose in albino Wistar rats (Siddique et al., 2015).

Following, hydrocortisone and hydroxytyrosol co-loaded chitosan nanoparticles were successfully upscaled by ionic gelation method using an overhead spinning-disc mixer, without changing its physicochemical characteristics. Besides, the co-loaded chitosan nanoparticles 28-day application showed no signs of local irritation, redness, and toxicity on healthy human skin, as well as the blood hematology, blood biochemistry, and adrenal cortico-thyroid hormone level did not indicate systemic toxicity in female Malaysian volunteers (Siddique et al., 2019). The clinical efficacy of co-loaded chitosan nanoparticles was demonstrated in a double-blind, randomized controlled study which had subjects of mild to moderate AD (EASI score of <18). The 6-weeks treatment with the nanoformulation provided a TEWL and erythema intensity decreased while melanin level was not significant reduced. In addition, no changes were found in the liver enzymes, fasting blood sugar and serum cortisol level in the nanoparticle-treated patients. In contrast, in the treatment with hydrocortisone commercial formulation the TEWL was not reduced as with co-loaded chitosan nanoparticles, and an increased blood cortisol level was observed in the group treated with the commercial formulation (Siddique et al., 2021). This set of studies demonstrated that hydrocortisone and hydroxytyrosol-loaded chitosan nanoparticles are superior to the hydrocortisone commercial formulation and did not reach the systemic circulation, preventing side effects.

In a different strategy to improve the solubility and skin permeation of tacrolimus, this drug was associated to nicotinamide into chitosan nanoparticles. The addition of nicotinamide, a water-soluble derivative of vitamin B3 and hydrotropic agent, improved the entrapment efficiency of tacrolimus and decreased the nanocarriers particle size. Besides, *in vitro* and *in vivo* permeation studies showed a synergistic effect between chitosan nanoparticles and nicotinamide. The total tacrolimus amount retained in the skin was ordered as follows: nanoparticles containing nicotinamide and tacrolimus association > tacrolimus and nicotinamide solution > commercial formulation ≈ tacrolimus suspension. Likewise, *in vivo* evaluations demonstrated that tacrolimus and nicotinamide association into chitosan nanoparticles presented higher efficacy in ameliorating the AD symptoms than commercial formulation and tacrolimus+nicotinamide solution, reducing epidermal thickness, mast cell accumulation and IgE levels at approximately one-third the dose of commercial formulation in DNBC-induced AD-like clinical symptoms on BABL/c mice (Yu et al., 2018).

Another promising approach to treat AD includes coating nanoparticles with hyaluronic acid, which can provide sustained release and improved dermal targeting to drugs. Pandey and co-workers developed betamethasone valerate-loaded chitosan nanoparticles coated with hyaluronic acid. These nanoparticles presented average diameter around 300 nm, positive zeta potential and entrapment efficiency around 86%. Besides, coated nanoparticles provided a more controlled release profile to betamethasone than non-coated nanoparticles. Furthermore, the drug release from coated-nanoparticles was pH-triggered, showing higher rates of drug released at pH 5.5 than at pH 7.4. Because of its mucoadhesive properties the coating with hyaluronic acid provided lower betamethasone permeation flux and higher drug deposition in the epidermis and the dermis than non-coated nanoparticles (Pandey et al., 2019). In another study, hyaluronic acid-coated chitosan nanoparticles with size of about 223 nm were produced for tacrolimus delivery. In addition to controlling release and improving skin retention, AD induced by 2,4-dinitroflourobenzene on NC/Nga mice was mitigated by the topical treatment with these nanoparticles, being the anti-dermatitis efficacy more pronounced for coated nanoparticles (Zhuo et al., 2018).

Non-pharmacological therapies such as skin regenerators also have their effectiveness improved by nanoencapsulation. Chitosan-coated PLGA nanoparticles loaded with ceramide were developed and presented mean diameter of 211 nm and a controlled release profile, which was pH and temperature-dependent. Additionally, the nanoparticles were labeled with fluorescein isothiocyanate for skin penetration observation. As required for correct ceramide action, nanoparticles penetrated into SC accumulating in the epidermis without reaching the dermis. *In vivo* studies were performed by application of 10% sodium dodecyl sulfate on rats with 4-week-old, simulating AD in infants, children, and adolescents. The treatment with coated nanoparticles containing ceramides quickly regenerated the epidermis, and presented FLG filaments well-dispersed (Jung et al., 2015).

Also, the encapsulation of natural substances into matrix-type polymeric nanoparticles has been reported. Dictamnine, a Chinese herbal medicine widely used on skin inflammations, was encapsulated into PLGA nanoparticles by antisolvent flash precipitation method. Dictamnine-loaded nanoparticles were spherical and presented approximately 186 nm, encapsulation efficiency of about 93% and controlled release. The nanoparticles notably improved the apparent epidermal regeneration, presented the CD^{3+} and CD^{45+} cell infiltration and the proinflammatory component COX-2 reduced in oxazolone-induced AD on mouse. In addition, the atopic mouse skin treated with free or nanoencapsulated dictamnine blended with fluorescent dye was evaluated in intravital two-photon microscopy and proved that nanoencapsulated dictamnine reached the dermal tissue layer while free drug showed a sparse fluorescence on the superficial epidermis and most fluorescence was found on residual hairs. Moreover, dictamnine-loaded nanoparticles significantly reduced TSLP, IL-1β and TNF-α expression in comparison to free dictamnine (Lin et al., 2021).

Nanocapsules are also advantageous for drugs targeting the skin immune system, providing a localized effect. Different cyclosporine A-loaded PLGA nanocapsules were prepared by varying the oil core Permeation studies showed that nanocapsules increased the cyclosporine A penetration through the skin, without reaching the receptor compartment. Besides, nanoencapsulated cyclosporine A presented higher accumulation in SC and epidermis than dermis. Because of the higher drug encapsulation efficiency, the oleic:labrafil oil core was selected for efficacy studies. The reduction of cell proliferation and IL-2 secretion and suppression of pro-inflammatory cytokines were shown in *in vitro* and *ex vivo* studies, respectively. Moreover, cyclosporine A-loaded nanocapsules meliorated cutaneous inflammatory reactions induced by ovalbumin on BALB/c mice, reducing the allergen-specific immune responses of serum ovalbumin-specific IgE and the Th2 cytokines, as well as preserved skin integrity (Badihi et al., 2020).

Moreover, considering that AD is an inflammatory skin disease, non-steroidal anti-inflammatories have also been studied to treat this eczema. In this sense, Weber and colleagues associated meloxicam with PCL and Miglyol® 810 nanocapsules, aiming to improve the drug solubility and to investigate the effects of the nanoformulation in mitigating the signs of AD. Nanocapsule suspensions presented negative zeta potential and particle diameter of about 247 nm. In DNBC-induced dermatitis model, meloxicam-loaded nanocapsules reduced skin severity scores, scratching behavior, edema, and myeloperoxidase activity in the ears of mice. Contrary, unloaded nanocapsules and non-nanoencapsulated meloxicam presented no effect in these parameters (Weber et al., 2018).

Recently, films containing pomegranate oil nanocapsules were evaluated in AD-like skin lesions induced by DNBC. Nanocapsules were prepared by the interfacial precipitation of preformed polymer method using Eudragit® RS100 as polymer and presented size around 181 nm. In the *in vivo* study, films containing the nanocapsules showed an oil pure-like reduction in dermatitis severity, while pomegranate oil nanoemulsions film had no effect in this parameter. In the biochemical analysis of the excised skin, only the nanocapsules formulation showed a reduction in reactive species and myelo-peroxidase activity and an increase in superoxide dismutase activity. The better *in vivo* performance observed for the film containing nanocapsules was suggested to be related to the bioadhesive characteristic of Eudragit® RS100, providing higher oil residence time in the skin tissue, which increased and prolonged its effect (Cervi et al., 2021).

Although topical therapy is the focus of studies involving nanocarriers for AD treatment, the systemic administration of nanocapsules has also been evaluated. Tacrolimus-loaded PCL nanocapsule suspensions were prepared by interfacial deposition of preformed polymer method using medium-chain triglycerides as oil core and presented drug encapsulation efficiency of 99.39%, mean diameter of 226 nm and controlled release profile. The efficacy of subcutaneously administered nanoformulations was demonstrated in AD model induced by topical application of 12-O-tetradecanoylphorbol-13-acetate on ear of mice. Tacrolimus-loaded nanocapsules demonstrated better inflammation control than the pure drug, with a marked reduction in serum fibrinogen, inflammatory infiltrate and in the epidermis thickness of the ear (Camargo et al., 2021).

8.3.2.2 POLYMERIC MICELLES

In recent years, polymeric micelles have emerged as promising drug delivery nanocarriers. The use of amphiphilic polymers above the critical micellar concentration enables micelles formation through molecular self-assembly resulting in a structure formed by a hydrophobic core and hydrophilic shell. Because of their self-assemble formation, these micelles present an easier preparation and a higher scale-up feasibility than lipid-based nanocarriers and polymeric nanoparticles (Ghezzi et al., 2021). Besides, the unique characteristics of polymeric micelles allows the formation of smaller-sized particles (10–200 nm) providing a more efficient cellular internalization. In addition, the lipophilic core gives adequate solubilization of hydrophobic drugs, while the hydrophilic shell provides a prolonged blood circulation time (Pepić, Lovrić & Filipović-Grčić, 2013).

Transdermal micelles were designed to improve hydrocortisone absorption through the skin and to provide a safe treatment for AD with reduced side effects. Micelles were produced with monomethyl poly(ethylene glycol)-poly(ε-caprolactone) by thin-film hydration method. The optimized formulation with drug ratio of 10% presented a mean diameter of 25.3 nm and significantly increased the hydrocortisone permeation through the skin at a low dose, presenting 9-fold increase in the drug cumulative quantity transferred compared with hydrocortisone cream. The skin penetration was confirmed by fluorescent images of tissue sections in which was visualized that the micelles helped to transport the encapsulated dye to the epidermis and dermis, while non-encapsulated dye reached in lower intensity the epidermis without reaching the dermis. Additionally, the nanoformulation presented higher reduction in inflammatory response (epidermal thickness, cell infiltration and level of IL-6) and lower systemic effects than hydrocortisone cream on a mouse model of AD induced by 1-fluoro-2,4-dinitrobenzene (Yuan et al., 2020).

The AD treatment with a localized effect and minimal systemic absorption can also be achieved with a correct management of nanocarrier size based on the choice of formulation constituents and their proportions. Assem and co-workers (2019) developed mixed micelles with Pluronic® L121/Pluronic® F127 to carry beclomethasone dipropionate. The micelles presented size around 120 nm and caused a higher local accumulation efficiency (amount retained versus amount permeated) than micelles prepared with Pluronic® L121/Poloxamer P84 mixture with 48 nm of size. The micelle with highest dermal deposition was incorporated into hydroxypropyl methylcellulose gels which have increased the drug local accumulation efficiency. In addition, Pluronic® L121/Pluronic® F127 micelles into gels were almost 40 times higher deposited into skin than the commercial formula (Beclozone®) causing a faster and efficacious healing of skin tissue as evaluated on sub-chronic dermatitis induced by 12-otetradecanoylphorbol 13-acetate in Wister rats (Assem et al., 2019).

8.3.2.3 NANOFIBERS

Polymeric nanofibers are an interesting class of nanomaterials composed by fibers with diameters in sub-micrometer range and produced using synthetic or natural polymers (Hu et al., 2014). Nanofibers present large surface area, high porosity and small pore size. These unique features provide a superior mechanical property and favor high skin adhesion compared with any other material (Kamble et al., 2017).

In recent studies, nanofibers have been considered as drug carriers for AD treatment. Nanofibers containing tacrolimus dispersed into self-microemulsifying drug delivery system (SMEDDS) were optimized by electrospinning process using different ratios of polyvinyl alcohol and SMEDDS. The optimized nanofiber formulation consisted of 90:10 ratio due to its tacrolimus sustained release. In DNBC-induced AD model, nanofibers showed a thinning of the cornified layer of epidermis similar to tacrolimus commercial ointment (Protopic®). However, nanofibrous membranes were applied every 48 h, while Protopic® was applied daily, proving the benefits of sustained drug release (Shams et al., 2021). The association of a non-traditional drug into nanofibers for dermal and transdermal delivery have also been reported. Pioglitazone-loaded polyvinylpyrrolidone nanofibers were produced by electrospinning method in comparison to a casted film. Polyvinylpyrrolidone-based nanofibers showed a high swelling degree which led to faster release of pioglitazone from nanofibers than from the casted film. Moreover, the higher surface area of nanofibers structure led to a greater skin permeation of pioglitazone than the casted film (Obaidat et al., 2022).

8.3.3 INORGANIC NANOCARRIERS

Inorganic-based nanocarriers have been investigated for skin disease treatment due to their large surface area, biocompatibility, and stability, as well as by their unique features as optical and superparamagnetic properties. For skin application, the main inorganic nanocarriers are: (i) metallic nanoparticles (iron oxide, gold, and silver and titanium dioxide (TiO_2) and zinc oxide (ZnO)); (ii) mineral-based nanoparticles (natural clay minerals, layered double hydroxides, mesoporous silica); and (iii) quantum dots (Sa et al., 2018). For the treatment of AD, some studies have demonstrated the benefits of inorganic nanoparticles, as metallic nanoparticles and mesoporous silica nanoparticles (MSNs).

MSNs presented tunable size (50–200 nm) and shape. Pore diameter and volume can influence the drug loading and the release profile. Additionally, MSNs can have their surface chemically functionalized through by different organic functional groups (Vallet-Regí et al., 2018). Aiming to improve solubility and skin retention of tacrolimus for AD control, a mesoporous silica nanoparticle-based gel was produced. Nanoparticles were synthesized and functionalized with amino or phosphonate groups using sol-gel technique. The optimized formulation consisted of phosphonate functionalized MSNs which presented size in the 300–350 nm range and increased by 7 folds the tacrolimus solubility. Also, these nanoparticles significantly improved the drug amount retained into skin, which may have contributed for the good performance on 1-fluoro-2,4-dinitrobenzene induced dermatitis in Balb/c mice. Tacrolimus-loaded nanoparticles reduced the mice ear thickness and the hyperkeratosis as well as presented low degree of inflammatory infiltration cells. Moreover, the formulation reduced acanthosis formation contrary to observed for free tacrolimus treatment in the irritation test (Parekh et al., 2021).

Iron oxide nanoparticles are iron-based magnetic materials, such as maghemite, magnetite, and hematite. Maghemite nanoparticles are preferred for biomedical applications because of their stable, biocompatible, and non-toxic characteristics (Łazarczyk et al., 2019). For AD management, Lee and co-workers (2021) produced maghemite nanoparticles using various Fe^{2+}: Fe^{3+} molar ratios (1:1, 1:2, and 2:3) by co-precipitation from ferrous/ferric salts which presented size around 16 nm. *In vitro* antioxidant assay showed that the 1:2 ratio presented higher 2,2-diphenyl-1-picrylhydrazyl scavenging activity than other ratios. In addition, topical application of maghemite nanoparticles presented anti-inflammatory and immunomodulatory effects dependents on the proportion of Fe^{3+} which were evaluated in *Dermatophagoides farinae* extract/DNBC-sensitized BALB/c mice. The greatest proportions of Fe^{3+} showed better inhibition of Th1, Th2 cytokines and inflammation-related proteins (COX-2, iNOS, and TNF-α) (Lee et al., 2021). Following, this same research group coated maghemite nanoparticles with hederagenin, a natural compound with anti-inflammatory effects. These nanoparticles presented higher *in vivo* efficacy than both non-coated maghemite nanoparticles and ceramide in AD-like lesions. Besides, only nanoparticles with hederagenin ameliorated the enlarged lymph nodes demonstrating the immunomodulatory effect of this novel formulation (Lee et al., 2022).

In another study, Ilves and colleagues compared the skin penetration and biological effects of ZnO nanoparticles and pure ZnO on mechanically damaged mouse skin with or without ovalbumin and staphylococcal enterotoxin B sensitization. The nanoparticles presented increased skin penetration in both damaged and allergic skin, as well as presented a greater reduction in the Th2-type cytokines expression than pure ZnO. However, ZnO nanoparticles presented an aggravation of IgE-antibody secretion, signaling an alert for the use of sunscreen containing these nanoparticles in patients with allergic skin (Ilves et al., 2014).

Indeed, some inorganic nanomaterials can exhibit significant immunomodulatory effects to penetrate or damaged skin (Yoshioka et al., 2017). Some studies report the aggravation of atopic effects after skin exposure with certain inorganic nanomaterials. For example, the reduction of amorphous silica nanoparticles from 1,000 nm to 30 nm increased the ear thickness and induced total-IgE, IL-18 and TSLP production after their intradermal co-administration with mite allergen extract using the same animal model (Hirai et al., 2012). Also, contrary to what was observed for 100 nm silver nanoparticles (AgNPs), 5 nm nanoparticles induced the ROS generation and granule release in mast cell *in vitro*, as well as increased the skin lesions and IgE serum levels after their co-administration with mite *in vivo* (Kang et al., 2017).

8.4 FINAL DOSAGE FORMS CONTAINING NANOSTRUCTURES

As previously commented, nanocarriers for topical and/or transdermal drug delivery have been extensively studied in AD management. However, most of these nanocarriers are obtained as aqueous dispersions which makes it difficult for the formulation to remain on the skin and complicates accurate dose administration Thus, for effective topical delivery in AD treatment, the incorporation of nanocarriers into appropriate dosage forms has been reported (Eroğlu et al., 2016; Kang et al., 2010; Kong et al., 2016; Pople & Singh, 2010). However, the development of formulations as vehicle for nanocarriers is complex. The appropriate topical dosage form must consider the flexibility of nanocarriers and solubility of both nanosystem and drug encapsulated (Pohlmann et al., 2016). Additionally, the integrity of nanocarriers after their incorporation into a final formulation needs to be evaluated, as well as the vehicle must attend to specific needs of the diseased skin (Boisgard et al., 2017; Stefanov & Andonova, 2021). In AD, the vehicle interaction with the compromised skin barrier may promote its restoration, presenting therapeutic value (Danby et al., 2022).

One of the most explored and promising strategies to increase the contact and residence time of the nanocarriers in the skin surface is to incorporate them in semisolid vehicles such as hydrogels (Liu et al., 2020; Pohlmann et al., 2016). In this case, the water generally used to form the hydrogel is partially or completely substituted by the nanocarriers aqueous dispersion (Pohlmann et al., 2016). Gel formulations are suitable for all AD lesions (Danby et al., 2022). Nano-based hydrogels have been produced for AD treatment using bioadhesive gelling agents of natural (e.g., chitosan), and or synthetic (e.g., carbomers) origin. Table 8.2 summarizes the nanocarrier type and gelling agents used as final formulation for AD treatment.

TABLE 8.2 Hydrogels Containing Nanocarriers for AD Treatment

Gelling Agent	Nanocarrier Type	References
Chitosan	Liposomes	(Eroğlu et al. 2016)
Hydroxpropyl methylcellulose	Polymeric micelles	(Assem et al. 2019)
Carboxymethylcellulose sodium	Liposomes	(Kang et al. 2010)
Carbopol 934	Solid lipid nanoparticle, niosomes, ethosomes	(Akhtar et al. 2017; Akhtar et al. 2018; Saini et al. 2022)
Carbopol 980	Solid lipid nanoparticle	(Pople and Singh, 2010)
Carbopol 940	Microemulsions, polymeric nanoparticles	(Wang et al. 2019; Weber et al. 2018)
Carbopol 941	Polymeric micelles	(Yuan et al. 2020)

The gelling agent type may influence the accumulation of the drug on skin. Aiming to develop an innovative nano-based topical formulation to act as vehicle for AD and psoriasis treatment, Boisgard and co-workers tested five semisolid formulations as vehicle for poly(lactic acid) (PLA) nanoparticles: (i) the viscosity modulator Avicel® RC-591; (ii) the oil-in water emulsion base Pentravan®; (iii) the gel-forming thickening agent Lutrol® F127; (iv) the thickening-emulsifying Sepineo™ P600; and (v) the carrageenan gel polymer Viscarin® GP 209F. The spreadability and rheological behavior showed that only Avicel®, Pentravan®, and Viscarin® presented adequate spreadability (threshold > 10 cm^2). However, Pentravan® formulation destabilized the nanoparticle structure, as observed by electron microscopy. Avicel® and Viscarin® formulations were evaluated in *in vivo* studies carried out in mice for 8 consecutive days and no irritation was observed on mouse skin. In addition, the incorporation of PLA-nanoparticles into Avicel® or Viscarin® semisolids decreased dye skin penetration while did not modify dye retention through mouse inflamed skin, suggesting a local delivery without systemic absorption (Boisgard et al., 2017).

Besides hydrogels, emulsions, such as creams, have also been used as vehicle for nanocarriers in AD treatment. In this semisolid, nanocarriers may added to pre-formulated base cream (Kang et al., 2010; Keck et al., 2014; Kumar et al., 2021a, b; Siddique et al., 2015; Yilmaz & Borchert, 2006). The cream composition may influence the drug release and *in vivo* performance. Katas and colleagues evaluated the skin permeation of hydrocortisone-loaded chitosan nanoparticles incorporated into two different creams, QV, and aqueous cream. QV-cream is composed of higher contents of light liquid paraffin, white soft paraffin, and glycerol than the aqueous cream. Besides, this hydrophobic cream contains natural oils and other lipids which improve their occlusive and bioadhesive properties. The researchers observed that aqueous cream presented a sustained release while nanoencapsulated hydrocortisone was quickly released from QV-cream, probably due to the better hydrocortisone dissolution in the hydrophobic base and to glycerol presence (Katas et al., 2012). Although no differences were observed in immunological parameters between different tested creams, the QV-based nanoformulation was more effective in the dermatitis index reduction (Hussain et al., 2014).

Besides, the ointment may be a convenient strategy for incorporation of lipid nanoparticles containing hydrophobic drugs. It was demonstrated that W/O ointment was more appropriate for the topical use of betamethasone dipropionate-loaded NLCs than carbopol emulgel in AD control. The ointment increased the skin retention and decreased skin penetration amount of betamethasone dipropionate-loaded NLCs. This probably happened due to the high affinity of both ointment and hydrophobic drug with the SC lipids, inducing retention. In contrast, the more hydrophilic feature of the carbopol reduces the drug affinity with the vehicle, increasing its skin penetration which may increase the adverse effects induced by systemic absorption (Kong et al., 2016).

Another dosage form that has been studied as vehicle for the treatment of skin diseases is polymeric films. They can be composed by natural or synthetic polymers, being a solid and flexible dosage form, which may promote a longer residence time at the action site. In contrast with semisolid formulations, polymeric films are less associated to easy removal, uncertainty of the dose applied and sticky sensation during administration (Karki et al., 2016). Besides, polymeric films have shown promising benefits for the incorporation of aqueous formulations such as nanoparticles, improving their stability and assisting in the drug sustained release (Dhal & Mishra, 2020; Gehrcke et al., 2021; Shahzad et al., 2019). For AD treatment, films have showed important features such as controlled release, high swelling behavior and occlusive properties (Alves et al., 2016; Jeong et al., 2019; Voss et al., 2020). When associated to nanoparticles or nanoemulsions for application on atopic skin, the *in vitro* occlusive properties of polymeric films increased and in the *in vivo* performance they proved to be a promising vehicle for nanocarriers (Cervi et al., 2021), encouraging further studies with this association.

8.5 PERFORMANCE EVALUATION OF FORMULATIONS IN ATOPIC DERMATITIS (AD)

8.5.1 SKIN PERMEATION/PENETRATION EVALUATION

Both drug physicochemical properties and formulation type influence in skin retention and permeation of active substances. Besides, the skin conditions (health or damaged) can also alter the skin retention and permeation, especially when are attended by skin barrier disruption (*see* Figure 8.3) (Vogt et al., 2016). It is anticipated that the drug permeation in atopic skin is greater than healthy skin which can result in systemic toxicity, being an aggravating factor mainly for transdermal formulations. Besides, for local AD treatment, it must be ensured that the active substance will reach the deeper layers of the epidermis and the dermis to exert its therapeutic effect by controlling the immunoinflammatory effects of the disease (Fang et al., 2016). Therefore, it is essential to evaluate this parameter in different skin conditions in the early stage of development of nano-based formulations since nanocarriers modulate the dermal retention/penetration/permeation of drugs across the skin.

The effect of cutaneous barrier disrupted simulating atopic skin condition on drug-loaded nanocarriers penetration may evaluated using skin biopsy after *in vivo* induction of the damage and allergic response in animal model (Ilves et al., 2014; Try et al., 2016). However, *in vitro* mechanical damage of SC is a well-established method to obtain an impaired skin barrier simulating atopic skin. The mechanical damage can be performed by tape-stripping technique in which the skin impairment is achieved by the SC removing using tape pieces (Fullerton, 2007). The mechanical skin barrier disruption by abrasion can also be used. In this case, a sponge with an aluminum coating is used to remove part of SC by smooth motion over the skin surface (Schlupp et al., 2014). Both mechanical skin barrier disruption showed to be a suitable alternative method to predict the drug permeation/penetration across the atopic skin and may serve as screening for topical nano-based formulations.

8.5.2 ANIMAL MODELS OF ATOPIC DERMATITIS (AD)

In addition to achieve in therapeutic concentrations the target layer of skin, the anti-dermatitis efficacy of drug-loaded nanocarriers must be evaluated.

A suitable model of human AD should present both relevant cytokine networks and epidermal impairment. However, to date no single animal model simulate these two aspects (Ewald et al., 2017). Although the skin structure and pathologic mechanism of AD are different between murine and human species, animal models for preclinical evaluation of new formulations for AD are widely used. The murine models are considered easy to manipulate, low cost, and have the availability of genetically manipulated strains (Gilhar et al., 2021).

Actually, there are three murine models for AD evaluation: (i) spontaneous mutation; (ii) transgenic mice; and (iii) epicutaneous sensitization (Jin et al., 2009). In the first model, an inbred mouse strain (Nc/Nga mice) present skin barrier abnormality, development atopic-dermatitis-like lesion spontaneously after allergens exposure, such as oxazolone, DNBC and mites (*Dermatophagoides farinae*) (Matsumoto et al., 2004; Yamada et al., 2016). In this model is possible to observe scratching behavior, skin dryness and erythematous and erosive lesions with hemorrhage occurrence. Besides, skin histological examination shows infiltration of mast cells and eosinophils and hyperkeratose and hyperplasia. Increased IgE production and induction of Th2 responses are also observed in this model (Matsuda et al., 1997). On the order hand, the second model uses transgenic mice overexpressing a single gene, such as IL-4, IL-31, TSLP, caspase-1 or apolipoprotein C1. According to transgenic mouse chosen, a factor associated with AD will be observed, contradicting the complexity of human AD. Besides, this model is time-consuming, and therefore it is not used much (Jin et al., 2009).

The third model involves hapten-induced mice which are commonly used to produce AD-like lesions. In this model multiple challenges with haptens on the skin of hairless mice were carried out, usually BALB/c or C57BL/6 mice strains, over a prolonged period. The haptens more used to induce AD-like lesions are ovalbumin, dinitrofluorobenzene, oxazolone, dinitrochlorobenzene, mite allergen, and exotoxins of *Staphylococcus aureus* (Gilhar et al., 2021). The challenge with these haptens induces Th2 immune response with mast cell and eosinophil infiltrations. Besides, ovalbumin-sensitized mice may present specific IgE and IgG1 antibody responses (Man et al., 2007).

8.6 CONCLUSION

The knowledge of pathophysiology of AD reveals the complex and heterogeneous nature of this eczema with numerous aspects to consider for its treatment. Traditional treatments for atopic eczema include topical and systemic therapeutic agents, which are used as single or combined therapy depending on the injury severity. However, both topical and systemic treatments present limited effectiveness and relevant side effects. Additionally, to date does not exist a unique formulation that combines immunoinflammatory effects with skin barrier recovery effects. All these aspects make the treatment of patients difficult and result in low adherence to the proposed therapy. To overcome limitations and challenges of traditional treatment, DDSs based on nanotechnology (Keservani et al., 2017a, 2018; Baig et al., 2018) have shown a promising strategy for AD management.

This chapter reported numerous research have shown the benefits of nanocarriers for atopic eczema treatment. The studies conducted demonstrated the superiority of nano-based formulations to penetrate the skin and to improve the immune response while having little side effects as compared to classical topical treatment of AD. The action and selectivity into inflamed skin may influenced by both type and physicochemical features (size, charge, and flexibility) of nanocarriers. Besides, depending on the nanocarrier composition it is possible to obtain a synergistic effect of high hydration and recovery of the skin barrier with immunoinflammatory effects. In addition to nanocarriers composition, the vehicle used to facilitate their application on the skin may also influence the final biological effect, and the correct development and evaluation of this final formulation is important. However, although studies demonstrate the positive potential of nanocarriers for the treatment of AD, more in-depth research is still needed. There is a lack of investigation regarding the large-scale production and stability of these nanocarriers. Also, there is still a need for a better understanding of the penetration of nanocarriers through atopic skin, as well as their effects on the skin after repeated applications. Moreover, existing animal models for the preclinical evaluation of new formulations in AD do not involve the complexity and phenotypic variability that occurs in humans. Thus, further clinical studies in different patients are required to investigate the effects of nanocarriers in preventing atopic eczema progression. Despite these shortcomings, nano-based formulations demonstrated excellent results and represent a promising future option in AD treatment.

KEYWORDS

- **atopic dermatitis**
- **inorganic nanocarriers**
- **lipid nanoparticles**
- **nanostructures**
- **polymeric micelles**
- **skin permeation**
- **topical therapy**

REFERENCES

Abdel-Mottaleb, M. M. A., & Lamprecht, A., (2016). Polymeric nano (and micro) particles as carriers for enhanced skin penetration. In: *Percutaneous Penetration Enhancers Chemical Methods in Penetration Enhancement: Nanocarriers, 187.*

Abdulbaqi, I. M., Darwis, Y., Khan, N. A. K., Assi, R. A., & Khan, A. A., (2016). Ethosomal nanocarriers: The impact of constituents and formulation techniques on ethosomal properties, *In vivo* studies, and clinical trials. *Int. J. Nanomedicine, 11*, 2279–2304.

Akhtar, N., Verma, A., & Pathak, K., (2017). Feasibility of binary composition in development of nanoethosomal glycolic vesicles of triamcinolone acetonide using box-Behnken design: *In vitro* and *ex vivo* characterization. *Artif. Cells, Nanomedicine, Biotechnol., 45*(6), 1123–1131.

Akhtar, N., Verma, A., & Pathak, K., (2018). Investigating the penetrating potential of nanocomposite β-cycloethosomes: Development using central composite design, *in vitro* and *ex vivo* characterization. *J. Liposome Res., 28*(1), 35–48.

Alam, S., Ali, S., Alam, N., Siddiqui, M. R., Shamim, M., & Safhi, M. M., (2013). *In vivo* study of clobetasol propionate loaded nanoemulsion for topical application in psoriasis and atopic dermatitis. *Drug Invent. Today, 5*(1), 8–12.

Alves, N. O., Gabriela, T., Weber, D. M., Luchese, C., Wilhelm, E. A., & Fajardo, A. R., (2016). Chitosan/poly (vinyl alcohol)/bovine bone powder biocomposites: A potential biomaterial for the treatment of atopic dermatitis-like skin lesions. *Carbohydr. Polym., 148*, 115–124.

Assem, M., Khowessah, O. M., & Ghorab, D., (2019). Optimization and evaluation of beclomethasone dipropionate micelles incorporated into biocompatible hydrogel using a sub-chronic dermatitis animal model. *AAPS PharmSci, 20*(152), 1–12.

Badihi, A., Fru, M., Soroka, Y., Benhamron, S., Tzur, T., Nassar, T., & Benita, S., (2018). Topical nano-encapsulated cyclosporine formulation for atopic dermatitis treatment. *Nanomed.: Nanotechnol. Biol. Med., 24*, 102140.

Baig, M. S., Keservani, R. K., Ahmad, M. F., & Baig, M. E., (2018). Smart delivery of nanobiomaterials in drug delivery. In: *Nanobiomaterials* (pp. 241–287). Apple Academic Press. ISBN: 9781771885911.

Berger, T. G., Bergman, J. N., Chamlin, S. L., Cooper, K. D., Feldman, S. R., Hanifin, J. M., Krol, A., et al., (2014). Guidelines of care for the management of atopic dermatitis and systemic agents. *J. Am. Dermatology, 71*(2), 327–349.

Bernardi, D. S., Pereira, T. A., Maciel, N. R., Bortoloto, J., Viera, G. S., Oliveira, G. C., & Rocha-Filho, P. A., (2011). Formation and stability of oil-in-water nanoemulsions containing rice bran oil: *In vitro* and *in vivo* assessments. *J. Nanobiotechnology, 9*(44), 1–9.

Bertino, L., Guarneri, F., Patrizia, S., Casciaro, M., Pioggia, G., & Gangemi, S., (2020). Oxidative stress and atopic dermatitis. *Antioxidants, 5*, 1–15.

Bieber, T., (2017). How to define atopic dermatitis? *Dermatol. Clin., 35*(3), 275–281.

Boisgard, A., Lamrayah, M., Dzikowski, M., Salmon, D., Kirilov, P., Primard, C., Pirot, F., Fromy, B., & Verrier, B., (2017). Innovative drug vehicle for local treatment of inflammatory skin diseases: *Ex vivo* and *in vivo* screening of five topical formulations containing poly (lactic acid) (PLA) nanoparticles. *Eur. J. Pharm. Biopharm., 116*, 51–60.

Bouchemal, K., Briançon, S., Perrier, E., & Fessi, H., (2004). Nano-emulsion formulation using spontaneous emulsification: Solvent, oil and surfactant optimization. *Int. J. Pharm., 280*, 241–251.

Camargo, A., Ferreira, L., Jos, D., Lyra, A. M., Barboza, F. M., Carletto, B., Koga, A. Y., et al., (2021). Characterization and *in vitro* and *in vivo* evaluation of tacrolimus-loaded poly (ε -caprolactone) nanocapsules for the management of atopic dermatitis. *Pharmaceutics, 13*, 1–19.

Carreras, J. J., Tapia-ramirez, W. E., Sala, A., Guillot, A. J., Garrigues, T. M., & Melero, A., (2020). Ultraflexible lipid vesicles allow topical absorption of cyclosporin A. *Drug Deliv. Transl. Res., 10*, 486–497.

Carroll, C. L., & Fleischer, A. B., (2015). Tacrolimus ointment: The treatment of atopic dermatitis and other inflammatory cutaneous disease. *Expert Opin. Pharmacother, 5*, 2127–2237.

Cervi, V. F., Saccol, C. P., Sari, M. H. M., Martins, C. C., Rosa, L. S. Da., Ilha, B. D., Soares, F. Z., et al., (2021). Pullulan film incorporated with nanocapsules improves pomegranate seed oil anti-inflammatory and antioxidant effects in the treatment of atopic dermatitis in mice. *Int. J. Pharm., 609*, 121144.

Danby, S. G., Draelos, Z. D., Gold, L. F. S., Cha, A., Aikman, L., Sanders, P., Wu-linhares, D., et al., (2022). Vehicles for atopic dermatitis therapies: More than just a placebo. *J. Dermatolog. Treat., 33*(2), 685–698.

Deo, M., Yung, A., Hill, S., & Rademaker, M., (2014). Methotrexate for treatment of atopic dermatitis in children and adolescents. *Pharmacol. Ther., 53*, 1037–1041.

Dhal, C., & Mishra, R., (2020). *In vitro* and *in vivo* evaluation of gentamicin sulphate-loaded PLGA nanoparticle-based film for the treatment of surgical site infection. *Drug Deliv. Transl. Res., 10*, 1032–1043.

Dinshaw, I. J., Ahmad, N., Salim, N., & Leo, B. F., (2021). Nanoemulsions: A review on the conceptualization of treatment for psoriasis using a 'green' surfactant with low-energy emulsification method. *Pharmaceutics, 13*, 1–34.

El-telbany, D. F. A., El-telbany, R. F. A., Zakaria, S., Ahmed, K. A., & El-feky, Y. A., (2021). Formulation and assessment of hydroxyzine HCL Solid lipid nanoparticles by dual emulsification technique for transdermal delivery. *Biomed. Pharmacother., 143*, 112130.

Eroğlu, İ., Azizoğlu, E., Özyazıcı, M., Nenni, M., Gürer, H., Özbal, S., Tekmen, I., et al., (2016). Effective topical delivery systems for corticosteroids: Dermatological and histological evaluations effective topical delivery systems for corticosteroids: Dermatological and histological evaluations. *Drug Deliv.*, *23*(5), 1502–1513.

Espinoza, L. C., Vera-garc, R., Silva-abreu, M., Dom, Ò., Badia, J., Rodr, J., & Clares, B., (2020). Topical pioglitazone nanoformulation for the treatment of atopic dermatitis: Design, characterization and efficacy in hairless mouse model. *Pharmaceutics, 12*(3), 1–18.

Ewald, D. A., Noda, S., Oliva, M., & Litman, T., (2017). Major differences between human atopic dermatitis and murine models, as determined by using global transcriptomic profiling. *J. Allergy Clin. Immunol.*, *139*(2), 562–571.

Fang, Y., Yang, S., Lee, C., Aljuffali, I. A., Kao, H., & Fang, J., (2016). What is the discrepancy between drug permeation into/across intact and diseased skins? Atopic dermatitis as a model. *Int. J. Pharm.*, *497*, 277–286.

Ferreira, S., & Torres, T., (2018). Dupilumab for the treatment of atopic dermatitis. *Expert Rev. Clin. Pharmacol., 1*(5), 467–474.

Fullerton, L. S. A., (2007). Development of an *in vitro* skin permeation model simulating atopic dermatitis skin for the evaluation of dermatological products. *Skin Pharmacol. Physiol.*, *20*, 230–236.

Gehrcke, M., Brum, T. De. B., Da Rosa, L. S., Ilha, B. D., Soares, F. Z. M., & Cruz, L., (2021). Incorporation of nanocapsules into Gellan gum films: A strategy to improve the stability and prolong the cutaneous release of silibinin. *Mater. Sci. Eng. C*, *119*, 111624.

Ghezzi, M., Pescina, S., Padula, C., Santi, P., Favero, E. D., Cantù, L., & Nicoli, S., (2021). Polymeric micelles in drug delivery: An insight of the techniques for their characterization and assessment in biorelevant conditions. *J. Control. Release, 332*, 312–336.

Ghosalkar, S., Prabha, M., & Padmini, S., (2022). Emerging *Topical Drug Delivery Approaches for the Treatment of Atopic Dermatitis, 21*(2), 536–549.

Gilhar, A., Reich, K., Keren, A., Kabashima, K., Steinhoff, M., & Paus, R., (2021). Mouse models of atopic dermatitis: A critical reappraisal. *Exp. Dermatol.*, *30*, 319–336.

Goindi, S., Kumar, G., Kumar, N., & Kaur, A., (2013). Development of novel elastic vesicle-based topical formulation of cetirizine dihydrochloride for treatment of atopic dermatitis. *AAPS PharmSciTech, 14*(4), 1284–1293.

Hemrajani, C., Negi, P., Parashar, A., Gupta, G., Jha, N. K., Singh, S. K., Chellappan, D. K., & Dua, K., (2022). Overcoming drug delivery barriers and challenges in topical therapy of atopic dermatitis: A nanotechnological perspective. *Biomed. Pharmacother.*, *147*, 112633.

Hirai, T., Yoshikawa, T., Nabeshi, H., Yoshida, T., Tochigi, S., Ichihashi, K., Uji, M., et al., (2012). Amorphous silica nanoparticles size-dependently aggravate atopic dermatitis-like skin lesions following an intradermal injection. *Part. Fibre Toxicol.*, *9*(3), 1–11.

Ho, P. J., Sung, J. J., Cheon, K. K., & Tae, H. J., (2018). Phytomedicine anti-inflammatory effect of *Centella asiatica* phytosome in a mouse model of phthalic anhydride-induced atopic dermatitis. *Phytomedicine, 43*, 110–119.

Hu, X., Liu, S., Zhou, G., Huang, Y., Xie, Z., & Jing, X., (2014). Electrospinning of polymeric nanofibers for drug delivery applications. *J. Control. Release, 185*, 12–21.

Huang, X., & Xu, B., (2015). Efficacy and safety of tacrolimus versus pimecrolimus for the treatment of atopic dermatitis in children: A network meta-analysis. *Dermatology, 231*, 41–49.

Hussain, Z., Katas, H., Cairul, M., Mohd, I., Kumolosasi, E., & Sahudin, S., (2014). Downregulation of immunological mediators dermatitis-like skin lesions by hydrocortisone-loaded chitosan nanoparticles. *Int. J. Nanomedicine, 9*, 5143–5156.

Hussain, Z., Katas, H., Cairul, M., Mohd, I., Kumolosasi, E., Buang, F., & Sahudin, S., (2013). Self-assembled polymeric nanoparticles for percutaneous co-delivery of hydrocortisone/hydroxytyrosol: An *ex vivo* and *in vivo* study using an NC/Nga mouse model. *Int. J. Pharm.*, *444*, 109–119.

Hussain, Z., Katas, H., Cairul, M., Mohd, I., Kumulosasi, E., & Sahudin, S., (2013). Antidermatitic perspective of hydrocortisone as chitosan nanocarriers: An *ex vivo* and *in vivo* assessment using an NC/Nga mouse model. *J. Pharm. Sci.*, *102*(3), 1063–1075.

Ilves, M., Palomäki, J., Vippola, M., Lehto, M., Savolainen, K., Savinko, T., & Alenius, H., (2014). Topically applied ZnO nanoparticles suppress allergen induced skin inflammation but induce vigorous IgE production in the atopic dermatitis mouse model. *Part. Fiber Toxicol.*, *11*(38), 1–12.

Jeong, J. H., Back, S. K., An, J. H., Lee, N., Kim, D., Na, C. S., Jeong, Y., & Han, S. Y., (2019). Topical film prepared with *Rhus verniciflua* extract-loaded pullulan hydrogel for atopic dermatitis treatment. *J. Biomed. Mater. Res.*, *107*(7), 1–10.

Ji, H., & Li, X., (2016). Oxidative stress in atopic dermatitis. *Oxid. Med. Cell. Longev.*, *2016*, 1–8.

Jin, H., He, R., Oyoshi, M., & Geha, R. S., (2009). Animal models of atopic dermatitis. *J. Invest. Dermatol.*, *129*(1), 31–40.

Jung, S., Yoon, G. H., Lee, H. C., Jung, M. H., & Yu, S. I., (2015). Thermodynamic insights and conceptual design of skin-sensitive chitosan coated ceramide/PLGA nanodrug for regeneration of *Stratum corneum* on atopic dermatitis. *Sci. Rep.*, *5*, 1–12.

Kahraman, E., Güngör, S., & Özsoy, Y., (2017). Potential enhancement and targeting strategies of polymeric and lipid-based nanocarriers in dermal drug delivery. *Ther. Deliv.*, *8*(11), 967–985.

Kamble, P., Sadarani, B., Majumdar, A., & Bhullar, S., (2017). Nanofiber based drug delivery systems for skin: A promising therapeutic approach. *J. Drug Deliv. Sci. Technol.*, *41*, 124–133.

Kang, H., Kim, S., Lee, K. H., Jin, S., Kim, S. H., Lee, K., Jeon, H., et al., (2017). 5 Nm silver nanoparticles amplify clinical features of atopic dermatitis in mice by activating mast cells. *Adv. Sci. New*, *13*, 1–10.

Kang, M. J., Eum, J. Y., Jeong, M. S., Choi, S. E., Park, S. H., Cho, H. I., Cho, C. S., et al., (2010). Facilitated skin permeation of oregonin by elastic liposomal formulations and suppression of atopic dermatitis in NC/Nga mice. *Biol. Pharm. Bull*, *33*(1), 100–106.

Kang, M. J., Eum, J. Y., Park, S. H., Kang, M. H., Park, K. H., Choi, S. E., Lee, M. W., et al., (2010). Pep-1 peptide-conjugated elastic liposomal formulation of taxifolin glycoside for the treatment of atopic dermatitis in NC/Nga mice. *Int. J. Pharm.*, *402*(1, 2), 198–204.

Karki, S., Kim, H., Na, S., Shin, D., Jo, K., & Lee, J., (2016). Thin films as an emerging platform for drug delivery. *Asian J. Pharm. Sci.*, *11*, 559–574.

Katas, H., Hussain, Z., & Ling, T. C., (2012). Chitosan nanoparticles as a percutaneous drug delivery system for hydrocortisone. *J. Nanomater.*, *2012*, 1–11.

Keck, C. M., & Schwabe, K., (2009). Silver-nanolipid complex for application to atopic dermatitis skin: Rheological characterization, *in vivo* efficiency and theory of action. *J. Biomed. Nanotechnol.*, *5*, 428–436.

Keck, C. M., Anantaworasakul, P., Patel, M., Okonogi, S., Singh, K. K., & Roessner, D., (2014). A new concept for the treatment of atopic dermatitis: Silver – nanolipid complex (SNLC). *Int. J. Pharm.*, *462*(1, 2), 44–51.

Keservani, R. K., & Gautam, S. P., (2020). Formulation and evaluation of baclofen liposome vesicles using lecithin. *ARS Pharmaceutica, 61*(3), 175–180.

Keservani, R. K., & Gautam, S. P., (2022). Skeletal muscle relaxant activity of different formulation of span 60 niosome. *ARS Pharmaceutica, 63*(91), 32–44.

Keservani, R. K., Bandopadhyay, S., Bandyopadhyay, N., & Sharma, A. K., (2020a). Design and fabrication of transdermal/skin drug-delivery system. In: *Drug Delivery Systems* (pp. 131–178). Academic Press.

Keservani, R. K., Kesharwani, R. K., & Sharma, A. K., (2017a). Introduction to nanotechnology in drug delivery. In: *Drug Delivery Approaches and Nanosystems* (pp. 1–19). Apple Academic Press. ISBN: 9781771885836.

Keservani, R. K., Sharma, A. K., & Kesharwani, R. K., (2018). Nanoparticulate nanocarriers in drug delivery. In: *Nanobiomaterials* (pp. 3–22). Apple Academic Press. ISBN: 9781771885911.

Keservani, R. K., Sharma, A. K., & Ramteke, S., (2010). Novel vesicular approach for topical delivery of baclofen via niosomes. *Lat. Am. J. Pharm, 29*, 1364–1370.

Kildaci, I., Budama-kilinc, Y., Kecel-gunduz, S., & Altuntas, E., (2021). Linseed oil nanoemulsions for treatment of atopic dermatitis disease: Formulation, characterization, *in vitro* and *in silico* evaluations. *J. Drug Deliv. Sci. Technol., 64*, 102652.

Kong, X., Zhao, Y., Quan, P., & Fang, L., (2016). Development of a topical ointment of betamethasone dipropionate loaded nanostructured lipid carrier. *Asian J. Pharm. Sci., 11*(2), 248–254.

Kumar, P., Sharma, D. K., & Ashawat, M. S., (2021). Development of phospholipids vesicular nanocarrier for topical delivery of tea tree oil in management of atopic dermatitis using BALB/c mice model. *Eur. J. Lipid Sci. Technol., 123*, 1–12.

Kumar, P., Sharma, D. K., & Ashawat, M. S., (2021). Topical creams of piperine loaded lipid nanocarriers for management of atopic dermatitis: Development, characterization, and *in vivo* investigation using BALB/c mice model. *J. Liposome Res., 32*(1), 62–31.

Kushwaha, P., Saxena, S., & Shukla, B., (2021). A recent overview on dermatological applications of liposomes. *Recent Pat. Nanotechnol., 15*(4), 310–321.

Łazarczyk, A., Hałubiec, P., & Duli, J., (2019). Superparamagnetic iron oxide nanoparticles – current and prospective medical applications. *Materials, 12*(617), 1–26.

Lee, K., Patrick, K., Ulrich, N., Kim, G., Choi, J. W., Kim, J., Kim, E., & An, J. H., (2021). Fe_2: Fe^{3+} molar ratio influences the immunomodulatory properties of maghemite (γ -Fe_2O_3) nanoparticles in an atopic dermatitis model. *ACS Appl. Bio Mater., 4*, 1252–1267.

Lee, K., Ratih, K., Kim, G., Lee, Y., Shin, J., Chung, K., Choi, E., et al., (2022). Immunomodulatory and anti-inflammatory efficacy of hederagenin-coated maghemite (γ -Fe_2O_3) nanoparticles in an atopic dermatitis model. *Colloids Surf. B: Biointerfaces, 210*, 112244.

Li, G., Fan, C., Li, X., Fan, Y., Wang, X., Li, M., & Liu, Y., (2012). Preparation and *in vitro* evaluation of tacrolimus-loaded ethosomes. *Sci. World J., 2012*, 1–6.

Limongi, T., Susa, F., Marini, M., Allione, M., Torre, B., Pisano, R., & Fabrizio, E., (2021). Lipid-based nanovesicular drug delivery systems. *Nanomaterials, 11*, 1–38.

Lin, C., Hsieh, Y., Yi, L., Yang, T., Maeda, T., Chang, T., & Huang, H., (2021). Dictamnine delivered by PLGA nanocarriers ameliorated inflammation in an oxazolone-induced dermatitis mouse model. *J. Control. Release, 329*, 731–742.

Liu, M., Wen, I., & Sharma, M., (2020). Solid lipid nanoparticles for topical drug delivery: Mechanisms, dosage form perspectives, and translational status. *Curr. Pharm. Des., 6128*, 3203–3217.

Malik, K., & Heitmiller, K. D., (2017). An update on the pathophysiology of atopic dermatitis. *Dermatol. Clin.*, *35*(3), 317–326.

Man, M., Hatano, Y., Lee, S. H., Man, M., Chang, S., Feingold, K. R., Leung, D. Y. M., et al., (2007). Characterization of a hapten-induced, murine model with multiple features of atopic dermatitis: Structural, immunologic, and biochemical changes following single versus multiple oxazolone challenges. *J. Invest. Dermatol.*, *128*, 79–86.

Mancuso, J. B., Lee, S. S., Paller, A. S., & Ohya, Y., (2021). Management of severe atopic dermatitis in pediatric patients. *J. Allergy Clin. Immunol. Pract.*, *9*(4), 1462–1471.

Mariyate, J., & Bera, A., (2022). A critical review on selection of microemulsions or nanoemulsions for enhanced oil recovery. *J. Mol. Liq.*, *353*, 118791.

Matsuda, H., Watanabe, N., Geba, G. P., Sperl, J., Tsudzuki, M., Hiroi, J., Matsumoto, M., et al., (1997). Development of atopic dermatitis-like skin lesion with IgE hyperproduction in NC/Nga mice. *Int. Immunol.*, *9*(3), 461–466.

Matsumoto, K., Mizukoshi, K., Oyobikawa, M., & Ohshima, H., (2004). Establishment of an atopic dermatitis-like skin model in a hairless mouse by repeated elicitation of contact hypersensitivity that enables to conduct functional analyses of the *Stratum corneum* with various non-invasive biophysical instruments. *Ski. Res. Technol.*, *10*, 122–129.

Meggitt, S. J., & Reynolds, N. J., (2001). Azathioprine for atopic dermatitis. *Clin. Dermatology*, *26*, 369–375.

Misery, L., Huet, F., Gouin, O., Deleuran, M., & Sta, S., (2019). Current pharmaceutical developments in atopic dermatitis. *Curr. Opin. Pharmacol.*, *46*, 7–13.

Mora-Huertas, C. E., Fessi, H., & Elaissari, A., (2010). Polymer-based nanocapsules for drug delivery. *Int. J. Pharm.*, *385*, 113–142.

Nastiti, C. M. R. R., Ponto, T., Abd, E., Grice, J. E., Benson, H. A. E., & Roberts, M. S., (2017). Topical nano and microemulsions for skin delivery. *Pharmaceutics, 9*(37), 1–25.

Neuber, K., Schwartz, I., Itschert, G., & Tom, D. A., (2000). Treatment of atopic eczema with oral mycophenolate mofetil. *Br. J. Dermatol.*, *143*, 385–391.

Obaidat, R., Shameh, A. A., Aljarrah, M., & Hamed, R., (2022). Preparation and evaluation of polyvinylpyrrolidone electrospun nanofiber patches of pioglitazone for the treatment of atopic dermatitis. *AAPS PharmSciTech, 23*(51), 1–19.

Paiva-Santos, A. C., Gama, M., Peixoto, D., Sousa-Oliveira, I., Ferreira-Faria, I., Zeinali, M., Abbaspour-Ravasjani, S., et al., (2022). Nanocarrier-based dermopharmaceutical formulations for the topical management of atopic dermatitis. *Int. J. Pharm.*, *618*, 121656.

Paiva-santos, A. C., Silva, A. L., Guerra, C., Peixoto, D., Pereira-silva, M., Zeinali, M., Mascarenhas-melo, F., & Castro, R., (2021). Ethosomes as nanocarriers for the development of skin delivery formulations. *Pharm. Res.*, *38*, 947–970.

Pal, R. R., Maurya, A. K., Parashar, P., & Saraf, S. A., (2021). A comparative study of levocetirizine loaded vesicular and matrix type system for topical application: Appraisal of therapeutic potential against atopic dermatitis. *J. Pharm. Innov.*, *16*, 469–480.

Pandey, M., Choudhury, H., Gunasegaran, T. A. P., Nathan, S. S., Md, S., Gorain, B., Tripathy, M., & Hussain, Z., (2019). Hyaluronic acid-modified betamethasone encapsulated polymeric nanoparticles: Fabrication, characterization, *in vitro* release kinetics, and dermal targeting. *Drug Deliv. Transl. Res., 9*, 520–533.

Parekh, K., Hariharan, K., Qu, Z., Rewatkar, P., & Cao, Y., (2021). Tacrolimus encapsulated mesoporous silica nanoparticles embedded hydrogel for the treatment of atopic dermatitis. *Int. J. Pharm.*, *608*, 121079.

Pepić, I., Lovrić, J., & Filipović-Grčić, J., (2013). How do polymeric micelles cross epithelial barriers? *Eur. J. Pharm. Sci.*, *50*, 42–55.

Pohlmann, A. R., Detoni, C. B., Paese, K., Coradini, K., Beck, R. C. R., & Guterres, S. S., (2016). *Polymeric Nanocapsules for Topical Delivery*. In: *Percutaneous Penetration Enhancers Chemical Methods in Penetration Enhancement: Nanocarriers* (p. 201).

Pople, P. V., & Singh, K. K., (2010). Targeting tacrolimus to deeper layers of skin with improved safety for treatment of atopic dermatitis. *Int. J. Pharm.*, *398*(1, 2), 165–178.

Pople, P. V., & Singh, K. K., (2012). Targeting tacrolimus to deeper layers of skin with improved safety for treatment of atopic dermatitis – part II: *In vivo* assessment of dermatopharmacokinetics, biodistribution and efficacy. *Int. J. Pharm.*, *434*(1, 2), 70–79.

Prado, V. C., Sari, M. H. M., Borin, B. C., Pinheiro, R. Do. C., Cruz, L., Schuch, A., Nogueira, C. W., & Zeni, G., (2021). Development of a nanotechnological-based hydrogel containing a novel benzofuroazepine compound in association with vitamin E: An *in Vitro* biological safety and photoprotective hydrogel. *Colloids Surf. B: Biointerfaces.*, *199*, 111555.

Quintanar-Guerrero, D., Allémann, E., Fessi, H., & Doelker, E., (1998). Preparation techniques and mechanisms of formation of biodegradable nanoparticles from preformed polymers. *Drug Dev. Ind. Pharm.*, 1113–1128.

Ramanunny, A. K., Wadhwa, S., Gulati, M., Singh, S. K., Kapoor, B., Dureja, H., KumarChellappan, D., et al., (2021). Nanocarriers for treatment of dermatological diseases principle, perspective and practices. *Eur. J. Pharmacol.*, *890*(5), 173691.

Rerknimitr, P., Otsuka, A., Nakashima, C., & Kabashima, K., (2017). The etiopathogenesis of atopic dermatitis: Barrier disruption, immunological derangement, and pruritus. *Inflamm. Regen.*, *37*(14), 1–15.

Roberts, M. S., Mohammed, Y., Pastore, M. N., Namjoshi, S., Yousef, S., Alinaghi, A., Haridass, I. N., & Abd, E., (2017). Topical and cutaneous delivery using nanosystems. *J. Control. Release, 247*, 86–105.

Rullo, V. E. V., Segato, A., Kirsh, A., & Sole, D., (2008). Severity scoring of atopic dermatitis: A comparison of two scoring systems. *Allergol. Immunopathol. (Madr).*, *36*(4), 205–211.

Sa, R., Cerezo, P., Carazo, E., Aguzzi, C., & Viseras, C., (2018). Advanced inorganic nanosystems for skin drug delivery. *Chem. Rec.*, *18*, 891–899.

Saini, K., Modgill, N., Singh, K. K., & Kakkar, V., (2022). Tetrahydrocurcumin lipid nanoparticle based gel promotes penetration into deeper skin layers and alleviates atopic dermatitis in 2,4-dinitrochlorobenzene (DNCB) mouse model. *Nanomaterials, 12*, 1–20.

Schlupp, P., Weber, M., Schmidts, T., Geiger, K., & Runkel, F., (2014). Development and validation of an alternative disturbed skin model by mechanical abrasion to study drug penetration. *Results Pharma Sci.*, *4*, 26–33.

Schmitt, J., Schmitt, N., & Meurer, M., (2007). Cyclosporin in the treatment of patients with atopic eczema – a systematic review and meta-analysis. *J. Eur. Acad. Dermatol. Venereol.*, *21*(5) 606–619.

Sengar, V., Jyoti, K., Jain, U. K., Katare, O. P., Chandra, R., & Madan, J., (2018). Lipid nanoparticles for topical and transdermal delivery of pharmaceuticals and cosmeceuticals: A glorious victory. In: Grumezescu, A. M., (ed.), *Lipid Nanocarriers for Drug Targeting* (p. 413). William Andrew Publishing.

Shahzad, A., Khan, A., Afzal, Z., Farooq, M., Khan, J., & Majid, G., (2019). Formulation development and characterization of cefazolin nanoparticles-loaded cross-linked films of sodium alginate and pectin as wound dressings. *Int. J. Biol. Macromol.*, *124*, 255–269.

Shams, G., Nayeri, A., Safdarian, M., Rezaie, A., Bavarsad, N., & Abbaspour, M., (2021). Self-microemulsification-assisted incorporation of tacrolimus into hydrophilic nanofibers for facilitated treatment of 2,4-dinitrochlorobenzene induced atopic dermatitis like lesions. *J. Drug Deliv. Sci. Technol.*, *62*, 102326.

Sibbald, C., & Drucker, A. M., (2017). Patient burden of atopic dermatitis. *Dermatol. Clin.*, *35*(3), 303–316.

Siddique, M. I., Katas, H., Cairul, M., Mohd, I., Ng, S., Hanif, M., & Jamil, A., (2016). *In-vivo* dermal pharmacokinetics, efficacy, and safety of skin targeting nanoparticles for corticosteroid treatment of atopic dermatitis. *Int. J. Pharm.*, *507*, 72–82.

Siddique, M. I., Katas, H., Cairul, M., Mohd, I., Ng, S., Zulfakar, M. H., Buang, F., & Jamil, A., (2015). Minimization of local and systemic adverse effects of topical glucocorticoids by nanoencapsulation: *In vivo* safety of hydrocortisone – hydroxytyrosol loaded chitosan nanoparticles. *J. Pharm. Sci.*, *104*(12), 4276–4286.

Siddique, M. I., Katas, H., Jamil, A., Cairul, M., Mohd, I., Ng, S., & Zulfakar, M. H., (2019). Potential treatment of atopic dermatitis: Tolerability and safety of cream containing nanoparticles loaded with hydrocortisone and hydroxytyrosol in human subjects. *Drug Deliv. Transl. Res.*, *9*, 469–481.

Siddique, M. I., Katas, H., Sarfraz, M., Ali, T., Jamil, A., Cairul, M., & Mohd, I., (2021). Clinical insights into topically applied multipronged nanoparticles in subjects with atopic dermatitis. *J. Drug Deliv. Sci. Technol.*, *65*,102744.

Silva, M. I., Barbosa, A. I., Lima, S. A. C., Costa, P., Torres, T., & Reis, S., (2020). Freeze-dried Softisan® 649-based lipid nanoparticles for enhanced skin delivery of cyclosporine A. *Nanomaterials, 10*(5), 1–15.

Simpson, E. L., Bruin-weller, M., Flohr, C., Bieber, T., Vestergaard, C., Brown, S. J., Foelster-Holst, R., et al., (2017). When does atopic dermatitis warrant systemic therapy? Recommendations from an expert panel of the international eczema council. *J. Am. Dermatology, 77*(4), 623–633.

Singh, S., Behl, T., Sharma, N., Zahoor, I., Chigurupati, S., Yadav, S., Rachamalla, M., et al., (2022). Targeting therapeutic approaches and highlighting the potential role of nanotechnology in atopic dermatitis. *Environ. Sci. Pollut. Res.* Epub ahead of print. PMID: 35195869.

Smeden, J. V., & Bouwstra, J. A., (2016). Stratum corneum lipids: Their role for the skin barrier function in healthy subjects and atopic dermatitis patients. *Curr. Probl. Dermatol.*, *49*, 8–26.

Souto, E. B., Macedo, A. S., Dias-Ferreira, J., Cano, A., Zielinska, A., & Matos, C. M., (2021). Elastic and ultradeformable liposomes for transdermal delivery of active pharmaceutical ingredients (APIs). *Int. J. Mol. Sci.*, *22*, 1–14.

Stefanov, S. R., & Andonova, V. Y., (2021). Lipid nanoparticulate drug delivery systems: Recent advances in the treatment of skin disorders. *Pharmaceuticals, 14*, 1–29.

Tier, H. L., Balogh, E. A., Bashyam, A. M., Fleischer, A. B., Spergel, J. M., Masicampo, E. J., Kammrath, L. K., et al., (2021). Tolerability of and adherence to topical treatments in atopic dermatitis: A narrative review. *Dermatol. Ther. (Heidelb).*, *11*(2), 415–431.

Togni, S., Riva, A., Maramaldi, G., Cesarone, M. R., & Belcaro, G., (2019). Oral curcumin (Meriva®) reduces symptoms and recurrence rates in subjects with atopic dermatitis. *Esperienze Dermatologiche, 21*, 42–46.

Tokura, Y., (2010). Extrinsic and intrinsic types of atopic dermatitis. *J. Dermatol. Sci.*, *58*(1), 1–7.

Try, C., Moulari, B., Béduneau, A., Fantini, O., Pin, D., Pellequer, Y., & Lamprecht, A., (2016). Size dependent skin penetration of nanoparticles in murine and porcine dermatitis models. *Eur. J. Pharm. Biopharm.*, *100*, 101–108.

Vallet-Regí, M., Colilla, M., Izquierdo-Barba, I., & Manzano, M., (2018). Mesoporous silica nanoparticles for drug delivery: Current insights. *Molecules, 23*(47), 1–19.

Vogt, A., Wischke, C., Neffe, A. T., Ma, N., Alexiev, U., & Lendlein, A., (2016). Nanocarriers for drug delivery into and through the skin — Do existing technologies match clinical challenges? *J. Control. Release, 242*, 3–15.

Voss, G. T., Gularte, M. S., Oliveira, R. L. De., Luchese, C., Fajardo, A. R., & Wilhelm, E. A., (2020). Biopolymeric films as delivery vehicles for controlled release of hydrocortisone: Promising devices to treat chronic skin diseases. *Mater. Sci. Eng. C, 114*, 111074.

Wang, Y., Cao, S., Yu, K., Yang, F., Yu, X., Zhai, Y., Wu, C., & Xu, Y., (2019). Integrating tacrolimus into eutectic oil-based microemulsion for atopic dermatitis: Simultaneously enhancing percutaneous delivery and treatment efficacy with relieving side effects. *Int. J. of Nanomedicine, 14*, 5849–5863.

Weber, D. M., Voss, G. T., Oliveira, R. L. De., Fonseca, C. A. R. Da., Paltian, J., Rodrigues, K. C., Ianiski, F. R., Vaucher, R. A., Luchese, C., & Wilhelm, E. A., (2018). Topic application of meloxicam-loaded polymeric nanocapsules as a technological alternative for treatment of the atopic dermatitis in mice. *J. Appl. Biomed. J.*, *16*, 337–343.

Wickett, R. R., & Visscher, M. O., (2006). Structure and function of the epidermal barrier. *Am. J. Infect. Control, 34*(10), 98–110.

Yamada, Y., Ueda, Y., Nakamura, A., Kanayama, S., Tamura, R., Hashimoto, K., Kido, H., et al., (2016). Biphasic increase in scratching behavior induced by topical application of *Dermatophagoides farinae* extract in NC/Nga mice. *Exp. Dermatol.*, *25*, 611–617.

Yang, G., Lee, H. E., Shin, S. W., Um, S. H., Lee, J. D., Kim, K. B., Kang, H. C., et al., (2018). Efficient transdermal delivery of DNA nanostructures alleviates atopic dermatitis symptoms in NC/Nga mice. *Adv. Funct. Mater.*, *28*, 1–9.

Yang, G., Seok, J. K., Kang, H. C., Cho, Y., Lee, H. S., & Lee, J. Y., (2020). Skin barrier abnormalities and immune dysfunction in atopic dermatitis. *Int. J. Mol. Sci.*, *21*(8), 1–14.

Yilmaz, E., & Borchert, H., (2006). Effect of lipid-containing, positively charged nanoemulsions on skin hydration, elasticity, and erythema – an *in vivo* study. *Int. J. Pharm.*, *307*, 232–238.

Yoshioka, Y., Kuroda, E., Hirai, T., Tsutsumi, Y., & Ishii, K. J., (2017). Allergic responses induced by the immunomodulatory effects of nanomaterials upon skin exposure. *Front. Immunol.*, *8*(169), 1–11.

Yu, K., Wang, Y., Wan, T., Zhai, Y., Cao, S., Ruan, W., Wu, C., & Xu, Y., (2018). Tacrolimus nanoparticles based on chitosan combined with nicotinamide: Enhancing percutaneous delivery and treatment efficacy for atopic dermatitis and reducing dose. *Int. J. Nanomedicine*, 129–142.

Yuan, L., Pan, M., Lei, M., Zhou, X., Hu, D., Liu, Q., Chen, Y., et al., (2020). A novel composite of micelles and hydrogel for improving skin delivery of hydrocortisone and application in atopic dermatitis therapy. *Appl. Mater. Today, 19*, 100593.

Zhuo, F., Abourehab, M. A. S., & Hussain, Z., (2018). Hyaluronic acid decorated tacrolimus-loaded nanoparticles: Efficient approach to maximize dermal targeting and anti-dermatitis efficacy. *Carbohydr. Polym. J.*, *197*, 478–489.

CHAPTER 9

Polymeric Nanoparticles Applied to Skin Diseases

GRAZIELA SCHEUER GOMES,[1] TALITA PIZZA ANUNCIATO CASARINI,[1] RAFAELA GAZZI,[1] TANIRA ALESSANDRA SILVEIRA AGUIRRE,[2] KARINA PAESE,[1] and RENATA VIDOR CONTRI[1]

[1]*Pharmaceutical Sciences Graduate Program, Federal University of Rio Grande do Sul, Brazil*

[2]*Biosciences Graduate Program, Federal University of Health Sciences of Porto Alegre (UFCSPA), Brazil*

ABSTRACT

Skin diseases occur with high frequency (HF) and can impact the daily routine and quality of life, imposing significant challenges to patients. There is an extensive number of medications available for the treatment of skin disorders on the market. However, such medications often present attributes that limit the therapeutic, including greasiness and low spreadability of the products, adverse effects, and insufficient stability and skin penetration of the active substances, leading to a low efficiency after topical administration. So, recently, innovative nanotechnological approaches based on polymeric nanoparticles for topical treatment of skin diseases have been proposed. These delivery systems provide novel mechanisms for targeted drug delivery, maximizing therapeutic effects while minimizing side effects. The most commonly described nanoparticles include nanospheres, nanocapsules, and polymeric micelles, obtained with synthetic or natural polymers. Here we discuss the use of polymeric nanoparticles as a strategy to improve the topical treatment of skin diseases such as acne, melasma, atopic dermatitis (AD), psoriasis, rosacea, mycoses, and skin cancer.

Novel Nanocarriers forSkin Diseases: Advances and Applications.
Raj K. Keservani and Júlia Scherer Santos (Eds.)

9.1 INTRODUCTION

The skin, in addition to sensory and immunological functions, acts as a primary biological barrier between the body and the environment (Foldvari, 2000). Disorders and diseases that affect the skin are extremely common worldwide and due to their visibility, often result in severe suffering and stigma for patients (Bodeker et al., 2017). On a global level, skin conditions are among the most prevalent non-fatal diseases. The impact of these diseases is enormous in both high and low-income countries. The prevention and treatment of skin diseases are relevant to future global health strategies (Ferreira et al., 2017). The main dermatological diseases that affect the population are hyperpigmentation disorders, such as melasma, inflammatory diseases such as acne, dermatitis, rosacea, and psoriasis, infectious diseases caused by fungi, viruses, and bacteria, as well as skin cancer (Verhoeven et al., 2008).

Among the treatment options for the diseases mentioned is the topical administration of drugs or cosmetic actives. Topical drug delivery is a minimally invasive and patient-friendly route. This route is capable of providing greater drug bioavailability and drug targeting, minimizing drug interactions and adverse effects, in addition to providing flexible administration, promoting an improvement in patient compliance (Paudel et al., 2010; McMurtry et al., 2015). The demand for new strategies drives the increase in studies using topical formulations based on nanotechnology.

Nanotechnology used in topical formulations is capable of promoting drug delivery to skin structures (Keservani et al., 2017a, 2018, 2020a), such as follicles, or interacting with cutaneous lipids to mediate transport and provide an increase in percutaneous drug permeation. In addition, nanoparticles are able to create a deposit of the substance in the skin providing a controlled release, which is desirable for diseases that affect the skin. These advantages, arising from the use of nanometer-sized systems, can help to reduce the dose and frequency of application, minimize its side effects and the possible toxicity that drugs can present in healthy tissues, in addition to vectoring the delivery of drug and actives, improving treatment efficacy (Schaffazick et al., 2003; Guterres et al., 2007; Contri et al., 2014; Venturini et al., 2015).

Polymeric nanoparticles have received great attention as potential systems for the topical route of administration. As examples of polymeric nanoparticles studied for the topical route, nanospheres (also called polymeric nanoparticles by authors), nanocapsules, and micelles can be mentioned (Figure 9.1). Nanospheres are matrix carriers, formed by polymer and stabilized by surfactant. The active substance can be retained or adsorbed in the polymer matrix. Nanocapsules are vesicular carriers, which have a polymeric outer layer that is around an oily core, stabilized by surfactant. The substance can be dissolved in the core and/or adsorbed to the polymeric wall. Polymeric micelles are nanometric drug delivery systems (DDSs) characterized by a core-shell structure originating from the self-assembly of amphiphilic block copolymers in an aqueous solution (Schaffazick et al., 2003; Ghezzi et al., 2021).

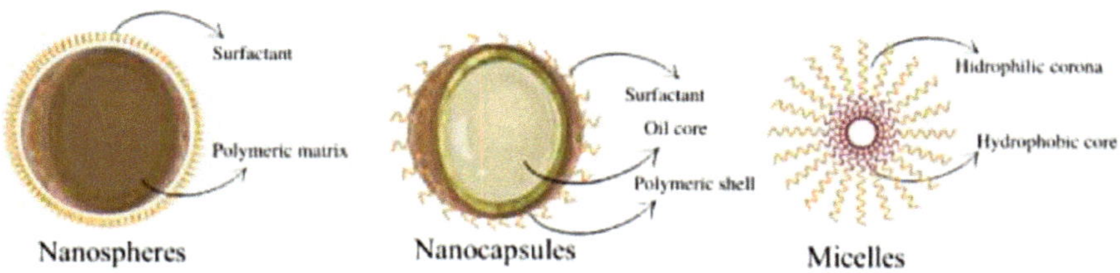

FIGURE 9.1 Main types of polymeric nanoparticles applied to skin diseases.

The main characteristics of polymeric nanoparticles are the considerable stability in biological fluids, and the flexibility for structure modification, including functionalization of their surfaces and the modulation of the entrapped compounds release as a function of specific stimuli (Guterres et al., 2007). Polymer-based nanoparticles can be made up of natural or synthetic polymers. The use of biodegradable polymers stands out as a consequence of their notable biocompatibility and biosafety. Biodegradable polymers include synthetic polymers such as poly(D,l-lactide) (PLA), co-polymer poly(lactide-co-glycolide) (PLGA), poly-ε-caprolactone (PCL); amphiphilic polymers, such as poly(ethylene glycol) (PEG), methoxy-poly(ethylene glycol), and D-α-tocopheryl polyethylene glycol succinate (TPGS); and natural polymers such as chitosan and gelatin (Gagliardi et al., 2021). Non-biodegradable polymers, such as polyacrylates, can also be applied on the skin (Zhang et al., 2013).

Polymeric nanoparticles may differ in composition and components concentration, as well as in physical properties, such as size, shape, surface properties, crystallinity or dispersion state. Depending on the type of drug to be loaded into the polymeric nanoparticles and their requirements for a particular administration route, different methods can be used for the production of the particles. Nanospheres are possible to be produced using techniques such as solvent evaporation, emulsification/solvent diffusion, emulsification/reverse salting-out, and nanoprecipitation. For polymeric micelles, the easiest preparation method is the self-assembling of amphiphilic polymers (Bennet & Kim, 2014; Ghezzi et al., 2021). The drug concentration in the nanoparticle's suspensions is usually low, near 1 mg/mL or less, which can be modulated according to the type and amount of components. Also, the elimination of water (drying of particles) can improve the percentage of drug related to final weight of nanoparticles, also improving the stability of the system (Marin et al., 2013). Polymeric nanoparticles are frequently incorporated into hydrogels in order to facilitate skin application (Ebrahimi et al., 2021).

The nanoparticles properties are usually assessed by several methods. Electron microscopy, dynamic light scattering, or photon correlation spectroscopy, Near-infrared spectroscopy, electrophoresis, and chromatography are a few of the most commonly used techniques (Carbone et al., 2018). Properties evaluated include particle distribution profile (average particle size and polydispersity – PDI), zeta potential, morphology, pH of the suspensions, drug encapsulation efficiency, drug release profile and stability (Schaffazick et al., 2003).

In this chapter, the use of polymeric nanoparticles as a possibility to improve the topical treatment of skin conditions such as acne, melasma, atopic dermatitis (AD), psoriasis, rosacea, mycoses, and skin cancer is discussed.

9.2 ACNE

Acne vulgaris is a chronic inflammatory disease of the pilosebaceous units with multifactorial pathogenesis. It is considered the most common dermatological disease. The major pathogenic factors include genetic predisposition, high sebaceous gland secretion, hyperkeratinization of the hair follicle, follicular hyperproliferation, proliferation of *Cutibacterium acnes* (*C. acnes*) and inflammatory response initiated by bacterial antigens and cytokines (Scholz & Kilian, 2016; Dréno, 2017).

Topical therapy for the treatment of acne vulgaris aims at reducing sebum production and proliferation of *C. acnes*, reversing hyperkeratinization of the hair follicle, and decreasing or preventing the release of inflammatory mediators. In mild to moderate cases, acne is often treated with topical retinoids or antibiotics, benzoyl peroxide, keratolytics, and alpha-hydroxy acids (Ourique et al., 2011; Patel & Prabhu, 2020). It is worth noting that many of the substances used for the treatment of acne, such as topical retinoids, present some side effects: local skin irritation, chemical instability and limited penetration into the skin, more specifically into the pilosebaceous unit (Ourique et al., 2008). The nanoencapsulation of these substances has been studied and applied in recent years in order to reduce and/or reverse these negative effects (Table 9.1).

The improvement of photostability in tretinoin-loaded nanocapsules has already been confirmed. Tretinoin nanoencapsulation in lipid-core nanocapsules (a type of nanocapsules composed by a dispersion of sorbitan monostearate and medium chain triacylglycerol, in the core, surrounded by a polymeric wall of PCL) increased degradation half-life time from 40 to 100 minutes after the formulation was exposed to UVC radiation, compared to the tretinoin methanolic solution (Ourique et al., 2008). The presence of a polymeric wall in the nanostructures has also proven to be important, considering that the half-life time observed for tretinoin nanoemulsion was 82 minutes. Higher photostability of tretinoin-loaded nanocapsules compared to nanoemulsion may be associated with the polymer crystallinity and the greater capacity of these nanocarriers to scatter light, reducing the interaction of light with the encapsulated substance (Ourique et al., 2011). Higher photostability in tretinoin-loaded lipid-corenanocapsules was maintained after adding the suspension in a final semi-solid formulation. After 8-hour exposure to UVA radiation, the photodegradation of nanoencapsulated tretinoin and unencapsulated form of the active in semisolid form was about 25% and 70%, respectively (Ourique et al., 2011). In order to increase microbiological stability, spray-drying can be used to dry the polymeric nanoparticle suspensions. This process does not interfere in the increase of photostability caused by nanoencapsulation. After 60-min exposure to UVA radiation, the nanoencapsulated tretinoin submitted to the spray-drying process degraded approximately 30%, lower than the tretinoin methanolic solution, which degraded around 60% (Marchiori et al., 2012).

Besides the chemical instability, retinoids are substances that can trigger skin irritation. The nanoencapsulation of these substances may decrease induced irritation after topical administration. The irritancy of the nanoencapsulated adapalene in tyrosine-derived nanospheres (tyrospheres) was determined by the mitochondrial activity and the concentration of inflammatory mediators in medium (IL-1α and IL-8), in an *in vitro* skin model. After 24-hour exposure to nanoencapsulated adapalene, tissue viability was higher and less secretion of IL-1α and IL-8 was detected compared to treatment

TABLE 9.1 Polymeric Nanoparticles for Acne Treatment

Nanoparticle Type*	Method of Nanoparticle Production	Polymer	Drug	Particle Size and PDI	References
Nanocapsules	Interfacial deposition of preformed polymers.	PCL	Tretinoin	228 nm, PDI 0.16	Ourique et al. (2008)
Lipid-core nanocapsules	Interfacial deposition of preformed polymers.	PCL	Tretinoin	200–250 nm, PDI below 0.25.	Ourique et al. (2011)
Lipid-core nanocapsules	Interfacial deposition of preformed polymers.	PCL	Tretinoin	220 nm, PDI 0.12	Marchiori et al. (2012)
Tyrospheres	Self-assembly of the polymers into nanospheres induced by addition of copolymer.	ABA triblock copolymer PEG5K-b-oligo (desaminotyrosyl-tyrosine octyl ester suberate)-b-PEG5K.	Adapalene	64.7–81.6 PDI below 0.2	Ramezanli et al. (2017)
Lipid-core nanocapsules	Interfacial deposition of preformed polymer.	PCL	Adapalene and dapsone.	194.9 nm, PDI 0.12	Pereira et al. (2016)
Nanoparticles	Nanoprecipitation or solvent displacement.	PCL or Eudragit® EL	Spironolactone	102.7–180.0 nm, PDI 0.09–0.11	Ferreira-Nunes et al. (2021)
Nanoparticles	Ionotropic gelation	Chitosan or hyaluronic acid.	Clindamycin	362.0–417.4 nm, PDI 0.46	Tolentino et al. (2021)
Micelles	Thin film hydration.	PCL-PEG-PCL copolymer.	Lauric acid	27–89 nm, PDI 0.21–0.33	Tran et al. (2016)
Micelles	Thin film hydration.	Pluronic® F127	Benzoyl peroxide	24.8–25.9 nm, PDI 0.176–0.216	Kahraman et al. (2016)
Nanoparticles	Emulsification–diffusion by solvent displacement.	Eudragit® E 100	Triclosan	147 nm	Domínguez-Delgado et al. (2011)
Nanospheres	Emulsification-solvent displacement.	Eudragit® RL 100	Triclosan	261 nm	Rodríguez-Cruz et al. (2013)
Micelles	Solvent evaporation	MPEG-dihexPLA copolymer (methoxy-poly(ethylene glycol) di-(hexyl-substituted polylactide)).	Retinoic acid	Below 20 nm	Lapteva et al. (2015)

*As described by authors.

with commercial formulations (Ramezanli et al., 2017). Other formulations of polymeric nanoparticles containing adapalene and dapsone (Pereira et al., 2016), spironolactone (Ferreira-Nunes et al., 2021) and clindamycin (Tolentino et al., 2021) were found to be non-irritating by an *in vitro* model (HET-CAM assay).

Improved antimicrobial activity of substances against *C. acnes* has also been evidenced after nanoencapsulation. The association of lauric acid, a saturated medium-chain fatty acid with antimicrobial activity, to PCL-PEG-PCL polymeric micelles showed a reduction in the minimal inhibitory concentration (MIC) compared to lauric acid solution. The minimum inhibitory concentration (MIC) of unencapsulated lauric acid was 20 μg/mL, while the MIC of lauric acid associated with the formulation with higher encapsulation efficiency was 10 μg/mL. Additionally, the minimum bactericidal concentration (MBC) was also lower after the treatment with lauric acid-loaded micelles compared to the lauric acid solution, decreasing MBC values from 80 μg/mL to 40 μg/mL (Tran et al., 2016).

Among the numerous advantages of the cutaneous administration of substances associated in polymeric nanoparticles for the treatment of acne, the increase in skin penetration of nanoencapsulated substances stands out. Moreover, studies have demonstrated that the use of polymeric nanoparticles allows higher deposition of active ingredients in hair follicles when compared to conventional formulations. These structures are considered an ideal target for the delivery of active substances for the treatment of this skin disorder.

Improved skin delivery of benzoyl peroxide when loaded into polymeric micelles composed of Pluronic® F127 has been proven. Skin penetration/permeation was examined *in vitro*. After 24-hour evaluation, skin permeation of the substance was not detected, however, the skin penetration of encapsulated benzoyl peroxide was three-fold higher compared to commercial formulations. Enhanced penetration of this formulation is due to the nanometric size of the micelles, which provides an increase in the contact surface, and to the role of these micelles as benzoyl peroxide reservoirs (Kahraman et al., 2016). This reservoir effect has also been observed in triclosan encapsulated in both Eudragit® E 100 (Domínguez-Delgado et al., 2011) and Eudragit® RL100 nanoparticles (Rodríguez-Cruz et al., 2013). Both studies have evaluated skin permeation/penetration *in vitro* using pig skin.

A higher deposition of tretinoin in hair follicles when nanoencapsulated in polymeric micelles of methoxy-poly(ethylene glycol) di-(hexyl-substituted polylactide) has already been evidenced. Delivery effectiveness into the pilosebaceous unit of human skin was higher for nanoencapsulated tretinoin (10.4 ± 3.2%) compared to commercial formulations (0.6 ± 0.2%) (Lapteva et al., 2015). The relationship between particle size and hair follicle deposition has been evaluated in recent studies. Particle size has a significant role in the development of nanotechnological formulations targeting the delivery to the pilosebaceous units for the treatment of acne. Most recently, PCL and Eudragit® E100 nanoparticles were produced by obtaining formulations with different mean particle sizes (102, 126, and 180 nm) to evaluate the impact of these sizes on the amount of spironolactone deposited in hair follicles. After 24-hour *in vitro* evaluation using pig ear skin models, the follicular contents were removed, and the retained drug was quantified. The larger nanoparticles (180 nm) produced with PCL increased 5-fold the amount of spironolactone in hair follicles compared to control solution; 2.1-fold compared to nanoparticles produced with the same polymer (PCL), but with a smaller size (126 nm); and 4.9-fold when compared to 102 nm Eudragit® E100 nanoparticles (Ferreira-Nunes et al., 2021).

The polymeric material used in the production of nanoparticles was also evaluated, comparing chitosan (nanoparticles with zeta potential of +27.7 mV) and hyaluronic acid (nanoparticles with zeta potential of – 30.2 mV) for follicular delivery of clindamycin. After 24-hour *in vitro* permeation using pig skin, the follicles were removed, and the amount of drug determined. The nature of the polymer did not influence the drug deposition in the pilosebaceous units, considering that the "follicular targeting factor" (amount of drug that penetrated the pilosebaceous structures divided by the total amount of drug permeate), was statistically equal for both nanoparticle formulations (52.9 ± 20.5% for chitosan nanoparticles and 77.0 ± 8.6% for hyaluronic acid nanoparticles). However, the nanoencapsulation had a positive effect on the deposition of clindamycin into the pilosebaceous unit, considering that the "follicular targeting factor" for commercial formulations (25.6 ± 9.6%) was lower than for nanotechnology-based formulations (Tolentino et al., 2021).

9.3 SKIN WHITENING

Skin whitening is a challenge. The main enzyme responsible for the production of melanin, our natural pigment, is tyrosinase. It is responsible for the first step in melanin production inside melanocytes, specialized dendritic cells presented in the lower layer of epidermis. Therefore, inhibiting tyrosinase activity is the most popular target of skin whitening substances

(Pillaiyar et al., 2017). Hydroquinone has been used as skin-whitening agent in dermatological formulations for almost 60 years but toxicological aspects such as damage to DNA and inhibition of apoptosis of mutated cells are cited in the literature. Because of concerns about hydroquinone, it was banned in 2006 by the FDA in the US market (Kooyers & Westerhof, 2004).

Other substances such as arbutin and azelaic acid have been proposed as safe approaches for melasma but many treatments fail because of some issues, such as substance instability when incorporated into dermatological vehicles, difficulty to reach the target cell in the skin – melanocyte, skin irritation, among others (Hatem et al., 2020). The development of systems based on polymeric nanoparticles have emerged in order to surpass the barriers inherent to the substances and achieve success in skin whitening treatment (Table 9.2).

TABLE 9.2 Polymeric Nanoparticles for Skin Whitening Treatment

Nanoparticle Type*	Method of Nanoparticle Production	Polymer	Drug	Particle Size and PDI	References
Nanoparticles	Ionotropic gelation	Chitosan	Arbutin	466.93 nm	Leelapornpisid et al. (2010)
Nanoparticles	Ionic cross-linking	Chitosan	α- and β-arbutin	α-arbutin: 147–274 nm; β-arbutin: 211–284 nm, PDI 0.2–0.3.	Ayumi et al. (2019)
Nanoparticles	Ionic gelation	Chitosan	α-Arbutin	340–570 nm, PDI 0.32–0.60	Hatem et al. (2022)
Nanosponges	Melt method	β-cyclodextrin	Azelaic acid	228.3 nm, PDI 0.141	Kumar & Rao (2021)
Nanoparticles	Interfacial polymer deposition.	PLA and PLGA	Ascorbyl palmitate	115–150 nm, PDI around 0.1	Tangsumranjit et al. (2006)
Nanoparticles	Nanoprecipitation	(PEG-PCL) diblock copolymer	AP736	50–200 nm, PDI 0.9–0.19	Shin et al. (2018)

*As described by authors.

Arbutin is one of the most popular active substances for skin whitening treatment. This molecule is formed by hydroquinone and D-glucose. β-Arbutin is called arbutin, and β-anomer of D-glucose is bound to hydroquinone. On the other hand, α-arbutin is a compound of hydroquinone and the α-anomer of D-glucose. These molecules are competitive inhibitors against both the monophenolase and diphenolase activities of tyrosinase enzyme (Boo, 2021). The first studies about arbutin as a skin lightening agent were conducted about 30 years ago (Akiu et al., 1991). Arbutin is highly hydrophilic (log P value = –1.49) and a hygroscopic substance, which results in poor skin permeation in order to reach melanocytes (Leelapornpisid et al., 2010).

To date, three studies focused on the nanoencapsulation of arbutin into polymeric structures. Different arbutin nanoparticles were developed by Leelapornpisid and co-workers (2010). Optimum formulations were obtained presenting around 400 nm of particle size, zeta potential of around +30 mV and loading efficiency of 41%. Arbutin from nanoparticles showed a slow-release profile and stability (evaluated by entrapment efficiency) under different storage conditions (45°C, room temperature, 4°C), for 3 months (Leelapornpisid et al., 2010). Ayumi and co-workers (2019) developed nanoparticles of α- and β-arbutin by ionic cross-linking of chitosan with tripolyphosphate. Different particle sizes were obtained and compared to α- and β-arbutin in their unencapsulated form, the nanoencapsulation resulted in a significantly higher percentage of drug release. Hatem and co-workers (2022) produced α-arbutin-loaded chitosan nanoparticles, which were further incorporated in a semisolid form, using Carbopol® 940 as the gelling agent, for clinical efficacy evaluation in patients with melasma. Compared to unencapsulated arbutin, hydrogel containing arbutin nanoparticles exhibited significantly better results in the following parameters: modified MASI (melasma area and severity index), epidermal MPSA (melanin particle size surface area) and number of epidermal monoclonal mouse anti-melanoma antigen recognized by T cells-1 (Hatem et al., 2020).

Although azelaic acid is a US FDA-approved compound for the treatment of mild to moderate inflammatory acne and rosacea, it is very popular as an off-label bleaching agent (Kumar & Rao, 2021). Two mechanisms of action are cited in the literature. First, azelaic acid can inhibit the energy production and/or DNA synthesis of hyperactive melanocytes, and secondly, it acts as a tyrosinase inhibitor, therefore stopping the processes of production of melanin (Breathnach, 1996). Due to low water-solubility of azelaic acid, Kumar & Rao (2021) developed cyclodextrin nanosponges (a porous nanocarrier system) with diphenyl carbonate as a cross-linker. Particle size was in the nano-range and the *in vitro* release study showed controlled and precise drug release when compared to unencapsulated azelaic acid. When *in vitro* tyrosinase assay was conducted, azelaic acid nanoparticles resulted in superior inhibition of tyrosinase activity, in all tested concentrations, compared to unencapsulated azelaic acid, as well as to kojic acid and ascorbic acid, other known enzyme inhibitors. Moreover, the nanoparticles presented suitable antioxidant activity and were considered safe, when assessed using Human Epidermal Keratinocyte cell lines.

Ascorbyl palmitate, the lipophilic derivative of ascorbic acid, has been widely used in cosmetics, including for skin whitening purposes. However, the substance instability is a challenge that can be overcome by nanoencapsulation. Two polymers were evaluated, PLA and PLGA. Both nanoparticles presented high encapsulation efficiency however, the nanoparticles obtained with PLA showed higher potential to stabilize the ascorbyl palmitate (Tangsumranjit et al., 2006).

A novel skin whitening substance has been proposed, AP736 (damantan-1-yl-N-(2,4-dihydroxybenzyl)-2,4-di methoxy-benzamide). A previous study showed that this molecule acts by suppression of the expression of tyrosinase, tyrosinase-related protein-1 and tyrosinase-related protein-2, among other targets involved in melanogenesis (Lee et al., 2013). Clinical efficacy of AP736 was reported by Jeong and co-workers (2016). In this study, the formulation with AP736 0.5% twice daily was significantly superior ($p<0.05$) than the vehicle control in reducing the appearance of pigmentation of volunteers.

AP736 has poor solubility and recrystallization can be observed in oil-in-water emulsions. In order to surpass this issue, polymeric nanoparticles encapsulating AP736 were developed employing the polymers PEG and PCL, with different PCL chain sizes and co-surfactants, resulting in nanoparticles with encapsulation efficiency up to 90%. As expected, with higher PCL chain length, higher particle size was observed. A permeation study with the membrane Strat-M™ (predictive of diffusion in human skin) showed a greater permeation capability when nanoparticles were formulated with Choleth-24 as a co-surfactant. In addition, the nanoformulation showed stability for 4 weeks, as seen by the maintenance of particle size and absence of precipitation.

9.4 ATOPIC DERMATITIS (AD)

Atopic dermatitis (AD) is a chronic non-contagious inflammatory and immunological skin disease. Among the causes of AD, there is a dysfunctional skin barrier and immune system abnormalities. Treatment of AD involves application of emollients to restore skin barrier and ameliorate skin hydration and the use of topical corticosteroids such as hydrocortisone and betamethasone valerate (Mayba & Gooderham, 2016). Immunomodulators such as tacrolimus and cyclosporine A are also used to treat AD. Although the topical treatment for AD is generally efficient to control the disease for maintaining clinical remission, the topical drug delivery can lead to systemic drug absorption due to disruption on skin barrier function on AD patients. In turn, this absorption profile can eventually lead to complications due to long-term treatment. Furthermore, local side effects of conventional treatments for AD may be due to repeated and direct contact of the drug with the skin. Thus, the main objectives employing polymeric nanoparticles as vehicles for topical drug delivery to manage AD (Table 9.3) is to obtain improved therapeutic efficacy by means of: (i) diminish contact of drugs and skin and improve the release profile of drug in order to minimize local and systemic side effects; and (ii) increase the retention of drugs in deeper layers of the skin regulating the epithelium permeability and bioavailability of drugs.

TABLE 9.3 Polymeric Nanoparticles for Atopic Dermatitis Treatment

Nanoparticle Type*	Method of Nanoparticle Production	Polymer	Drug	Particle Size and PDI	References
Nanoparticles	Modified solvent displacement.	PCL	Hydrocortisone	190–230 nm, PDI 0.010–0.030	Rosado et al. (2013)
Nanoparticles	Emulsification solvent evaporation.	PLGA (coated with chitosan)	Budesonide	324 nm, PDI 0.125	Campos et al. (2021)
Micelles	Dry film hydration.	Pluronic® L121/ Pluronic® F127	Beclomethasone dipropionate	20.4 nm, PDI 0.33	Assem et al. (2019)
Nanoparticles	High-pressure homogenization–solvent evaporation.	Chitosan	Betamethasone valerate	338 nm, PDI 0.321	Pandey et al. (2019)
Nanoparticles	Ionotropic gelation	Chitosan	Hydrocortisone	214 nm, PDI 0.321	Hussain et al. (2014)
Nanoparticles	Ionotropic gelation	Chitosan	Hydrocortisone	267 nm, PDI 0.46	Siddique et al. (2021)
Nanocapsules	Interfacial deposition of preformed polymer.	PCL	Meloxicam	247 nm, PDI 0.14	Weber et al. (2018)
Nanoparticles	Ionotropic gelation	Chitosan	Tacrolimus	110 nm, PDI 0.20	Yu et al. (2018)
Nanocapsules	Solvent displacement	PLGA	Cyclosporine A	162 nm, PDI 0.061	Badihi et al. (2020)

*As described by authors.

Topical corticosteroids have been used in the treatment of AD for many decades because of the anti-inflammatory, immunosuppressant, and proliferative activity (Badihi et al., 2020), however, skin dryness, burning, stinging sensation, itching, and reduction of water content are described after long periods of use (Mayba & Gooderham, 2016). A prolonged release of drugs, allowing that only a small amount of drug come into contact with the skin at a time, is an alternative to reduce those side effects. PCL-nanoparticles loaded with hydrocortisone released approximately 7% of drug over 24 h, and a similar amount permeated through an *in vitro* model of human epidermis over 12 h, resulting in a drug flux of approximately 30% lower than unencapsulated hydrocortisone (Rosado et al., 2013). The corticosteroid budesonide was encapsulated into chitosan coated PLGA nanocapsules, which were further incorporated into poloxamer 407 hydrogels. The nanoparticles released around 25% of budesonide and less than 5% of drug when incorporated into the hydrogels, over 30 h. These release profiles reflected on excised human skin percutaneous modulation of drug skin penetration. The nanoparticles caused a decrease of 21.5-fold on drug amount found on epidermis compared to unencapsulated drug, and an even more pronounced reduction was seen for the dermis. A skin penetration study demonstrated that both flux and lag time of budesonide from nanoparticles were higher when applied into intact compared to damaged skin, suggesting that, on AD patients, the drug flux may be higher, but the nanoparticles prevent the drug from percutaneous absorption and may decrease adverse effects (Campos et al., 2021).

An improved therapeutic efficacy of topical corticosteroids is also suggested to occur by increasing the retention of drugs in deeper layers of the skin. Penetration and accumulation of polymeric nanoparticles in inflamed skin of mice and pigs are size-dependent (Try et al., 2016). Beclomethasone dipropionate was incorporated into size-reduced polymeric micelles and formulated in hydroxypropyl methyl cellulose hydrogel. *Ex vivo* permeation across newly born CD-1 mice skin was 10-fold lower for drug encapsulated compared to a commercial product containing the drug. This led to an increase of more than three-fold on the amount of drug retained into the skin after 6 h, being further related to an increase of near to 40-fold on local accumulation efficiency for beclomethasone dipropionate into micelles compared to commercial formulation. Further, *in vivo* anti-inflammatory effect in terms of healing of tissues occurred 6 days earlier to drug into micelles compared to the commercial formula (Assem et al., 2019). Polymeric nanoparticles usually are larger structures compared to polymeric micelles; further coating of these structures may improve its penetration profile. For chitosan nanoparticles loaded with betamethasone valerate, the amount of drug retained into epidermis and dermis were increased by approximately 22 and 40%, respectively, after they were coated with hyaluronic acid (Pandey et al., 2019).

Chitosan nanoparticles loaded with hydrocortisone showed *ex vivo* drug accumulation in epidermis and dermis, besides anti-inflammatory and antifibrotic activity on AD-like skin lesions on NC/Nga mouse model, in terms of control of transepidermal water loss (TEWL), erythema reduction, mild classification of dermatitis index, and reduced dorsal skin thickness (Hussain et al., 2013). The immunomodulatory efficacy of nanoparticles loaded into lipophilic and aqueous cream was also shown, using the same animal model (Hussain et al., 2014). A clinical study in subjects with AD, carried over 42 days, confirmed the safety and tolerability of chitosan nanoparticles containing both hydrocortisone and hydrocortisol, showing further the clinical efficacy of the system. The authors reported that TEWL from patients suffering from AD enrolled in nanoparticles group decreased, indicating the recovery of the skin barrier function. In terms of erythema intensity, it decreased for nanoparticles and the commercial cream, however, for the vehicle cream (without drug), inflammation could still be seen at the affected area after 6 weeks of treatment, with no changes in erythema or redness. A decrease in melanin levels in AD patients was also reported. Moreover, improvement on nanoparticles group compared to commercial and vehicle groups were reported in terms of clinical observations such as eczema area severity index (EASI) scores and dermatology life quality index (DLQI) based on the subject assessment. By analyzing blood parameters, it was concluded that there was no systemic absorption of drugs from nanoparticle formulation, while an increase in cortisol levels from patients in the commercial cream group was noticed, possibly indicating systemic absorption of the drug (Siddique et al., 2021).

Alternatives to topical corticosteroids in AD treatment include non-steroidal anti-inflammatory and immunomodulators. Meloxicam presents low solubility and low skin permeation; thus, nanoparticles can overcome these physical properties. Topical administration of meloxicam-loaded nanocapsules incorporated into Carbopol® hydrogel in a 2,4-dinitrochlorobenzene (DNBC) induced AD on BALB/c mice reduced inflammatory response. A more than 40% reduction was observed on ears swelling, compared to unencapsulated drug, and the myeloperoxidase activity level was back to normal. Therefore, symptoms such as scratching behavior were improved. There is increasing evidence regarding the role of oxidative stress in AD (Parekh et al., 2021). The level of thiobarbituric acid reactive species in dorsal skin of mice increased significantly with DNBC, but the same did not happen with non-protein thiol. However, meloxicam, either encapsulated or not, had no effect on these parameters (Weber et al., 2018). Tacrolimus first complexed to nicotinamide and loaded into chitosan nanoparticles was mostly retained in the stratum corneum (SC) layer of Sprague Dawley rats, resulting in more than two-fold increase on skin drug retention compared to commercial formulation of the drug. Efficacy of tacrolimus-loaded nanoparticles were demonstrated on AD-like skin lesions induced by DNCB to BABL/c mice. The AD-like skin symptoms on mice were improved, evaluated by means of dermatitis score and ear thickness, after 28 days of treatment. Furthermore, it was possible to reduce the tacrolimus dose to one third when nanoencapsulated, showing similar effect to the commercial formulation. The nanoparticles also led to downregulating serum total IgE levels at lower dose compared to commercial formulation (Yu et al., 2018). Nanocapsules loaded with cyclosporine A and dispersed in an anhydrous formulation in order to prevent drug diffusion showed high drug levels in epidermis and dermis (pig skin). Drug loaded-nanoparticles were able to reduce IL-6 and IL-8 in human skin after LPS-induced inflammation. *In vivo* study of ovalbumin-induced AD on BALB/c mice showed that the cyclosporine A, when loaded into nanoparticles, significantly preserved skin integrity by reducing TEWL, prevented skin thickening, reduced INF-γ, OVA-IgE serum levels and IL-4 displaying the most effective results among samples tested (Badihi et al., 2020).

9.5 PSORIASIS

Psoriasis is a chronic inflammatory disease that affects mainly the skin (Zhai et al., 2011). The main psoriasis characteristic is the growth of skin cells in excess due to faulty signals produced by the immune system (Alvarez-Figueroa, 2001). Topical treatment is the most prescribed method since topical delivery of the drug is the first line of defense for psoriatic skin. These current treatments are useful in controlling mild and major disease types, but they lead to some adverse effects (Alvarez-Figueroa, 2001).

Different drugs are proposed for nanoparticles obtainment regarding the topical treatment of psoriasis. The polymeric nanostructures investigated for topical treatment of psoriasis include the application of cyclosporin-A (Jain et al., 2011; Lapteva et al., 2015; Prajapati et al., 2021), tacrolimus (Gabriel et al., 2016; Fereig et al., 2021), methotrexate (Asad et al., 2021; Panonnummal et al., 2018), paclitaxel (Kilfoyle et al., 2012), curcumin (Sun et al., 2017; Mao et al., 2017) and coal tar (Sunoqrot et al., 2022) (Table 9.4). The nanoparticles provide better therapeutic efficacy, less toxicity, dose reduction, and drug-specific targeting. Some studies are brought in detail in the sequence.

TABLE 9.4 Polymeric Nanoparticles for Psoriasis Treatment

Nanoparticle Type*	Method of Nanoparticle Production	Polymer	Drug	Particle Size and PDI	References
Nanoparticles	Emulsion-diffusion-evaporation.	PLGA	Cyclosporin-A	Around 163 nm, PDI 0.118	Jain et al. (2011)
Micelles	Solvent evaporation	MPEG-dihexPLA copolymer.	Cyclosporine-A	10–50 nm, PDI 0.580	Lapteva et al. (2015)
Nanospheres	Nanoprecipitation	Eudragit® L100	Cyclosporine-A	Around 100 nm	Prajapati et al. (2021)
Nanoparticles	Interfacial deposition	mPEGhexPLA	Tacrolimus	50 nm, PDI 0.150	Gabriel et al. (2016)
Nanoparticles	Modified solvent free ionic gelation	Chitosan	Tacrolimus	Around 140 nm	Fereig et al. (2021)
Nanoparticles	Stirring and sonication	Chitin	Methotrexate	Around 195 nm	Panonnummal et al. (2018)
Nanospheres	Emulsion-evaporation	Eudragit® E100	Methotrexate	Around 199 nm, PDI around 0.17	Asad et al. (2021)
Nanospheres	Self-assembly	PEG-β-oligo (DTR-XA)-β-PEG	Paclitaxel	55–122 nm, PDI 0.17–0.32	Kilfoyle et al. (2012)
Nanoparticles	Conventional anti-solvent	PLGA	Curcumin	Around 50 nm, PDI 0.11	Sun et al. (2017)
Nanoparticles	Dialysis	RRR-α-tocopheryl succinate-grafted-polylysine conjugate (VES-g-ε-PLL)	Curcumin	24.4 nm, PDI 0.18–0.21.	Mao et al. (2017)
Nanoparticles	Nanoprecipitation	PLGA	Coal tar	Around 133 nm, PDI 0.10	Sunoqrot et al. (2022)

*As described by authors.

Cyclosporin-A, an immunosuppressive drug, shows some limitations in its traditional route of administration, the oral, for example, nephrotoxicity, hypertension, hyperlipidemia, and hepatitis. A way to avoid these limitations is the topical route, however, skin permeation is not readily achieved due to its rigid cyclic structure and high molecular weight. To avoid these limitations, polymeric nanoparticles (Jain et al., 2011; Prajapati et al., 2021) and polymeric micelles of MPEGdihexPLA (Lapteva et al., 2015) have been developed. PLGA nanoparticles (Jain et al., 2011) and Eudragit L100 (Prajapati et al., 2021) loading cyclosporin-A exhibited increased penetration into the dermis and epidermis offering better accumulation in the skin, in comparison with unencapsulated drug, reducing systemic absorption and improving antipsoriatic effects of the drug. It was observed an antiproliferative activity for cyclosporin-A-loaded nanoparticles, showing a better effect on cell growth as compared to the free drug which was due to higher uptake by the cells. The cell viability diminished in a dose-dependent way (Prajapati et al., 2021). In another study, cyclosporin-A loaded into polymeric micelles increased skin permeation of the drug due to the encapsulation system, the increase in cutaneous drug levels was due to improved tacrolimus deposition in the SC, viable epidermis, and upper dermis (Lapteva et al., 2015). Given that there was no increase in the amount of cyclosporin-A in deeper skin layers or any transdermal permeation, the results suggested that it is possible to increase cyclosporin-A levels selectively in the target tissue without increasing systemic absorption and the risk of side effects *in vivo*.

Another important drug in psoriasis treatment is tacrolimus, its topical limitation is mainly related to patient acceptability and low permeation due to high molecular weight and hydrophobicity. The efficacy of tacrolimus-loaded mPEGhexPLGA nanoparticles in the treatment of psoriasis was evaluated, and the nanoencapsulation provided a delayed release of the drug into the skin thus enhancing the stability of the drug along with a significant reduction in the side effects as exhibited by the conventional formulations (Gabriel et al., 2016). Skin delivery of tacrolimus-loaded nanoparticles composite hydrogel in an imiquimod (IMQ)-induced psoriasis mouse model was found to be twice as high as for the commercial formulation, used as a benchmark. Tacrolimus nanoparticles composite hydrogel showed significant improvement in the *in vivo* and histopathological features of the IMQ-induced psoriasis model (Gabriel et al., 2016). Chitosan nanoparticles loading tacrolimus have also been developed, and it was observed a low skin permeation with higher skin retention of drug, indicating minimal systemic absorption. Also, it was observed that tacrolimus-loaded-chitosan nanoparticles provided faster and more efficient control of psoriatic manifestations, skin thickness, erythema, and scaling than tacrolimus ointment in the animal model of psoriasis (Fereig et al., 2021).

Methotrexate is known for its immunomodulatory efficacy, as well as being one of the most commonly available medicines for psoriasis treatment. However, its physicochemical characteristics, such as hydrophilicity, and its improper topical absorption, limits its topical use. The IMQ-induced psoriasis mouse model has been used to investigate the effectiveness of methotrexate-loaded chitin nanogel compared to unencapsulated drug in penetration into the skin. Significant anti-psoriatic efficacy on IMQ-induced model of psoriasis without any dermal and systemic toxicities suggests that it is an ideal delivery platform for topical delivery of methotrexate in psoriasis (Panonnummal & Sabitha, 2018). Methotrexate-loaded chitosan nanoparticles have also been developed (Asad et al., 2021), showing a sustained release from polymer-based diffusion control. A cell viability assay evaluating human lymphocytes showed that the nanoformulation was safe and biocompatible. Also, a low skin permeation and high deposition of drug in the epidermal skin layer of healthy mice has been observed (Asad et al., 2021).

Other substances have been incorporated into polymeric nanocapsules and evaluated for topical drug delivery, such as paclitaxel (Kilfoyle et al., 2012), curcumin (Mao et al., 2017; Sun et al., 2017), and Coal TAR (Sunoqrot et al., 2022). Paclitaxel shows low water solubility and many side effects by oral route, so the topical route is an alternative. The study with paclitaxel-loaded tyrospheres showed that the solubility of paclitaxel in tyrospheres was almost 4,000-fold higher than paclitaxel in PBS and enabled sustained-release under the condition of simulated skin penetration (Kilfoyle et al., 2012). Paclitaxel-tyrospheres, delivered to the epidermis, have enhanced the cytotoxicity of the drug to human keratinocytes, thereby providing a way for psoriasis treatment.

PLGA, and the amphiphilic polymer RRR-α-tocopheryl succinate-grafted-ε-polylysine conjugate, have shown promising results for topical delivery of curcumin (Mao et al., 2017; Sun et al., 2017). Curcumin is chemically unstable, showing limited permeation and accumulation due to poor aqueous solubility (Mao et al., 2017; Sun et al., 2017). Curcumin-nanoparticles showed significantly improved skin penetration and accumulation (Mao et al., 2017; Sun et al., 2017), a uniform distribution into skin after 48 h, and a high adhesivity when compared to its unencapsulated form (Mao et al., 2017). This improvement can be due to the characteristics of encapsulation, such as a small diameter (Mao et al., 2017; Sun et al., 2017), and positive surface charge (Mao et al., 2017). Polymeric nanoparticles can act as a reservoir accumulating in skin structures. Also, a large surface area may facilitate drug-loaded retention. In antiproliferative cell evaluation, drug encapsulation had an increase in curcumin effect, inducing apoptosis of keratinocytes, showing promising efficacy in psoriasis treatment (Sun et al., 2017). The psoriasis area severity index (PASI), an index used to express the severity of psoriasis, spleen weight, and bodyweight indicated a better therapeutic efficacy by the polymeric nanoparticles than those treated by unencapsulated curcumin (Sun et al., 2017) or clobetasol, a traditional drug in the psoriasis treatment (Mao et al., 2017). Besides that, the results indicate promisor results in terms of morphological evaluation, and biomarkers at mRNA and protein levels (Mao et al., 2017; Sun et al., 2017). Coal tar, a thick dark liquid that shows medical application, was encapsulated in PLGA particles (Sunoqrot et al., 2022). The nanoencapsulation of coal tar has shown the potential to reduce cytotoxicity in fibroblasts assay, besides improving skin accumulation of the substance, what can maximize effects. Also, it was observed a reduction in skin scaling and staining of clothes, some its limitations, due to encapsulation of coal tar (Sunoqrot et al., 2022).

9.6 ROSACEA

Rosacea is a chronic and inflammatory disease, characterized by facial skin manifestations, such as flushing, no transient erythema, papules/pustules, telangiectasia, itching, burning, and phymatous changes (Tan et al., 2017; Wang et al., 2020). The pathogenesis and pathophysiology of rosacea are not fully understood (Rainer et al., 2020), but immune dysfunction, Demodex infection, and exposure to ultraviolet (UV) radiation are contributing factors (Tan et al., 2017). In recent years, a variety of treatment options have been used for rosacea treatment including topical therapies, oral therapies, light devices, skincare, and lifestyle management (Thiboutot et al., 2020). However, treatment options for rosacea are still a challenge, because of their complexity. Another limitation is the physicochemical characteristics of the used drugs. One alternative to avoid the limitations is the polymeric nanoparticles. However, in the literature, there are no studies regarding polymeric nanoparticles focused specifically on rosacea treatment. It is important to notice that some nanoparticles presented in section "Acne" such as the ones loaded with adapalene (Ramezanli & Michniak-Kohn, 2018) and tretinoin (Ourique et al., 2008, 2011; Marchiori et al., 2012) can be applied to rosacea as well. The nanoencapsulation of these drugs aims to improve skin permeation, increase drug stability and reduce adverse effects that often result from the use of solvents to increase the solubility of lipophilic drugs leading to skin irritation.

9.7 SKIN MYCOSES

Skin mycoses (fungal infection of the skin) have become more common over the years, infecting also immunocompetent people (Ma et al., 2021). They are usually painless and superficial; however, they can become serious if the infection disseminates and invades deeper tissues (Bangia et al., 2019; Garg et al., 2020). Besides, social and psychological impacts are frequently observed among patients. The most common type of skin infection is dermatophytosis, also known as tinea infections, caused by dermatophytes (Bangia et al., 2019), affecting 20–25% of the population worldwide (Ma et al., 2021). Tricophyton, Microsporun, Epidermophyton, and Nanizzia are the genera of the dermatophytes, being *T. rubrum* and *T. mentagrophytes* the most common pathogens (Ma et al., 2021). Besides dermatophytosis, skin infection types include Dematiaceous infection, Mucormycosis, Candidiasis, Malassezia infection, Sporotrichosis, and Talaromycosis, all caused by different microorganisms (Garg et al., 2020; Ma et al., 2021).

Topical antifungals formulations are the first therapy option, however, the formulations available often contribute to treatment dropout and the topical drugs can cause irritation, burning, rashes among others (Bangia et al., 2019; De Souza et al., 2012). In addition, many topical antifungals present low or variable skin penetration capability (de Souza et al., 2012), therefore, frequent and high doses are needed (Garg et al., 2020), since the efficacy of the treatment depends on the delivery of the drug to the target at the desired concentrations (De Souza et al., 2012; Garg et al., 2020). Also, microbial resistance and recurrence after treatment is frequently observed (Bangia et al., 2019). Therefore, nanoparticles are interesting innovative tools for skin mycoses treatment, being capable of modulating skin penetration and decreasing side effects in a patient-friendly formulation.

Several different antifungal drugs have been incorporated into polymeric nanoparticles aiming improvement of mycoses treatment (Table 9.5), such as terbinafine hydrochloride (Pervaiz et al., 2021), econazole (Bachhav et al., 2011), clotrimazole (Kareem et al., 2019), miconazole nitrate (Abdel-Rashid et al., 2022), ketoconazole (Endo et al., 2020) and nystatin (Mohammadi et al., 2017), among others. Regarding the nanoparticle types, polymeric nanospheres, nanocapsules, nanosponges, and micelles can be found as delivery systems for skin fungal infection, obtained with different polymers alone or in association (either synthetic or natural). Most of the articles describe, besides the nanoparticle's properties, the influence of the particles on the *in vitro* skin permeation/retention of the drug and on the antifungal activity, especially in *Candida albicans* and different dermatophytes (disk diffusion or MIC). Some published articles are discussed in Table 9.5.

TABLE 9.5 Polymeric Nanoparticles for Skin Mycoses Treatment

Nanoparticle Type*	Method of Nanoparticle Production	Polymer	Drug	Particle Size and PDI	References
Nanoparticles	Polyelectrolyte complexation	Chitosan and xanthan gum.	Terbinafine hydrochloride.	213 nm	Pervaiz et al. (2021)
Nanoparticles	Emulsification probe sonication	PLGA	Butenafine	267 nm, PDI 0.227	Alshehri & Imam (2021)
Micelles	Solvent evaporation	(TPGS) copolymer	Terbinafine hydrochloride, amorolfine, and econazole.	Below 10 nm, PDI around 0.1	Gou et al. (2022)
Micelles	Co-solvent evaporation sonication.	Amphiphilic methoxy-poly(ethylene glycol)-hexyl substituted polylactide (MPEG-hexPLA) block copolymers.	Econazole	91 nm, PDI 0.16	Bachhav et al. (2011)
Micelles	Co-solvent evaporation	Poly(ethylene oxide)-block-poly(ε-caprolactone) block copolymers.	Clotrimazole	153 nm, PDI 0.256	Kareem et al. (2019)
Nanocapsules	Emulsification/ nanoprecipitation.	PCL	Miconazole nitrate	108 nm, PDI 0.33	Abdel-Rashid et al. (2022)
Nanoparticles	Nanoprecipitation with dropping.	PLA	Ketoconazole	188 nm, PDI 0.075	Endo et al. (2020)
Nanosponges	Emulsion solvent diffusion	Ethylcellulose and PVA	Luliconazole	300 nm, PDI 0.386	Kapileshwari et al. (2020)
Nanoparticles	Solvent evaporation	Ethylcellulose	Itraconazole	219 nm, PDI 0.109	Ho et al. (2020)
Nanoparticles	Spray drying	Chitosan	Voriconazole	210 nm	Shah et al. (2022)
Nanoparticles	Quasi emulsion solvent diffusion.	PLGA and Eudragit® RS100	Nystatin	128 nm	Mohammadi et al. (2017)

*As described by authors; PVA: polyvinyl alcohol.

Terbinafine hydrochloride is considered one of the most efficient drugs for skin mycoses, and local application is preferred due to protein binding and low bioavailability after oral use (Pervaiz et al., 2021). Terbinafine was incorporated into chitosan and xanthan gum nanoparticles, aiming to increase the retention time of the drug in the target site. By means of skin permeation through rat skin, a higher drug retention was observed, and by means of an *in vivo* antifungal evaluation (rats), a rapid and complete removal of the fungal burden was observed for the nanoparticle incorporated into Carbopol® gel, when compared to the control gel and marketed cream (Pervaiz et al., 2021). Another allylamine, butenafine hydrochloride, was loaded into PLGA nanoparticles and incorporated into a chitosan gel. The proposed nanoformulation increased drug skin permeation/skin retention, evaluated by an egg membrane, as well as increased antifungal efficacy after 48 h (zone of inhibition), due to several factors such as controlled release, nanoparticles size, improved solubility, and chitosan properties (Alshehri & Imam, 2021). The association of terbinafine with other antifungal agents (amorolfine and econazole) in polymeric micelles has been described, being called by the authors as a tri-therapy. Similar or higher skin deposition (porcine and human skin) was observed for the drugs, when compared to marketed formulations presenting 10 times higher dosage. Also, a deposition of the antifungal substances in pilosebaceous unit was noticed, which could improve the therapeutic effect (Gou et al., 2022).

Econazole, clotrimazole, miconazole, and ketoconazole are widely used azoles for skin fungal infections, being considered broad-spectrum substances. However, their incorporation into polymeric nanoparticles can increase their cutaneous bioavailability. The incorporation of econazole (Bachhav et al., 2011) and clotrimazole (Kareem et al., 2019) into polymeric micelles was proposed. It was observed that the skin deposition of econazole was improved 13-fold (porcine skin) or 7.5-fold (human skin) when applying the micelles, compared to a marketed liposomal formulation. The difference observed among skin membranes is due to a larger contribution of the follicular penetration pathway for porcine skin (Bachhav et al., 2011). Clotrimazole micelles increased antifungal activity of the drug against *Microsporumcanis*. when compared to the drug solution (agar tube dilution method). The authors hypothesize that the improvement in drug availability, drug stability, drug distribution homogeneity, and drug penetration into the fungus membrane, releasing drug content inside the fungal cell, were responsible for the increase in activity (Kareem et al., 2019). PLA nanoparticles containing ketoconazole (with encapsulation efficiency of 45%) increased ketoconazole activity against all tested fungi strains (*Candida* spp. and dermatophytes) compared to unencapsulated drug, with reductions from 2- to 8-fold in MIC values (microdilution technique). The nanoparticles' small size, sustained drug release, and improved solubility are likely reasons for improved drug efficacy (Endo et al., 2020). PCL nanocapsules containing miconazole nitrate showed slow biphasic release, high encapsulation efficiency, and improved stability. The formulation increased *in vitro* skin permeation (rat skin) and activity (zone of inhibition) against *C. albicans*, compared to the drug suspension. When compared to lipid nanocapsules, PCL nanocapsules, besides increasing antifungal efficacy, increased drug retention in the skin. The polymeric particles are probably capable of creating a reservoir on the skin, prolonging cutaneous residence time of the drug (Abdel-Rashid et al., 2022).

A novel topical antifungal drug, luliconazole, was also incorporated into nanosponges, which was further incorporated into a Carbopol® gel. Enhanced skin permeation rate and skin retention (rat skin) was observed for the novel nanocarriers compared to pure drug gel. Also, a greater activity against *C. albicans* (zone of inhibition) was described (Kapileshwari et al., 2020).

Itraconazole and voriconazole are not commonly used by the cutaneous route, therefore, the nanoparticles were applied as a way to enable topical application of the drugs. Ethylcellulose nanoparticles incorporating itraconazole were produced aiming for higher permeation through the skin. The nanoparticles were incorporated into a Carbopol® gel, and a sustained permeation (rat skin) of the drug was observed for over 24 h, besides a higher drug permeation and retention when compared to the gel containing itraconazole-saturated suspension. The developed nanoparticle gel exhibited better antifungal activity against *C. albicans* and *A. niger in vitro* (Ho et al., 2020). Voriconazole, a wide spectrum agent against several fungi species, including resistant strains, was incorporated into chitosan nanoparticles. It was observed that the nanoparticles were able to slowly transport voriconazole through rat's skin and that the skin permeation improvement is dependent on the nanoparticle's components. Also, the antifungal effect was improved (zone of inhibition) probably due to chitosan presence (Shah et al., 2022).

Two polymers (PLGA and Eudragit RS100) were used together in order to encapsulate the drug nystatin, a drug applied in skin infections. The formulation was developed as a strategy to overcome resistance against fungal infections. The antifungal efficacy (*C. albicans*, MIC values) of the nanoparticles were increased when compared to pure nystatin, especially with lower PLGA concentration, and the improvement in the activity could be attributed to the modified surface characteristics (positive zeta potential) (Mohammadi et al., 2017).

The majority of articles observed increased skin deposition and increased efficacy when incorporating antifungal drugs into polymeric nanoparticles. However, it is important to notice that due to the facility of testing antifungal activity *in vitro*, this technique was preferred by the authors. Caution should be taken when translating such *in vitro* results to an improved therapy *in vivo*.

9.8 SKIN CANCER

Skin cancer can be classified as – (i) nonmelanoma, which includes basal cell carcinoma (BCC), the most common type of skin cancer, and squamous cell carcinoma (SCC); and (ii) melanoma. Nonmelanoma cancer is limited to the epidermis, whereas melanoma can spread to the dermis and frequently metastasizes.

Two FDA-approved topical treatments are available for the treatment of superficial BCC. Efudex® cream 5% contains the antimetabolite drug 5-fluorouracil, and Aldara® cream contains 5% IMQ, an immune response modifier agent. Even though there are no FDA-approved topical treatments for melanoma, due to limited skin penetration, the efficacy of topical 5-fluorouracil and IMQ has been investigated for this ending (Burns & Brown, 2005; Florin et al., 2012). However, severe side effects, such as burning sensation, erythema, erosion, and dermatitis, are associated with these therapies (Bahner & Bordeaux, 2013).

Polymeric nanoparticles have been used for the topical delivery of synthetic and natural compounds for skin cancer treatment (Table 9.6). Such a strategy can improve the active ingredient penetration into the skin, therefore reaching the cancerous cells; and decrease the occurrence of side effects that might be involved. Polymeric nanocapsules, nanospheres, and polymeric micelles are the most described nanocarriers for the topical treatment of skin cancer, and some interesting findings are discussed in Table 9.6.

IMQ-loaded polymeric nanocapsules containing Eudragit® L100 as polymer and 0.25 mg/ml of drug were produced aiming to improve IMQ penetration into the skin and reduce its side effects (Dias et al., 2018). Higher retention in the dermis (*in vivo*, mice) was reported for nanoencapsulated IMQ. Even though a low dose of drug was used, nanoencapsulation promoted a decrease in papilloma multiplicity and size distribution compared to the non-encapsulated drug (*in vivo*, mice). Considering that nanoencapsulated IMQ could reach the dermis, it could be a potential treatment for melanoma.

TABLE 9.6 Polymeric Nanoparticles for Skin Cancer Treatment

Nanoparticle Type*	Method of Nanoparticle Production	Polymer	Drug	Particle Size and PDI	References
Nanoparticles	Nanoprecipitation of preformed polymer.	Eudragit® L100	Imiquimod	249 nm, PDI 0.123	Dias et al. (2018)
Nanocapsules	Interfacial deposition of preformed polymer.	PCL	Imiquimod	213 nm, PDI 0.12	Gazzi et al. (2020)
Nanocapsules	Interfacial condensation.	Poly(N-vinylpyrrolidone-*alt*-itaconic anhydride) copolymer.	5-fluorouracil	133 nm, PDI 0.33	Rata et al. (2021)
Nanocapsules	Interfacial deposition of preformed polymer.	PCL	Diphenyl diselenide	280 nm, PDI 0.282	Ferreira et al. (2020)
Nanocapsules	Interfacial deposition of preformed polymer.	PCL	Phloretin	252 nm, SPAN 1.68	Casarini et al. (2021)
Nanoparticles	Emulsion–diffusion–evaporation	PLGA	Alpha-mangostin	168.06 nm, PDI 0.201	Md et al. (2021)
Nanoparticles	Ionotropic gelation	Chitosan	Aminolevulinic acid derivatives (5-ALA, 8-ALA).	5-ALA 573 nm, PDI 0.37. 652 nm, PDI 0.32	Ferreira et al. (2013)
Micelles	Solvent evaporation	Methoxy-poly(ethylene glycol)-di-hexyl substituted-poly(lactic acid) copolymer.	Vismodegib	20–30 nm, PDI 0.175–0.33	Kandekar et al. (2019)
Micelles	Solvent evaporation	Methoxy poly(ethylene glycol)-poly(ethylene imine) polymer.	Paclitaxel	221.7 nm, PDI 0.252	Xu et al. (2020)
Micelles	Direct dissolution	D-alpha-tocopheryl polyethylene glycol 1000 succinate	Imiquimod	15.31 nm, PDI 0.57	Ghezzi et al. (2021)
Dendrimers	Dendrimers and ASO incubation in HEPES buffer (pH 7.4).	PAMAM	Human Bcl-2 ASO	84 nm, PDI 0.2	Venuganti et al. (2015)

*As described by authors; PAMAM: poly(amidoamine).

NC with higher IMQ concentration (0.5 mg/ml) were also reported (Gazzi et al., 2020). PCL was used as the polymeric wall and copaiba oil was used as the lipid core. This formulation was tested in SK-MEL-28 cell line (melanoma) and it was reported a 44% reduction in the cell viability after 72 hours of treatment in comparison to a 9% reduction after treatment with non-encapsulated IMQ. The *in vitro* skin permeation (porcine ear skin) of encapsulated IMQ was evaluated after incorporation of the nanocapsules in a pectin hydrogel, and high retention in the dermis was achieved.

Improvement of IMQ skin permeation was also investigated using polymeric micelles. Ghezzi and co-workers (2020) prepared micelles using d-alpha-tocopheryl polyethylene glycol 1000 succinate, a biodegradable amphiphilic polymer. The co-encapsulation of oleic acid improved IMQ loading into the nanocarrier, and stability studies showed that this formulation had stable size, pH, and drug concentration for six months. Skin permeation (porcine ear skin) was evaluated in comparison to the commercial cream. An improvement on the drug delivery efficiency by the micellar formulation was observed since similar drug retention in the epidermis and dermis was reported using a 40-fold lower drug concentration.

Aptamer-functionalized nanoparticles loaded with 5-fluorouracil were evaluated on a human BCC cell line (TE 354.T) (Rata et al., 2021). Higher percentages of preapoptotic, apoptotic, and death cells were reported after 48-hour treatment with the nanocarriers. Besides, the encapsulation of 5-fluorouracil was able to reduce the irritant effect of the drug on the skin, and also to improve skin permeation (*in vitro*, chicken skin and *in vivo*, mice). By producing fluorescein-marked nanocapsules, it was possible to observe their uptake by Langerhans cells in the epidermis and epithelial sheath of dermal hair follicles (*in vivo*, mice).

Besides IMQ and 5-fluorouracil, other drugs have been incorporated into polymeric nanocarriers (Baig et al., 2018; Keservani et al., 2019) and evaluated as potential new therapies for skin cancer (Jarouliya et al., 2018), such as diphenyl diselenide (Ferreira et al., 2020), vismodegib (Kandekar et al., 2019), paclitaxel (Xu et al., 2020) and aminolevulinic acid derivatives (Ferreira et al., 2013). Diphenyl diselenide is an organoselenium compound which presents antitumor activity, but toxicity is a limitation for its broader use. Ferreira and co-workers (2020) encapsulated this drug into PCL nanocapsules, and reported selective cytotoxicity against melanoma cells and higher antitumoral effect in comparison to the non-encapsulated compound. Nanoencapsulation could improve dermal delivery *in vitro* (human skin), however, the compound was retained mainly in the SC.

Vismodegib is an orally administered drug approved by the FDA for the treatment of BCC. However, such therapy is not selective for cancerous cells and is associated with severe systemic side effects (Kandekar et al., 2019). A topical formulation containing vismodegib-loaded polymeric micelles was proposed (Kandekar et al., 2019). The drug penetration in human skin was evaluated *in vitro* and supra-therapeutic amounts of drug were retained in the basal epidermis and deeper tissue. The antitumor activity of this formulation, however, was not yet evaluated. Polymeric micelles were also proposed for topical melanoma therapy with paclitaxel (Xu et al., 2020). The antitumor potential was evaluated *in vitro* (B16 melanoma cells) and *in vivo* (mice) in comparison to Taxol® (intravenous paclitaxel-loaded liposomes). *In vitro*, the polymeric micelles presented higher cytotoxicity; and *in vivo*, the best results were achieved by combining intravenous (Taxol®) and topical (paclitaxel micelles) treatments. For the skin permeation studies, coumarin-6 was used in the nanoparticles. Fluorescence intensity in the skin was higher when polymeric micelles were applied, especially after 12 hours, showing that this formulation improves skin penetration of the drug.

The use of natural compounds, such as phloretin (Casarini et al., 2021) and alpha-mangostin (Md et al., 2021), for topical skin cancer treatment may provide advantages over synthetic molecules, once they are, usually, less toxic and induce minor side effects. The flavonoid phloretin had its activity against melanoma evaluated after incorporation in PCL nanocapsules with copaiba oil core (Casarini et al., 2021). Nanoencapsulation did not improve the cytotoxicity on melanoma cells (SK-MEL-28) over an 8-hour period. However, after a 72-hour treatment, cells treated with the nanocapsules suspension presented lower proliferation rate and higher percentage of senescent cells. Skin permeation (porcine ear skin) was evaluated after incorporation of the nanocapsules in Lecigel®. Such semisolid formulation improved drug retention in the SC and in the epidermis, in comparison to the non-encapsulated phloretin.

Md and co-workers (2021) developed nanoparticles encapsulating alpha-mangostin, and an improvement in antitumor activity (melanoma cells, B16-F10) was observed specially after 48-hour treatment (18.5% of viable cells *versus* 80.87% for the unencapsulated compound group). *In vitro* skin permeation (rat skin) showed higher drug retention in the epidermis (6-fold higher) and dermis (10-fold higher) for the nanoencapsulated compound, compared to the non-encapsulated compound.

In a different approach, Venuganti (2015) combined antisense-oligonucleotide (ASO)-dendrimers nanocomplex and iontophoresis for the treatment of carcinoma. Iontophoresis technique was able to improve the epidermal delivery (pig ear skin) of the nanocomplex. The dendrimers, nanosized globular molecules with a well-defined unique 3D architecture, could efficiently protect ASO and improve its cellular uptake. This innovative topical treatment was evaluated *in vivo* in a skin cancer mouse model, and gene silencing and reduction in tumor volume were observed.

Other techniques, such as photodynamic therapy (PDT), can be associated with drug therapies in order to obtain a more efficient drug response (Ferreira et al., 2013; Da Silva et al., 2013). PDT uses a photosensitizer (e.g., 5-aminolevulinic acid (ALA)) and light to induce cell death, thus it can be applied for skin cancer treatment. Ferreira and co-workers (2013) reported improved skin penetration of aminolevulinic acid derivatives after incorporation into chitosan nanoparticles. Photocytotoxicity assay (treatment + light irradiation) in melanoma cells (B16-F10) showed that the nanoencapsulated aminolevulinic acid derivatives were more cytotoxic than the non-encapsulated pro-drug.

9.9 CONCLUDING REMARKS

Skin diseases caused by hyperpigmentation, inflammatory conditions or pathogens impose significant challenges and are emerging targets. Currently, a variety of drugs have been incorporated into polymeric nanoparticles and applied in the topical treatment of these skin disorders. The nanoencapsulation has the possibility to improve the therapeutic effect, due to an increase in skin penetration, and a decrease in adverse effects, among other advantages (Figure 9.2). In the last years, polymeric nanoparticles intended for cutaneous delivery, such as nanospheres, nanocapsules, lipid-core nanocapsules, polymeric micelles, tyrospheres, nanosponges, and dendrimers were developed with unique physicochemical properties such as selective targeting, controlled release and protection of encapsulated agents. Those properties seem to be mainly dependent on the chemical composition of ingredients, on the encapsulation mechanism, which, by consequence, influences the drug release mechanism, on the size of nanoparticles, on the surface charge, and on the viscosity of final formulations. Several challenges remain regarding the development and use of polymeric nanocapsules for skin diseases, such as the use of eco-friendly processes, avoiding or reducing organic solvents; the increase in production scale, since several methods are difficult to be applied to large volume batches; the increase in drug loading, which is usually limited; the increase in stability, since many formulations are obtained as liquid suspensions; and the need for more tests related to nanoparticles toxicity potential as well as clinical trials. Despite that, several authors have proven the great applicability of the polymeric nanoparticles for improving the treatment of acne, skin whitening, AD, psoriasis, mycoses, and skin cancer.

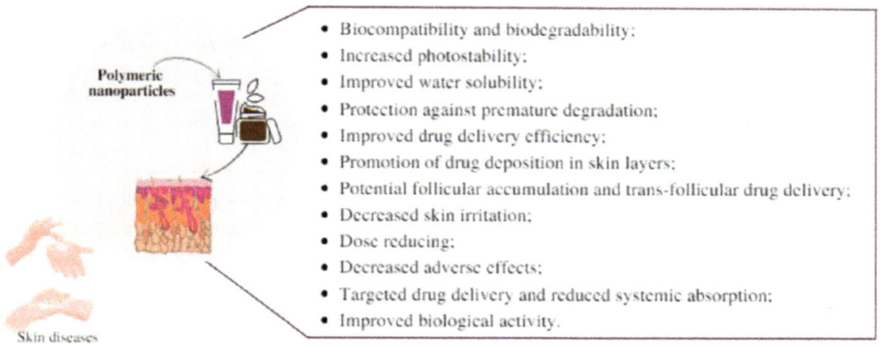

FIGURE 9.2 Main advantages observed with polymeric nanoparticles applied to skin diseases.

KEYWORDS

- **acne**
- **atopic dermatitis**
- **psoriasis**
- **rosacea**
- **skin cancer**
- **skin mycoses**

REFERENCES

Abdel-Rashid, R. S., Doaa, A. H., Alaa-Eldin, A. A., & Abdel-Monem, R., (2022). Polymeric versus lipid nanocapsules for miconazole nitrate enhanced topical delivery: *In vitro* and *ex vivo* evaluation. *Drug Delivery, 29*(1), 294–304. https://doi.org/10.1080/10717544.2022.2026535.

Akiu, S., Suzuki, Y., Asahara, T., Fujinuma, Y., & Fukuda, M., (1991). Inhibitory effect of arbutin on melanogenesis--biochemical study using cultured B16 melanoma cells. *Nihon Hifuka Gakkai Zasshi; The Japanese Journal of Dermatology, 101*(6), 609–613.

Alshehri, S., & Syed, S. I., (2021). Formulation and evaluation of butenafine loaded PLGA-nanoparticulate laden chitosan nano gel. *Drug Delivery, 28*(1), 2348–2360. https://doi.org/10.1080/10717544.2021.1995078.

Alvarez-Figueroa, M. J., (2001). Transdermal delivery of methotrexate: Iontophoretic delivery from hydrogels and passive delivery from microemulsions. *International Journal of Pharmaceutics, 215*, 57–65.

Asad, M. I., Khan, D., Rehman, A. U., Elaissari, A., & Ahmed, N., (2021). Development and *in vitro_in vivo* evaluation of PH-sensitive polymeric nanoparticles loaded hydrogel for the management of psoriasis. *Nanomaterials, 11*(12), 3433.

Assem, M., Omneya, M. K., & Dalia, G., (2019). Optimization and evaluation of beclomethasone dipropionate micelles incorporated into biocompatible hydrogel using a sub-chronic dermatitis animal model. *AAPS PharmSciTech, 20*(4). https://doi.org/10.1208/s12249-019-1355-6.

Ayumi, N. S., Shariza, S., Zahid, H., Mumtaz, H., & Nor, H. A. S., (2019). Polymeric nanoparticles for topical delivery of alpha and beta arbutin: Preparation and characterization. *Drug Delivery and Translational Research, 9*(2), 482–496. https://doi.org/10.1007/s13346-018-0508-6.

Bachhav, Y. G., Mondon, K., Kalia, Y. N., Gurny, R., & Möller, M., (2011). Novel micelle formulations to increase cutaneous bioavailability of azole antifungals. *Journal of Controlled Release, 153*(2), 126–132. https://doi.org/10.1016/j.jconrel.2011.03.003.

Badihi, A., Frušić-Zlotkin, M., Yoram, S., Sandrine, B., Tomer, T., Taher, N., & Simon, B., (2020). Topical nano-encapsulated cyclosporine formulation for atopic dermatitis treatment: Topical cyclosporine NCs for AD. *Nanomedicine: Nanotechnology, Biology, and Medicine, 24*. https://doi.org/10.1016/j.nano.2019.102140.

Bahner, J. D., & Jeremy, S. B., (2013). Non-melanoma skin cancers: Photodynamic therapy, cryotherapy, 5-fluorouracil, imiquimod, diclofenac, or what? Facts and controversies. *Clinics in Dermatology, 31*(6), 792–798. https://doi.org/10.1016/j.clindermatol.2013.08.020.

Baig, M. S., Keservani, R. K., Ahmad, M. F., & Baig, M. E., (2018). Smart delivery of nanobiomaterials in drug delivery. In: *Nanobiomaterials* (pp. 241–287). Apple Academic Press. ISBN: 9781771885911.

Bangia, R., Gajanand, S., Sunil, D., & Om Prakash, K., (2019). Nanotechnological interventions in dermatophytosis: From oral to topical, a fresh perspective. *Expert Opinion on Drug Delivery, 16*(4), 377–396. https://doi.org/10.1080/17425247.2019.1593962.

Bennet, D., & Sanghyo, K., (2014). Polymer nanoparticles for smart drug delivery. In: Ali, D. S., (ed.), *Application of Nanotechnology in Drug Delivery.*.Rijeka: IntechOpen. https://doi.org/10.5772/58422.

Bodeker, G., Terence, J. R., Adva, V., Jahnavi, H., & Gemma, B., (2017). Integrative skin care: Dermatology and traditional and complementary medicine. *Journal of Alternative and Complementary Medicine (New York, N.Y.) 23*(6), 479–486. https://doi.org/10.1089/acm.2016.0405.

Boo, Y. C., (2021). Arbutin as a skin depigmenting agent with anti-melanogenic and antioxidant properties. *Antioxidants, 10*(7), 1129. https://doi.org/10.3390/antiox10071129.

Breathnach, A. S., (1996). Melanin hyperpigmentation of skin: Melasma, topical treatment with azelaic acid, and other therapies. *Cutis, 57*(1 Suppl), 36–45.

Brian, E. K., Larisa, S., Zheng, Z., Marissa, L., Joachim, K., & Michniak-Kohn, B. B., (2012). Development of paclitaxel-tyrospheres for topical skin treatment. *J. Control Release, 163*(1), 18–24. https://doi.org/10.1016/j.jconrel.2012.06.021.Development.

Burns, C. A., & Marc, D. B., (2005). Imiquimod for the treatment of skin cancer. *Dermatologic Clinics, 23*(1), 151–64, vii. https://doi.org/10.1016/j.det.2004.08.007.

Campos, E. V. R., Patricia, L. F. P., Tais, G. D. C., Renata De, L., Sarah, H., Leonardo, F. F., & Daniele R. De. A., (2021). Hydrogels containing budesonide-loaded nanoparticles to facilitate percutaneous absorption for atopic dermatitis treatment applications. *ACS Applied Polymer Materials, 3*(9), 4436–4449. https://doi.org/10.1021/acsapm.1c00021.

Carbone, C., Martins-Gomes, C., Pepe, V., Silva, A. M., Musumeci, T., Puglisi, G., Furneri, P. M., & Souto, E. B., (2018). Repurposing itraconazole to the benefit of skin cancer treatment: A combined Azole-DDAB nanoencapsulation strategy. *Colloids and Surfaces. B, Biointerfaces, 167*, 337–344. https://doi.org/10.1016/j.colsurfb.2018.04.031.

Casarini, T. P. A., Luiza, A. F., Tainara, B., Giovana, O., Adriana, R. P., & Silvia, S. G., (2021). Innovative hydrogel containing polymeric nanocapsules loaded with phloretin: Enhanced SKIN penetration and adhesion. *Materials Science and Engineering C, 120*. https://doi.org/10.1016/j.msec.2020.111681.

Contri, R. V., Luiza, A. F., Moacir, K., Adriana, R. P., & Silvia, S. G., (2014). The use of nanoencapsulation to decrease human skin irritation caused by capsaicinoids. *International Journal of Nanomedicine, 9*, 951–962. https://doi.org/10.2147/IJN.S56579.

Dias, M. F., Bruna, C. P. De. F., Teixeira-Neto, J., Maria, C. A. G., Silvia, L. F., & Armando, S. C., (2018). *In vivo* evaluation of antitumoral and antiangiogenic effect of imiquimod-loaded polymeric nanoparticles. *Biomedicine and Pharmacotherapy, 103*, 1107–1114. https://doi.org/10.1016/j.biopha.2018.04.079.

Domínguez-Delgado, C. L., Rodríguez-Cruz, I. M., Escobar-Chávez, J. J., Calderón-Lojero, I. O., Quintanar-Guerrero, D., & Adriana, G., (2011). Preparation and characterization of triclosan nanoparticles intended to be used for the treatment of acne. *European Journal of Pharmaceutics and Biopharmaceutics, 79*(1), 102–107. https://doi.org/10.1016/j.ejpb.2011.01.017.

Dréno, B., (2017). What is new in the pathophysiology of acne, an overview. *Journal of the European Academy of Dermatology and Venereology*. Blackwell Publishing Ltd. https://doi.org/10.1111/jdv.14374.

Endo, E. H., Makimori, R. Y., Companhoni, M. V. P., Ueda-Nakamura, T., Nakamura, C. V., & Dias, F. B. P., (2020). Ketoconazole-loaded poly-(lactic acid) nanoparticles: Characterization and improvement of antifungal efficacy *in vitro* against candida and dermatophytes. *Journal de Mycologie Medicale, 30*(3), 101003. https://doi.org/10.1016/j.mycmed.2020.101003.

Fereig, S. A., El-zaafarany, G. M., Mona, G. A., & Mona, M. A. Abdel-Mottaleb., (2021). Tacrolimus-loaded chitosan nanoparticles for enhanced skin deposition and management of plaque psoriasis. *Carbohydrate Polymers Journal, 268*.

Ferreira, L. M., Marcel, H. M. S., Juliana, H. A., Elita, F. D. S., Verônica, F. C., Marila, C. L. M., Maria-Engler, S. S., et al., (2020). Xanthan gum-based hydrogel containing nanocapsules for cutaneous diphenyl diselenide delivery in melanoma therapy. *Investigational New Drugs, 38*(3), 662–674. https://doi.org/10.1007/s10637-019-00823-2.

Ferreira, M., Luísa, B., Marcela, A. S., Tiago, T., Manuela, S., Sofia, A. C. L., & Salette, R., (2017). Topical co-delivery of methotrexate and etanercept using lipid nanoparticles: A targeted approach for psoriasis management. *Colloids and Surfaces B: Biointerfaces, 159*, 23–29. https://doi.org/10.1016/j.colsurfb.2017.07.080.

Ferreira-Nunes, R., Cunha-Filho, M., Gratieri, T., & Guilherme, M. G., (2021). Follicular-targeted delivery of spironolactone provided by polymeric nanoparticles. *Colloids and Surfaces B: Biointerfaces, 208*. https://doi.org/10.1016/j.colsurfb.2021.112101.

Florin, V., Eve, D., Vercambre-Darras, S., & Laurent, M., (2012). Topical treatment of cutaneous metastases of malignant melanoma using combined imiquimod and 5-fluorouracil. *Investigational New Drugs, 30*(4), 1641–1645. https://doi.org/10.1007/s10637-011-9717-2.

Foldvari, M., (2000). Non-invasive administration of drugs through the skin: Challenges in delivery system design. *Pharmaceutical Science & Technology Today, 3*(12), 417–425. https://doi.org/10.1016/s1461-5347(00)00317-5.

Gabriel, D., Thibault, M., Herve, C., Niki, K., Maria, C. D., & Michael, M., (2016). Improved topical delivery of tacrolimus: A novel composite hydrogel formulation for the treatment of psoriasis. *Journal of Controlled Release*. https://doi.org/10.1016/j.jconrel.2016.09.007.

Gagliardi, A., Elena, G., Eeda, V., Massimo, F., Stefania, B., Vibhudutta, A., & Donato, C., (2021). Biodegradable polymeric nanoparticles for drug delivery to solid tumors. *Frontiers in Pharmacology, 12*, 1–24. https://doi.org/10.3389/fphar.2021.601626.

Garg, A., Ganti, S. S., Amit, K. G., Goutam, G., Sudam, C. S., & Goutam, R., (2020). Recent advances in topical carriers of anti-fungal agents. *Heliyon, 6*(8), e04663. https://doi.org/10.1016/j.heliyon.2020.e04663.

Gazzi, R. P., Frank, L. A., Onzi, G., Pohlmann, A. R., & Silvia, S. G., (2020). New pectin-based hydrogel containing imiquimod-loaded polymeric nanocapsules for melanoma treatment. *Drug Delivery and Translational Research, 10*(6), 1829–1840. https://doi.org/10.1007/s13346-020-00805-5.

Ghezzi, M., Pescina, S.,Padula, C., Santi, P., Del Favero, E., Cantù, L., & Nicoli, S., (2021). Polymeric micelles in drug delivery: An insight of the techniques for their characterization and assessment in biorelevant conditions. *Journal of Controlled Release: Official Journal of the Controlled Release Society, 332*, 312–336. https://doi.org/10.1016/j.jconrel.2021.02.031.

Gou, S., Michel, M., Denis, S., & Yogeshvar, N. K., (2022). Simultaneous delivery of econazole, terbinafine and amorolfine with improved cutaneous bioavailability: A novel micelle-based antifungal 'tri-therapy.' *Pharmaceutics, 14*(2). https://doi.org/10.3390/pharmaceutics14020271.

Guterres, S. S., Marta, P. A., & Adriana, R. P., (2007). Polymeric nanoparticles, nanospheres and nanocapsules, for cutaneous applications. *Drug Target Insights, 2*, 147–157.

Hatem, S., Nada, M. El. H., Reham, S. E., Maha, N., Amany, O. K., & Seham, A. E., (2020). Background and different treatment modalities for melasma: Conventional and nanotechnology-based approaches. *Journal of Drug Delivery Science and Technology, 60*, 101984. https://doi.org/10.1016/j.jddst.2020.101984.

Hatem, S., Seham, A. E., Amany, O. K., Maha, N., Noha, H. M., Maha, H. R., Reham, S. E., & Nada, M. El. H., (2022). Functionalized chitosan nanoparticles for cutaneous delivery of a skin whitening agent: An approach to clinically augment the therapeutic efficacy for melasma treatment. *Drug Delivery, 29*(1), 1212–1231. https://doi.org/10.1080/10717544.2022.2058652.

Ho, H. N., Thien, G. L., Thi Thanh, T. D., Thi, H. L., Thi Thanh, H. D., Dang, H. N., Trinh, C. T., & Chien, N. N., (2020). Development of itraconazole-loaded polymeric nanoparticle dermal gel for enhanced antifungal efficacy. *Journal of Nanomaterials.* https://doi.org/10.1155/2020/8894541.

Hussain, Z., Haliza, K., Mohd, C. I. M. A., Endang, K., & Shariza, S., (2014). Downregulation of immunological mediators in 2,4-dinitrofluorobenzene-induced atopic dermatitis-like skin lesions by hydrocortisoneloaded chitosan nanoparticles. *International Journal of Nanomedicine, 9*(1), 5143–5156. https://doi.org/10.2147/IJN.S71543.

Hussain, Z., Haliza, K., Mohd, C. I. M. A., Endang, K., & Shariza, S., (2013). Antidermatitic perspective of hydrocortisone as chitosan nanocarriers: An *ex vivo* and *in vivo* assessment using an NC/Nga mouse model. *Journal of Pharmaceutical Sciences, 102*(3), 1063–1075. https://doi.org/10.1002/jps.23446.

Hussain, Z., Haliza, K., Mohd, C., Iqbal, M., & Endang, K., (2014). *Efficient Immuno-Modulation of T_{H1} / T_{H2} Biomarkers in 2, 4-Dinitrofluorobenzene-Induced Atopic Dermatitis: Nanocarrier-Mediated Transcutaneous Co-Delivery of Anti-Inflammatory and Antioxidant Drugs, 9*(11). https://doi.org/10.1371/journal.pone.0113143.

Jain, S., Ankit, M., & Amit, K. J., (2011). Enhanced topical delivery of cyclosporin-a using PLGA nanoparticles as carrier. *Current Nanoscience, 7*(4), 524–530. https://doi.org/10.2174/157341311796196835.

Jarouliya, U., Kesharwani, R. K., & Kesharwani, R. K., (2018). Advances of nanotechnology in cancer therapy. In: *Nanobiomaterials* (pp. 291–328). Apple Academic Press. ISBN: 9781771885911.

Kahraman, E., Gül, Ö., Yıldız, Ö., & Sevgi, G., (2016). Polymeric micellar nanocarriers of benzoyl peroxide as potential follicular targeting approach for acne treatment. *Colloids and Surfaces B: Biointerfaces, 146*, 692–699. https://doi.org/10.1016/j.colsurfb.2016.07.029.

Kandekar, S. G., Mayank, S., Kiran, B. S., & Yogeshvar, N. K., (2019). Polymeric micelle nanocarriers for targeted epidermal delivery of the hedgehog pathway inhibitor vismodegib: Formulation development and cutaneous biodistribution in human skin. *Expert Opinion on Drug Delivery, 16*(6), 667–674. https://doi.org/10.1080/17425247.2019.1609449.

Kapileshwari, G. R., Apoorva, R. B., Lalit, K., Prashant, J. B., Madhusudan, J., & Rupesh, K. S., (2020). Novel drug delivery system of luliconazole – formulation and characterization. *Journal of Drug Delivery Science and Technology, 55*, 101302. https://doi.org/10.1016/j.jddst.2019.101302.

Kareem, F., Adnan, M. B., Muhammad, I., Muhammad, R. S., Khalid, M. K., & Muhammad, I. M., (2019). Enhanced therapeutic efficacy of clotrimazole by delivery through poly(ethylene oxide)-block-poly(ε-caprolactone) copolymer-based micelles. *Journal of Applied Polymer Science, 136*(28), 1–9. https://doi.org/10.1002/app.47769.

Keservani, R. K., Bandopadhyay, S., Bandyopadhyay, N., & Sharma, A. K., (2020a). Design and fabrication of transdermal/skin drug-delivery system. In: *Drug Delivery Systems* (pp. 131–178). Academic Press.

Keservani, R. K., Kesharwani, R. K., & Sharma, A. K., (2017a). Introduction to nanotechnology in drug delivery. In: *Drug Delivery Approaches and Nanosystems* (pp. 1–19). Apple Academic Press. ISBN: 9781771885836.

Keservani, R. K., Sharma, A. K., & Kesharwani, R. K., (2018). Nanoparticulate nanocarriers in drug delivery. In: *Nanobiomaterials* (pp. 3–22). Apple Academic Press. ISBN: 9781771885911.

Keservani, R. K., Sharma, A. K., & Kesharwani, R. K., (2019). *Nanocarriers for Brain Targeting: Principles and Applications.* CRC Press. ISBN:9781771887304.

Kooyers, T. J., & W, W., (2004). Toxicological aspects and health risks associated with hydroquinone in skin bleaching formula. *Nederlands Tijdschrift Voor Geneeskunde, 148*(16), 768–771.

Kumar, A., & Rekha, R., (2021). Enhancing efficacy and safety of azelaic acid via encapsulation in cyclodextrin nanosponges: Development, characterization and evaluation. *Polymer Bulletin, 78*(9), 5275–5302. https://doi.org/10.1007/s00289-020-03366-2.

Lapteva, M., Michael, M., Robert, G., & Yogeshvar, N. K., (2015). Self-assembled polymeric nanocarriers for the targeted delivery of retinoic acid to the hair follicle. *Nanoscale, 7*(44), 18651–18662. https://doi.org/10.1039/c5nr04770f.

Lee, C. S., Won-Hee, J., Miyoung, P., Kyoungmi, J., Heung, S. B., Yung, H. J., Young-Ho, P., & Kyung-Min, L., (2013). A novel adamantyl benzylbenzamide derivative, AP736, suppresses melanogenesis through the inhibition of CAMP-PKA-CREB-activated microphthalmia-associated transcription factor and tyrosinase expression. *Experimental Dermatology, 22*(11), 762–764. https://doi.org/10.1111/exd.12248.

Leelapornpisid, P., Phuriwat, L., Surapol, N., & Porjai, R., (2010). Application of chitosan for preparation of arbutin nanoparticles as skin whitening characterization of the mucilages extracted from hibiscus rosa-sinensis linn and hibiscus mutabilis linn and their skin moisturizing effect original article view project OXPIRT: Ontology-based expert system for production of a generic immediate release tablet view project application of chitosan for preparation of arbutin nanoparticles as skin whitening. *Journal of Metals, Materials and Minerals*, 20. https://www.researchgate.net/publication/267255182.

Luiza, R. De. S., A., Charlene, P. K., Fernanda, K. D. S., Gabriela, M. Da. L., Hilris, R. E. S., Marlus, C., & Maria, P. D. G., (2012). Nanotechnology-based drug delivery systems for dermatomycosis treatment. *Current Nanoscience, 8*(4), 512–519. https://doi.org/10.2174/157341312801784311.

M. Ferreira, D., Saga, Y. Y., Sarduy, E., & Tedesco, A. C., (2013). Chitosan nanoparticles for melanoma cancer treatment by photodynamic therapy and electrochemotherapy using aminolevulinic acid derivatives. *Current Medicinal Chemistry, 20*(14), 1904–1911. https://doi.org/10.2174/092986731132014000.

Ma, Y., Xiaowen, W., & Ruoyu, L., (2021). Cutaneous and subcutaneous fungal infections: Recent developments on host–fungus interactions. *Current Opinion in Microbiology, 62*, 93–102. https://doi.org/10.1016/j.mib.2021.05.005.

Mao, Kai-Li., Zi-liang, F., Jian-dong, Y., Pian-pian, C., Jing-jing, Y., & Jie, X., (2017). Colloids and surfaces B: Biointerfaces skin-penetrating polymeric nanoparticles incorporated in silk fibroin hydrogel for topical delivery of curcumin to improve its therapeutic effect on psoriasis mouse model. *Colloids and Surfaces B: Biointerfaces, 160*, 704–714. https://doi.org/10.1016/j.colsurfb.2017.10.029.

Marchiori, M. C. L., Ourique, A. F., De B. Da. Silva, C., Raffin, R. P., Pohlmann, A. R., Guterres, S. S., & Beck, R. C. R., (2012). Spray-dried powders containing tretinoin-loaded engineered lipid-core nanocapsules: Development and photostability study. *Journal of Nanoscience and Nanotechnology, 12*(3), 2059–2067. https://doi.org/10.1166/jnn.2012.5192.

Maria, L., Michael, M., Robert, G., & Yogeshvar, N. K., (2015). Self-assembled polymeric nanocarriers for the targeted delivery of retinoic acid to the hair follicle. *Royal Society of Chemistry, 7*.

Marin, E., Maria, I. B., & Catherina, C., (2013). Critical evaluation of biodegradable polymers used in nanodrugs. *International Journal of Nanomedicine, 8*, 3071–3091.

Mayba, J. N., & Melinda, J. G., (2016). *Review of Atopic Dermatitis and Topical Therapies*. https://doi.org/10.1177/1203475416685077.

McMurtry, C. M., Rebecca, P. R., Anna, T., Nicole, R., Gordon, J. G. A., Melanie, N., Christine, T. C., & Vibhuti, S., (2015). Far from 'just a poke': Common painful needle procedures and the development of needle fear. *Clinical Journal of Pain, 31*(10), S3–11. https://doi.org/10.1097/AJP.0000000000000272.

Md, S., Nabil, A. A., Thikryat, N., Samah, A., Md Ali, M., Yassine, R., Ammu, K. R., Habibullah, K., Manish, G., & Md Habban, A., (2021). Development, characterization, and evaluation of α-mangostin-loaded polymeric nanoparticle gel for topical therapy in skin cancer. *Gels (Basel, Switzerland), 7*(4). https://doi.org/10.3390/gels7040230.

Mohammadi, G., Elham, N., Ali, M., Pardis, M., & Khosro, A., (2017). Preparation, physicochemical characterization and anti-fungal evaluation of the nystatin-loaded Eudragit RS100/PLGA nanoparticles. *Journal of Drug Delivery Science and Technology, 38*, 90–96. https://doi.org/10.1016/j.jddst.2017.02.004.

Ourique, A. F., Pohlmann, A. R., Guterres, S. S., & Beck, R. C. R., (2008). Tretinoin-loaded nanocapsules: Preparation, physicochemical, characterization, and photostability study. *International Journal of Pharmaceutics, 352*(1, 2), 1–4. https://doi.org/10.1016/j.ijpharm.2007.12.035.

Ourique, Melero, Silva, Schaefer, Pohlmann, Guterres, Lehr, Kostka, & Beck. (2011). Improved photostability and reduced skin permeation of tretinoin: Development of a semisolid nanomedicine. *European Journal of Pharmaceutics and Biopharmaceutics, 79*(1), 95–101. https://doi.org/10.1016/j.ejpb.2011.03.008.

Pandey, M., Hira, C., Tarakini, A. P. G., Saranyah, S. N., Shadab, M., Bapi, G., Minaketan, T., & Zahid, H., (2019). Hyaluronic acid-modified betamethasone encapsulated polymeric nanoparticles: Fabrication, Characterization, *in vitro* release kinetics, and dermal targeting. *Drug Delivery and Translational Research, 9*(2), 520–533. https://doi.org/10.1007/s13346-018-0480-1.

Panonnummal, R., & Sabitha, M., (2018). Anti-psoriatic and toxicity evaluation of methotrexate loaded chitin nanogel in imiquimod induced mice model. *International Journal of Biological Macromolecules, 110*, 245–258. https://doi.org/10.1016/j.ijbiomac.2017.10.112.

Parekh, K., Tejal, A. M., Namdev, D., Pavan, K., & Amirali, P., (2021). Emerging nanomedicines for the treatment of atopic dermatitis. *AAPS PharmSciTech*. Springer Science and Business Media Deutschland GmbH. https://doi.org/10.1208/s12249-021-01920-3.

Patel, R., & Priyanka, P., (2020). Nanocarriers as versatile delivery systems for effective management of acne. *International Journal of Pharmaceutics*. Elsevier B.V. https://doi.org/10.1016/j.ijpharm.2020.119140.

Paudel, K. S., Mikolaj, M., Courtney, L. S., Nicole, K. B., Priyanka, G., & Audra, L. S., (2010). Challenges and opportunities in dermal/transdermal delivery. *Therapeutic Delivery, 1*(1), 109–131. https://doi.org/10.4155/tde.10.16.

Pereira, R. L., Fernanda, I. L., Karina, P., Rafaela, M. S., Cecília, B. M., Silvia, S. G., & Elfrides, E. S. S., (2016). Hydrogel containing adapalene- and dapsone-loaded lipid-core nanocapsules for cutaneous application: Development, characterization, *in vitro* irritation, and permeation studies. *Drug Development and Industrial Pharmacy, 42*(12), 2001–2008. https://doi.org/10.1080/03639045.2016.1188110.

Pervaiz, F., Rabia, M., & Sobia, N., (2021). Formulation and optimization of terbinafine HCl loaded chitosan/xanthan gum nanoparticles containing gel: Ex-vivo permeation and *in-vivo* antifungal studies. *Journal of Drug Delivery Science and Technology, 66*, 102935. https://doi.org/10.1016/j.jddst.2021.102935.

Pillaiyar, T., Manoj, M., & Vigneshwaran, N., (2017). Skin whitening agents: Medicinal chemistry perspective of tyrosinase inhibitors. *Journal of Enzyme Inhibition and Medicinal Chemistry, 32*(1), 403–425. https://doi.org/10.1080/14756366.2016.1256882.

Prajapati, R., Jayvadan, P., & Anita, P., (2021). *Nanoparticles Containing Gel Formulation for the Treatment of Psoriasis, 11*(1), 76–81. https://doi.org/10.5530/ijpi.2021.1.14.

Prajapati, R., Se Eun, P., Hee, J. P., Hyun, A. J., & Jae, S. C., (2021). Identification of a potent and selective human monoamine oxidase – a inhibitor, glycitein, an iso flavone isolated from I flowers. *ACS Food Science & Technology, 4*, 538–550. https://doi.org/10.1021/acsfoodscitech.0c00152.

Rainer, B. M., Thompson, K. G., Antonescu, C., Florea, L., Mongodin, E. F., Bui, J., Fischer, A. H., et al., (2020). Characterization and analysis of the skin microbiota in rosacea: A case–control study. *American Journal of Clinical Dermatology, 21*, 139–147.

Ramezanli, T., & Michniak-Kohn, B. B., (2018). Development and characterization of a topical gel formulation of adapalene-tyrospheres and its clinical efficacy assessment development and characterization of a topical gel formulation of adapalene- tyrospheres and its clinical efficacy assessment Ernest. *Molecular Pharmaceutics*. https://doi.org/10.1021/acs.molpharmaceut.8b00318.

Ramezanli, T., Zheng, Z., & Michniak-Kohn, B. B., (2017). □□□□□□□□Development and characterization of polymeric nanoparticle-based formulation of adapalene for topical acne therapy□□□□□□□□□□□□□□□□□□□□□□□□□□□□□□□□□□□□□. *Nanomedicine: Nanotechnology, Biology, and Medicine, 13*(1), 143–152. https://doi.org/10.1016/j.nano.2016.08.008.

Rata, D. M., Anca, N. C., Leonard, I. A., Marcel, P., Cosmin, T. M., Carmen, S., Lacramioara, O., & Gabriela, V., (2021). Topical formulations containing aptamer-functionalized nanocapsules loaded with 5-fluorouracil – an innovative concept for the skin cancer therapy. *Materials Science and Engineering C, 119*(11), 111591. https://doi.org/10.1016/j.msec.2020.111591.

Rodríguez-Cruz, I. M., Virginia, M., Matilde, M., Octavio, D., Amparo, N., & Quintanar-Guerrero, D., (2013). Polymeric nanospheres as strategy to increase the amount of triclosan retained in the skin: Passive diffusion vs. iontophoresis. *Journal of Microencapsulation, 30*(1), 72–80. https://doi.org/10.3109/02652048.2012.700956.

Rosado, C., Catarina, S., & Catarina, P. R., (2013). Hydrocortisone-loaded poly(ε-caprolactone) nanoparticles for atopic dermatitis treatment. *Pharmaceutical Development and Technology, 18*(3), 710–718. https://doi.org/10.3109/10837450.2012.712537.

Saeed, E., Reza, M., Rasool, H., & Seyed, Y. V., (2021). Design and optimization of cationica nanocapsules for topical delivery of tretinoin: Application of the box-Behnken design, *in vitro* evaluation, and *ex vivo* skin deposition study. *Biomed Research International*, 13.

Schaffazick, S. R., Liane De, L. F., Adriana, R. P., & Silvia, S. G., (2003). Caracterização e estabilidade físico-química de sistemas poliméricos nanoparticulados para administração de fármacos. *Química Nova, 26*(5), 726–737.

Scholz, C. F. P., & Mogens, K., (2016). The natural history of cutaneous propionibacteria, and reclassification of selected species within the genus *Propionibacterium* to the proposed novel genera *Acidipropionibacterium* GEN. Nov., *Cutibacterium* gen. Nov. and *Pseudopropionibacterium* gen. Nov. *International Journal of Systematic and Evolutionary Microbiology, 66*(11), 4422–4432. https://doi.org/10.1099/ijsem.0.001367.

Shah, M. K. A., Abul, K. A., Asif, N., Shafi, U., Muhammad, S. L., Habibur, R., Khalaf, F. A., et al., (2022). Formulation development, characterization, and antifungal evaluation of chitosan NPs for topical delivery of voriconazole *in vitro* and *ex vivo*. *Polymers, 14*(1), 1–17. https://doi.org/10.3390/polym14010135.

Shin, H. J., Heung, S. B., Soo, I. K., Yung, H. J., & Joonho, C., (2018). Development and evaluation of topical formulations for a novel skin whitening agent (AP736) using Hansen solubility parameters and PEG-PCL polymers. *International Journal of Pharmaceutics, 552*(1, 2), 251–257. https://doi.org/10.1016/j.ijpharm.2018.09.064.

Siddique, M. I., Haliza, K., Muhammad, S., Tahir, A. C., Adawiyah, J., & Mohd, C. I. M. A., (2021). Clinical insights into topically applied multipronged nanoparticles in subjects with atopic dermatitis. *Journal of Drug Delivery Science and Technology, 65*. https://doi.org/10.1016/j.jddst.2021.102744.

Silva, C. L. D., Jose, O. D. C., Fabia, C. R., Maria, V. L. B. B., & Maria, B. R. P., (2013). PLGA Nanoparticles as delivery systems for protoporphyrin ix in topical Pdt: Cutaneous penetration of photosensitizer observed by fluorescence microscopy. *Journal of Nanoscience and Nanotechnology, 13*(10), 6533–6540. https://doi.org/10.1166/jnn.2013.7789.

Suhair, S., Mohammad, N., Al-Natour, M. A., Malak, J., & Abu-Qatouseh, L., (2022). Loading of coal tar in polymeric nanoparticles as a potential therapeutic modality for psoriasis. *ACS Omega, 7*, 7333–7340.

Sun, L., Zeyu, L., Lun, W., Dongmei, C., & Henry, H. Y. T., (2017). Enhanced topical penetration, system exposure and anti-psoriasis activity of two particle-sized, curcumin-loaded PLGA nanoparticles in hydrogel. *Journal of Cellualar Physiology*, (28), 44–54. https://doi.org/10.1016/j.jconrel.2017.03.385.

Tan, J., Almeida, L. M., Bewley, A., Cribier, B., Dlova, N. C., Gallo, R., Kautz, G., et al., (2017). Updating the diagnosis, classification and assessment of rosacea_ recommendations from the global rosacea consensus (ROSCO) panel _ enhanced reader.pdf. *British Journal of Dermatology, 176*, 283–284.

Tangsumranjit, A., Pellequer, Y., Lboutounne, H., Guillaume, Y. C., Lamprecht, A., & Millet, J., (2006). Enhanced ascorbyl palmitate stability by polymeric nanoparticles. *Journal of Drug Delivery Science and Technology, 16*(2), 161–163. https://doi.org/https://doi.org/10.1016/S1773-2247(06)50025-5.

Thiboutot, D., Rox, A., Cook-Bolden, F., Zoe, D., Richard, L. G., Richard, D. G., Sewon, K., Marian, M., Linda, S. G., & Jerry, T., (2020). Standard management options for rosacea: The 2019 update by the national rosacea society expert committee. *Journal of American Dermatology, 82*(6), 1501–1510. https://doi.org/10.1016/j.jaad.2020.01.077.

Tolentino, S., Maira, N. P., Cunha-Filho, M., Tais, G., & Guilherme, M. G., (2021). Targeted clindamycin delivery to pilosebaceous units by chitosan or hyaluronic acid nanoparticles for improved topical treatment of acne vulgaris. *Carbohydrate Polymers, 253*. https://doi.org/10.1016/j.carbpol.2020.117295.

Tran, T. Q. M., Ming Fa, H., Keng, L. C., Quoc, H. P., Van, C. N., Ching Yi, C., & Chun, M. H., (2016). Bactericidal effect of lauric acid-loaded PCL-PEG-PCL nano-sized micelles on skin commensal *Propionibacterium acnes*. *Polymers, 8*(9). https://doi.org/10.3390/polym8090321.

Try, C., Brice, M., Arnaud, B., Oscar, F., Didier, P., Yann, P., & Alf, L., (2016). Size dependent skin penetration of nanoparticles in murine and porcine dermatitis models. *European Journal of Pharmaceutics and Biopharmaceutics, 100*, 101–108. https://doi.org/10.1016/j.ejpb.2016.01.002.

Venturini, C. G., Franciele, A. B., Renata, V. C., Francisco, N. F., Luiza, A. F., Camilo, M. D., Renata, P. R., et al., (2015). Co-encapsulation of imiquimod and copaiba oil in novel nanostructured systems: Promising formulations against skin carcinoma. *European Journal of Pharmaceutical Sciences, 79*, 36–43. https://doi.org/10.1016/j.ejps.2015.08.016.

Venuganti, V. V. K., Manju, S., Chandradhar, D., Radhey, S. K., & Omathanu, P. P., (2015). Topical gene silencing by iontophoretic delivery of an antisense oligonucleotide-dendrimer nanocomplex: The proof of concept in a skin cancer mouse model. *Nanoscale, 7*(9), 3903–3914. https://doi.org/10.1039/c4nr05241b.

Verhoeven, E. W. M., Floor, W. K., Chris, V. W., Peter, C. M. V. De. K., Piet, D., Pieter, G. M. V. D. V., Henk, J. M. V. D. H., et al., (2008). Skin diseases in family medicine: Prevalence and health care use. *Annals of Family Medicine, 6*(4), 349–354. https://doi.org/10.1370/afm.861.

Wang, Y., Zhang, H., Fang, R., Tang, K., & Sun, Q., (2020). The top 100 most cited articles in rosacea: A bibliometric analysis. *European Academy of Dermatology and Venereology*, 2177–2182. https://doi.org/10.1111/jdv.16305.

Weber, D. M., Guilherme, T. V., Renata, L. De. O., Caren, A. R. Da. F., Jaini, P., Rodrigues, K. C., Francine, R. I., et al., (2018). Topic application of meloxicam-loaded polymeric nanocapsules as a technological alternative for treatment of the atopic dermatitis in mice. *Journal of Applied Biomedicine, 16*(4), 337–343. https://doi.org/10.1016/j.jab.2018.03.003.

Xu, H., Yi, W., Shiyu, C., Li, Z., Runliang, F., & Zhimei, S., (2020). Paclitaxel skin delivery by micelles-embedded Carbopol 940 hydrogel for local therapy of melanoma. *International Journal of Pharmaceutics, 587*, 119626. https://doi.org/10.1016/j.ijpharm.2020.119626.

Yu, K., Yixuan, W., Tao, W., Yuanhao, Z., Sisi, C., Wenyi, R., Chuanbin, W., & Yuehong, X., (2018). Tacrolimus nanoparticles based on chitosan combined with nicotinamide: Enhancing percutaneous delivery and treatment efficacy for atopic dermatitis and reducing dose. *International Journal of Nanomedicine, 13*, 129–142. https://doi.org/10.2147/IJN.S150319.

Zhai, J., Jianjun, G., Jin, Y., & Jiaqi, C., (2011). Tacrolimus in the treatment of ocular diseases. *BioDrugs: Clinical Immunotherapeutics, Biopharmaceuticals and Gene Therapy, 25*(2), 89–103. https://doi.org/10.2165/11587010-000000000-00000.

Zhang, Z., Pei-Chin, T., Tannaz, R., & Michniak-Kohn, B. B., (2013). Polymeric nanoparticles-based topical delivery systems for the treatment of dermatological diseases. *Wiley Interdisciplinary Reviews. Nanomedicine and Nanobiotechnology, 5*(3), 205–218. https://doi.org/10.1002/wnan.1211.

CHAPTER 10

Herbal Extracts Loaded-Nanocarriers to Skin Disease Treatment

RUTH MERI LUCINDA-SILVA, ANGELA MALHEIROS, ANNA CAROLINA FURAER DA ROCHA, DÓRYS ANGELA CORDENUNZZI, JENNY SUMARA SOZO, and OTTO MAURÍCIO SANTOS GERLACH

Graduate Program in Pharmaceutical Sciences, University of Vale do Itajaí, Itajaí, Santa Catarina, Brazil

ABSTRACT

Medicinal plants are considered a repository of numerous types of bioactive compounds that have various therapeutic properties. In recent decades, many scientific studies have directed the search for medicinal plants as a source of drugs for diseases with the greatest impact on society today, such as cancer, viral infection, multidrug-resistant microbial infections, diabetes, obesity, and cardiovascular disorders. The complex mixture of molecules present in herbal extracts difficult the improve their biopharmaceutical properties. Nanostructured drug delivery systems (DDSs) are platforms capable of carrying molecules with limited biological responses mainly due to low solubility and skin permeability. New systems have been developed as strategies for herbal medicines with improved physicochemical, pharmacokinetic, and pharmacodynamic properties. The recent development of nanometric platforms for the topical administration of promising plant extracts and phytochemicals, along with their therapeutic applications supported by experimental evidence is presented.

Novel Nanocarriers forSkin Diseases: Advances and Applications.
Raj K. Keservani and Júlia Scherer Santos (Eds.)

10.1 INTRODUCTION

Medicinal plants have been used by man since the beginning of history and long before the emergence of writing, humanity already used herbs for medicinal purposes (Barata, 2005; Toscano Rico, 2011; Mandal et al., 2015). Currently, medicinal plants are used by a large part of the world population, as an alternative medicinal resource for various disease treatments. Consequently, after several studies, several natural products isolated from higher plants became drugs (Newman & Cragg, 2020). The medicinal value of plants has been well documented in several traditional medicine systems such as Chinese Medicine and Ayurveda and is recognized by the World Health Organization (WHO). Medicinal properties of herbal derivatives offer the benefit of developing formulations that are non-toxic, non-irritating, and biocompatible.

Medicinal plants are thought to have a wide variety of bioactive chemicals with a range of therapeutic applications in the treatment of different diseases such as cancer, viral infections, multidrug-resistant microbial infections, diabetes, obesity, and cardiovascular problems (Caesar & Cech, 2019). The medicinal properties of natural product extracts have made them promising active ingredients in formulations for skin diseases. A wide range of therapeutic effects has been found in medicinal plants such as anti-inflammatory, antiviral, antitumor, antimalarial, and analgesic (Raina et al., 2014; Zhang et al., 2020).

The therapeutic response of herbal extracts is usually dependent on a complex mixture of bioactive compounds with action potentiated by synergistic effects with each other. However, this complex mixture of compounds causes challenges for formulations. The low solubility of phytoconstituents often influences bioavailability, requiring specific transport methods to improve some characteristics and performance. Among the challenges in the topical administration of herbal extracts (Sharma et al., 2020; Rane et al., 2020, 2020a, c) are low solubility (water/lipid), low cutaneous permeation, lack of targeting specificity, chemical instability, and short half-life, requiring repeated administration or higher dose, making these products weak drug candidates. To overcome this limitation, new therapeutic systems containing natural product derivatives have been developed (Ansari et al., 2012; Namdar et al., 2017).

In this context, the development of herbal medicines has used innovative technologies to enhance the therapeutic activity and safety of natural product derivatives. Several herbal extracts have been studied as a source of new drugs and incorporated into nanotechnology platforms to increase their therapeutic potential (Bidone, 2015; Chaiittianan & Sripanidlulchai, 2014).

Nanotechnology performs an important role in the development of formulations (Jarouliya et al., 2018; Baig et al., 2018). Nanostructured delivery systems have numerous advantages for drug delivery (Keservani et al., 2016, 2017), including the ability to protect active molecules against degradation in a physiological environment, drug-controlled release at the site of action, in addition, to allow the administration of hydrophobic drugs in aqueous dispersed systems. Drug biopharmaceutical properties of substances are significantly improved with the use of nanostructured carriers, leading to important changes in the pharmacokinetic processes of absorption, distribution, metabolism, and elimination, also allowing the reduction of the dose and their adverse effects (Pandey, 2021).

Although these systems have been developed for pure drugs, some nanostructured systems allow the incorporation of crude herbal extracts with high efficiencies, such as nanoemulsions, polymeric micro- and nanoparticles, solid lipid nanoparticles (SLNs), phytosomes, self-emulsifying drug delivery system (DDS), among others. This chapter will discuss the main carrier systems for herbal extracts and phytoconstituents and their respective applications in the treatment of skin diseases.

10.2 LIPID NANOPARTICLES

Lipid nanoparticles are highly promising DDSs for dermal treatments because combine several advantages, such as high load capacity, modified release, and targeted drug delivery. SLNs were described in the 1990s and since then have been widely used in skin delivery systems. Originally, they were developed as alternative nanocarriers for microemulsions, liposomes (Keservani & Gautam, 2020), and polymeric nanoparticles. They are safe, biocompatible, and biodegradable nanocarriers (Keservani et al., 2018; Silva et al., 2015; Wissing et al., 2001).

Lipid nanoparticles have been successfully used as drug carriers for the treatment of various skin diseases such as psoriasis, fungal, and atopic dermatitis (AD). The use of these nanotechnological systems improves drug performance and reduces the potential for adverse effects or skin irritation (Jyothi et al., 2022).

Based on their composition and structure, lipid nanoparticles are classified into SLNs and nanostructured lipid carriers (NLCs) (Figure 10.1). While SLN is made up of solid lipids, NLC is made up of a mixture of solid and liquid lipids (Müller et al., 2011).

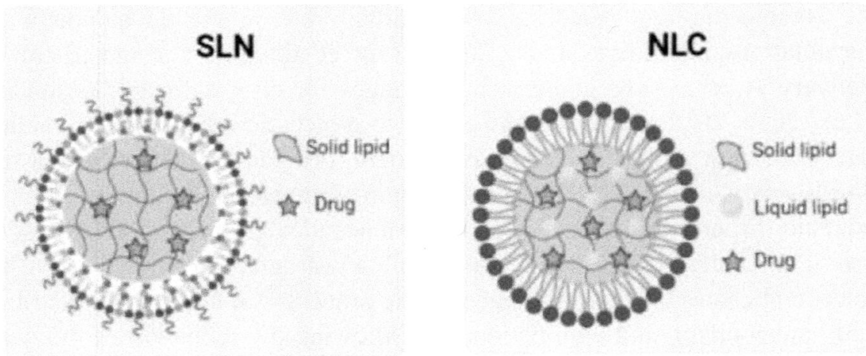

FIGURE 10.1 Structure of solid lipid nanoparticles (SLN) and nanostructured lipid carriers (NLC).

SLNs are carriers composed of biocompatible solid lipids and drugs, dispersed in a surfactant-stabilized matrix. These systems present properties such as biodegradability, low toxicity, protection of the drug against degradation, high load capacity, and scalability. The high permeation of drugs incorporated into SLNs is due to the interaction between the system and SC lipids (Pham et al., 2019). Although SLNs have high physical stability, crystalline reorganization of the lipid matrix can expel encapsulated drugs during storage (Zhang et al., 2016).

To overcome the SLN limitations, the second generation of lipid nanoparticles was developed. The NLCs are composed of a mixture of solid and liquid lipids, generally in a ratio of 7:3 to 9:1. The mixing of two distinct lipid types promotes a more disordered lipid matrix, which results in stable drug entrapment. The optimized composition of the matrix results in a higher drug loading capacity, better stability, and the ability to act at lower temperatures (Waghule et al., 2020).

After topical administration of lipid nanoparticles, a uniform film is formed on the SC. The high adherence and occlusion properties, and small size results in the lipid film, which guarantees greater oil/water partition coefficient and permeation of the drugs. This structure can also reduce water loss, increase hydration, and restore the skin's physical barrier. Lipid nanoparticles interact with sebum and specific skin lipids, causing a change in the natural arrangement of corneocytes. Thus, the encapsulated molecules are released, and their penetration into the epidermis and dermis is potentiated. The active delivery mechanism shows that the smaller particle size results in better skin penetration due to the greater occlusion and greater interaction of the nanoparticle with the skin (Zhai & Zhai, 2014).

A wide range of materials and processes can be used to obtain lipid nanocarriers (Keservani et al., 2019). Development and excipients must be closely correlated to the intended use. Likewise, the method of preparation is extremely important to maintain stability characteristics during the period of storage and administration. In the case of essential oils, methods that can avoid the loss of volatile compounds and degradation must also be taken into account. Examples of solid and liquid lipids and surfactants are shown in Table 10.1. The classic ingredients for the production of SLN include lipids such as triglycerides, fatty acids, steroids, and waxes, with the characteristic of remaining solid at room and body temperature. To provide stability of the lipid dispersion, water, and emulsifiers are used (Mehnert & Mäder, 2001; Assali & Zaid, 2022).

The most used methods in the production of lipid nanoparticles are high-pressure homogenization, high-shear homogenization, ultrasound, microemulsion (Behera et al., 2010), and solvent diffusion. Production methods for SLN and NLC are identical, only the matrix-forming excipients are different. The characterization of nanocarriers is important to ensure that the particles have an adequate sizer, homogeneous distribution, high encapsulation efficiency, zeta potential, and crystalline structure (Waghule et al., 2020; Assali & Zaid, 2022).

The use of lipid nanoparticles to carry actives of natural origin for topical administration is a very interesting strategy. These carriers can be used for both hydrophobic and hydrophilic drug encapsulation. Table 10.1 presents examples of herbal extracts and phytoconstituents incorporated into lipid nanoparticles.

Centella asiatica is an example of the extract incorporated into lipid nanoparticles. NLCs were able to increase the extract permeation to the epidermis and dermis, with a positive effect on the treatment of scleroderma (Rocha et al., 2019). Lipid nanoparticles containing the combination of two extracts, *Smilax china* and *Salix alba*, show promising results in the treatment of psoriasis. The NLCs showed small particle size, high encapsulation efficiency, sustained release, and increased dermal permeation (Qadir et al., 2020). With a topical anti-inflammatory effect, willow bark (*Salix alba*) extract was associated with the synthetic anti-inflammatory indomethacin in SLN, resulting in the gradual release of loaded drugs, an increase of antioxidant activity (oxygen-free radical scavenging exceeds 90%), and an increase of ability to reduce levels of inflammatory markers. This strategy can reduce the adverse effects of synthetic drugs in skin disease treatment related to inflammatory processes (Lacatusu et al., 2019).

TABLE 10.1 Herbal Extracts, Essential Oils, and Isolated Phytoconstituents Loaded in Lipid Nanoparticles

Herbal Material	System	Lipid	Surfactant	Method	Application	References
Centelha asiatica Dry and glycolic extract	NLC	Stearic acid Oleic acid	Lecithin Sodium taurodeoxycholate	Microemulsion	Scleroderma	Rocha et al. (2019)
Smilax china *Salix alba*	NLC	Glycerol monostearate. Acconon C6 (7:3)	Disodium lauryl sulfate Polyethylene glycol-400	Melt emulsification/ ultra-sonication	Psoriasis	Qadir et al. (2020)
Salix alba Willow bark extract	SLN	Glycerol monostearate Cetyl palmitate	Tween 20 and Poloxamer 188 Phosphatidylcholine	High-pressure homogenization	Anti-inflammatory Antioxidant	Lacatusu et al. (2019)
Punica granatum extract	SLN	Stearic acid	Tween 80 Lecithin	Hot homogenization/ ultra-sonication	Anticancer	Teaima et al. (2022)
Ridolfia segetum Essential oil	NLC	Precirol® ATO 5	Tween 80 Polyethylene glycol 400	Hot high-pressure homogenization.	Not reported	Miranda et al. (2019)
Rosmarinus officinalis Essential oil	NLC	Miglyol® and Precirol®	Poloxamer	Hot homogenization	Antibacterial Wound healing	Khezri et al. (2019)
Chamomile oil	SLN	Stearic acid	Tween 80	Hot homogenization	Wound healing	Gad et al. (2019)
Capsaicin	NLC	Compritol® 888 ATO Oleic acid	Phosphatidylcholine Poloxamer 188	Solvent diffusion	Psoriasis	Agrawal et al. (2015)
Sesamol	SLN	Glyceryl monostearate Cetyl alcohol	Phosphatidylcholine Sodium deoxycholate or Tween® 80	Microemulsion	Anticancer	Geetha et al. (2015)
Lycopene	NLC	Carnauba wax Oil palm	Tween® 80	Microemulsion	Not reported	Sharma et al. (2021)
Linalol	SLN	Myristyl myristate cetyl esters and cetyl palmitate.	Poloxamer 188	Sonication	Antiproliferative/ anticancer	Rodenak-Kladniewa et al. (2017)
Caffeine	SLN	Softisan® 100	Poloxamer 188	High-speed homogenization	Anticancer	Puglia et al. (2016)

The activity against Ehrlich ascites carcinoma of pomegranate extract-loaded SLN incorporated in transdermal emulgel was performed. *Ex vivo* permeation kinetic data showed non-Fickian diffusion transport. Histopathological investigation of treated mice showed that the application of the emulgel formulation containing the extract-loaded SLNs showed statistically significant anticancer effects against this specific type of carcinoma (Teaima et al., 2022).

Isolated compounds of natural products, many of them with hydrophobic characteristics, have been successfully transported in lipid nanoparticles for topical use. Caffeine is a naturally occurring alkaloid that has potential anti-cancer effects after oral and topical administration. Permeation properties of the caffeine-loaded SLN were studied and presented significantly higher permeation when compared to the control, overcoming the limitations of the molecule hydrophobicity (Puglia et al., 2016).

Capsaicin has also been studied in SLN and NLC carriers to assess topical delivery in psoriasis treatment. The amount of drug retained in the skin was higher for the NLC-type systems. Both carriers showed minimal or no skin irritation and had a good ability to increase capsaicin in the skin layers, being effective for the psoriasis treatment (Agrawal et al., 2015). Sesamol has an important apoptotic activity for melanoma treatments, but it has limited cutaneous bioavailability. Topical application of sesamol-loaded SLN showed greater retention and permeation in the skin, having an effect on cell normalization after melanoma induction (Geetha et al., 2015). Linanol is a monoterpene found in essential oils that has also been evaluated against melanoma. When carried in SLN, it showed controlled release with antiproliferative effects using *in vitro* model (Rodenak et al., 2017). Other studies of herbal derivatives topical application include alpha-pinene and citral-loaded NLC with anti-inflammatory and anti-cancer activity (Zielinska et al., 2018, 2019, 2020), limonene-loaded SLN as a potential anticancer drug (Souto et al., 2020), SLN and NLC containing resveratrol as an antioxidant (Gokce et al., 2012), and thymol-loaded NLC for psoriasis and inflammatory process (Pivetta et al., 2018).

Many studies have investigated the efficient use of lipid nanocarriers for successful intracellular delivery and protection of essential oils as therapeutic molecules for skin disorders. Miranda et al. (2019) incorporated *Ridolfia segetum* essential oil into the NLC, demonstrating that the essential oil can act both as a nanostructuring agent and as an active ingredient in formulations. Rosemary essential oil was carried in NLC to evaluate the antibacterial activity *in vitro* and the healing process of infected wounds *in vivo*, demonstrating that it has antibacterial properties and accelerates the healing of infected wounds (Khezri et al., 2019). Chamomile oil also has an important wound-healing effect; however, it has a low permeation potential. Thus, it was incorporated into SLN aiming to improve the healing effect. The results demonstrated that encapsulation improved the restoration of normal integument architecture, and promoted wound contraction, β1 growth factor transformation, and collagen deposition (Gad et al., 2019).

Studies show that lipid nanoparticles allow controlled permeation and release of herbal extracts and phytoconstituents, in safety systems for dermatological use. However, the efficiency of the medicine will depend on the selection of the appropriate lipid for each active ingredient, as well as the surfactants and production method, to maintain the therapeutic characteristics of the phytoconstituents.

10.3 NANOEMULSION

Nanoemulsions are stable colloidal dispersions with an average droplet size of 20–200 nm, formed by two immiscible liquids that are mixed using suitable surfactants to form a single phase (Bashir et al., 2021; Soliman et al., 2021; Sungpud et al., 2020). These systems have wide applicability in food, cosmetics, and medicines. The droplet sizes of nanoemulsions give characteristics of transparency or translucency to the naked eye, presenting a translucent appearance when the globule size is less than 200 nm or milky when the size is between 200 and 500 nm (Figure 10.2).

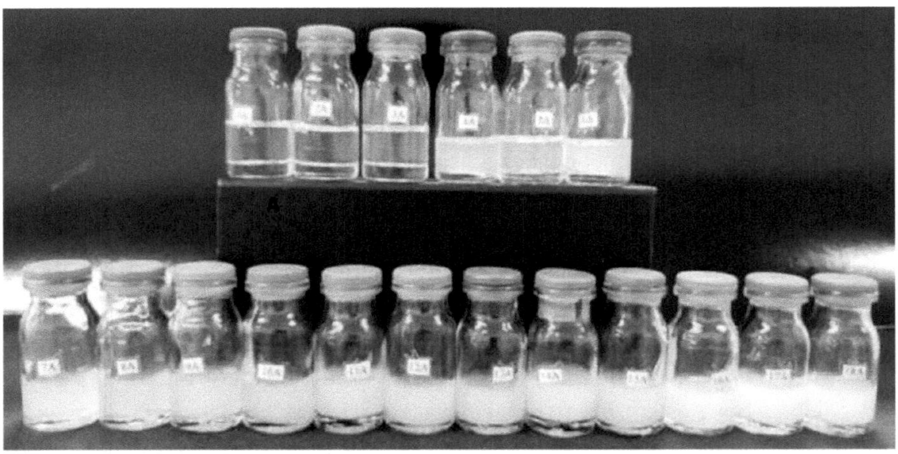

FIGURE 10.2 Visual aspect of nano-emulsified systems with different surfactant systems and internal phase size. (A) milky aspect with a size between 200 and 500 nm; and (B) translucent aspect with a size smaller than 200 nm.

Source: Authorized for publication by Rocha (2022).

When compared to conventional emulsions, nanoemulsions can improve topical and transdermal administration (Keservani et al., 2020a; Sharma et al., 2018), increasing the dissolution capacity of lipophilic compounds and promoting cutaneous absorption (Lewinska et al., 2020). Nanoemulsions are systems capable of increasing and controlling drug penetration through the skin. Main advantages of nanoemulsions as a vehicle for topical application are presented below (Cápek, 2004; Shah et al., 2010; Tadros et al., 2004; Chen & Inbaraj, 2019):

- The low interfacial tension promotes greater spreadability of the formulation and facilitates the penetration of globules through the roughness of the skin, allowing greater skin hydration and drug penetration.
- The fluidity of the system and the small size of the globules provide an even distribution of the product on the skin.
- The natural fluidity of the system (at low concentrations of the oil phase) gives a highly valued sensory aspect to products for topical application.
- Nanoemulsions can be alternatives to liposomes (which have low stability), and it is possible in some cases to obtain liquid-crystalline structures around the globules.
- They can be sterilized by filtration without changing their properties.
- The small size of the droplets reduces the action of the gravitational force and consequently, the Brownian motion. When the influence of the gravitational force is overcome, the flocculation process does not occur and the system remains dispersed, with no creaming or sedimentation processes occurring.

Low interfacial tension these systems, normally less than 1.0×10^{-6} N/m, are capable of dissolving and compartmentalizing numerous drugs (Rai et al., 2018; Wu et al., 2013). Such systems have peculiar physicochemical properties and are different from the dispersing medium, improving the solubility and increasing the drug absorption potential (Burger et al., 2017; Christofori et al., 2017). Generally, the high initial release is attributed to the fraction of the drug that is adsorbed or weakly bound on the immense interface area of the nanostructures. The most frequent nanoemulsion formulations are of the oil-in-water type, which is composed of the oil phase, surfactant, co-surfactant, and aqueous phase, with the lipophilic phase being dispersed in the form of colloidal droplets in the aqueous vehicle (Rai et al., 2018).

Nanoemulsions do not suffer conventional destabilization effects as a result of the force of gravity, such as creaming or sedimentation, due to their Brownian motion. Although the nanoemulsions are thermodynamically unstable, they have kinetic stability, visual transparency, and small droplet size (Rai et al., 2018). Such characteristics make nanoemulsions a system of practical interest. For the formation of nanoemulsions, the concentration of surfactants used is about 3 to 10%, while microemulsions require at least 20% of surfactants. Although emulsification in nanoemulsions is not a spontaneous process, its preparation can be performed using low or high energy depending on the excipients used and the stability of the drug to be incorporated (Christofori et al., 2017).

Several studies have shown increased skin permeation of hydrophilic and lipophilic drugs incorporated into nanoemulsions when compared to conventional emulsions. The development of new nanoemulsion systems for the release of natural compounds present in herbal extracts or fractions has increased in the last few years (Chen & Inbaraj, 2019).

The depigmenting action of nanoemulsions containing 0.02% (w/w) of *Artocarpus incises* extract was evaluated in an *in vivo* model. The dorsal area was irradiated with UVB light to cause cutaneous hyperpigmentation (melasma). After six weeks of topical treatment with the extract-loaded nanoemulsion or with the aqueous solution of free extract, the treatment using nanoemulsion resulted in a greater depigmenting action (Buranajaree et al., 2011).

Nanoemulsions containing 0.05% (w/w) of *Phyllanthus urinaria* dry extract were prepared by the self-emulsification method for application as antioxidant and anti-aging skin (Mahdi et al., 2011). Chaiittianan & Sripanidkulchai (2014) developed nanoemulsions by high-pressure homogenization containing 0.15% (w/w) of hydroalcoholic extract from the *Phyllanthus emblica* bark. The extract presents phenolic compounds including gallic acid, vanillic acid, and epicatechins, among others.

Nanoemulsions containing *Tagetes erecta* flower extract were obtained by the phase inversion method and evaluated for their regenerative potential for the skin. Nanoemulsions were incorporated into a gel base (Leelapornpisid et al., 2014). Comparing the gel containing the nano-emulsified extract with the gel containing the free extract, the authors reported greater *in vitro* antioxidant activity and better cutaneous retention of the major compound, quercetagetin, in the different skin layers for the gel containing the nanoemulsions. Furthermore, studies in volunteers showed an improvement in skin hydration and reduction of wrinkles after eight weeks of treatment with the gel containing the *T. erecta* extract-loaded nanoemulsion.

Achyrocline satureioides extract was incorporated into nanoemulsions obtained by spontaneous emulsification. The product was developed and proposed for application as an antiviral product (*Herpes simplex* virus)

(Bidone et al., 2014). *In vitro* permeation studies of the major flavonoids using esophageal mucosa and porcine ear were performed. The detection of all flavonoids of interest on the mucosal surface and in the epidermis up to eight hours after topical application showed the potential of the nanoemulsion as a carrier for topical administration of the extract (Bidone et al., 2015).

Nanoemulsion containing extract from the bark of *Rapanea ferruginea* was developed by Dal Mas et al. (2016), using the low-energy phase inversion method. In an *in vivo* animal model, extract-loaded nanoemulsion showed an increase in anti-inflammatory activity after topical administration. The nanoemulsion containing 0.13% of the extract showed an effect 1.6 times greater than conventional cream.

To analyze the influence of nanoemulsion as a carrier on the anti-inflammatory activity of the *Aleurites moluccanus* dry extract, the biological activity of nanoemulsions containing 0.1%, 0.3%, and 0.5% of the dry extract of the leaves was evaluated. Among the groups tested, the inhibition of edema, as indicative of anti-inflammatory activity, in the groups using dexamethasone 1 mg/g (0.1%), nanoemulsion containing 0.1% extract, nanoemulsion containing 0.3% extract, and nanoemulsion containing 0.5% of the extract was 63.77%, 52.8%, 69.25%, and 80.53%, respectively (Rocha, 2017). The highest concentration incorporated in the system showed activity superior to the conventional cream containing 1% of dry extract of *A. moluccanus.*

Scientific studies prove the efficiency of nanoemulsion systems as carriers that increase the drug permeability in the skin. The fluidity of nanoemulsions, although it is a characteristic that allows greater interaction with the skin surface, limits its application due to the easy flow. To solve this limitation, precursor or complementary systems to nanoemulsions have been developed, such as self-emulsifying systems and nanoemulgels.

10.4 NANOEMULGEL

Nanoemulgels are formulations resulting from the junction of nanoemulsion with hydrogel. Therefore, the development of this system requires the development of an aqueous nanoemulsion containing the lipophilic drug in the internal phase, and the subsequent incorporation of the nanoemulsion into the hydrogel, resulting in a formulation with high skin permeation of lipophilic drugs (Kaur et al., 2017; Malay et al., 2018).

To improve topical application and patient compliance, the viscosity of the nanoemulsion can be increased by adding a gelling agent forming the nanoemulgel (Nagaraja et al., 2021). Therefore, nanoemulgels are structured by the addition of an oil-in-water (o/w) nanoemulsion in a polymeric dispersion, a hydrogel. Nanoemulgels are developed in two steps. The first step is the preparation of the nanoemulsion, and the second step is the incorporation into the previously prepared hydrogel (Kaur et al., 2017).

Nanoemulgel is considered an appropriate candidate for dermal drug delivery of lipophilic molecules due to its dual characteristics, i.e., nanoemulsion and hydrogel. The main nanoemulgels advantages are increased physical stability of the nanoemulsion, high spreadability, high permeability, and consequent bioavailability favored by the internal phase nanodroplets, incorporation of hydro and lipophilic drugs, controlled release, and better patient compliance (Kaur et al., 2017; Malay et al., 2018). In addition to these properties, it has improved thixotropic and bioadhesive characteristics, a dual-release system, hydrogel, and nanoemulsion, and a nanometric internal phase that allows rapid skin permeation (Rao et al., 2021).

Hydrogels are formed by cross-linked polymeric networks. They have a high affinity for water due to the presence of hydrophilic groups. Therefore, the polymeric network acts as a reservoir, increasing the viscosity of the aqueous medium through gelation. The three-dimensional cross-linked polymeric network can be modified to meet different requirements, such as active or passive drug targeting, controlled release of bioactive components, mechanical strength, and physicochemical properties (Micale et al., 2020).

The purpose of using the gelling excipients in the nanoemulsion is to change its physical state from liquid to gel. The gelled structure influences the release of oil droplets from the internal phase to the external phase. The excipients used are synthetic polymers such as Carbopol® 940, Carbopol® 934, Carbopol® 971, Carbopol® 980, Polamaxer, and hypromellose (HPMC). Natural polymers such as chitosan, guar gum, tragacanth, and xanthan gum, also are used (Ting et al., 2020; Mikušová & Mikuš, 2022).

The combination of nanoemulgel systems with herbal derivatives is a great strategy for the administration of natural products. As the nanoemulsion is an amphiphilic system, the diversified composition of the herbal extracts, including hydro and lipophilic compounds, are easily incorporated into the internal and external phases of the nanoemulsion. Subsequently, this nanosystem is dispersed in the hydrogel, resulting in a dermatological product of high stability, cutaneous permeability, and consequent bioavailability of the molecules in the different cutaneous strata.

Herbal extracts with an anti-inflammatory, analgesic, antioxidant, antimicrobial, antitumor, and healing biological activity were incorporated into nanoemulgels, as shown in Table 10.2.

TABLE 10.2 Herbal Material Loaded in Nanoemulgel Systems

Herbal Material	Application	Oil/Surfactant/ Co-Surfactant	Hydrogel	References
Curcumin Roots	Anti-inflammatory, antioxidant, and antimicrobial	Tween® 80 Polyethylene glycol 400	Carbopol® 940	Algahtani et al. (2020)
		Tween® 80 Propylene glycol	Sodium carboxymethyl cellulose	Soliman et al. (2021)
Syzygium aromaticum L. Essential oil from flowers	Analgesic, antibacterial, antifungal, antiallergic, anti-inflammatory, anticarcinogenic, and antimutagenic	Tween® 80 Labrasol®	Chitosan/gum acacia/ guar gum	Aman et al. (2020)
Coriandrum sativum oil	Antimicrobial, anticancer	Tween® 80 Span® 80	Carbopol® 940	Eid et al. (2021)
Safrole oil Seeds	Antioxidant, antidiabetic, antimicrobial, and anticancer.	Tween® 80 Span® 80	Carbopol® 940	Eid & Hawash (2021)
Chrysin Flavone extracted from passion flowers.	Anti-cancer	Caproyl® 90 Tween® 80 Transcutol® HP	Pluronic® F-127	Nagaraja et al. (2021)
Eucalyptus Essential oil from leaves	Antioxidant and anti-inflammatory	Tocopheryl polyethylene glycol succinate Propylene glycol	Carbopol® 934	Rizg et al. (2022)
Garcinia mangostana Linn. Extracts from fruits	Antioxidant, antibacterial	Span® 20 Tween® 20	Acryloyldimethyltaurate	Sungpud et al. (2020)
Nigella sativa L. Oil from seeds	Antibacterial, antifungal, wound-healing, bone-healing, anti-inflammatory, antioxidant, and analgesic.	Polyethylene glycol	Methylcellulose	Sultan et al. (2022)
Piper betle L. Essential oil from leaves	Antioxidant	Soybean oil Tween® 80	Carbopol® 940	Ting et al. (2020)

Carbopol was the most cited hydrogel in obtaining nanoemulgels. Its favorable properties such as easy dispersion, low cost, and physical stability against different excipients and adjuvants, including ethyl alcohol, make this polymer one of the excipients of the first choice.

Nanoemulsion containing 0.13% of soft extract from the bark of *Rapanea ferruginea*, an anti-inflammatory extract, with an internal phase size of 100.6 nm, PDI of 0.171, and zeta potential of – 25.6 mV, was incorporated into Carbopol® and Aristoflex® hydrogels in 1:1 and 1:2 proportions. The internal phase size was maintained after incorporation into the hydrogel, being from 100.3 to 119.8 nm, for the Carbopol® 940 and Aristoflex® AVC hydrogels, respectively. In the physical resistance test by centrifugation, only the nanoemulsion containing extract showed physical instability, while the nanoemulgel systems remained stable against mechanical stress. The nanoemulgels showed non-Newtonian, pseudoplastic, and thixotropic rheological behavior. The incorporation of the nanoemulsion in the nanoemulgel resulted in an increase in the average viscosity from 374.90 mPa.s to 1297.67 mPa.s, 1446.35 mPa.s, 12110.82 mPa.s, and 14105.56 mPa.s for the prepared nanoemulgels, with Aristoflex® 1:1 and 1:2 and Carbopol® 1:1 and 1:2, respectively (Dionysio, 2019).

Therefore, nanoemulgel systems are carriers that allow the physical stabilization of nanoemulsions containing plant extracts, probably by increasing the stabilization of the interface by the steric mechanism characteristic of polymeric dispersions. Studies present evidence that these are viable systems for topical application of herbal extracts.

10.5 SELF-EMULSIFYING SYSTEMS

Self-emulsifying drug delivery systems (SEDDS) are isotropic mixtures of oils and surfactants, thermodynamically stable, with the potential ability to act as a carrier in the drug cutaneous permeation. After administration, the formulation disperses immediately in aqueous body fluids, creating micro- or nano-emulsions, assuming the dissolution of the active ingredient and its absorption effectively. In recent years there has been an increase in the study of self-emulsifying systems, as it is one of the most interesting approaches to improving the solubility, dissolution rate, and absorption of various drugs, administered by different routes such as oral, rectal, vaginal, ocular, and nasal (Pendey, 2021). The topical route remains relatively unexplored in the use of these systems. However, the self-emulsification capacity of some surfactants leads to the formation of supramolecular structures with multilayer emulsions that have demonstrated potential for *in vivo* applications in topical treatments. These multilayer emulsions showed greater drug delivery to the skin with long-lasting release when compared to conventional emulsions (Forouz et al., 2020).

Self-emulsifying systems can be classified as liquid-SEDDS (L-SEDDS), semi-solid SEDDS, and solid SEDDS (S-SEDDS). Depending on the globule size after biological dispersion, SEDDS can be categorized as self-micro-emulsifying drug delivery systems (SMEDDS) with a globule size ranging from 150 to 200 nm, or self-nanoemulsifying drug delivery systems (SNEDDS) with a globule size of less than 100 nm (Prameelarani et al., 2020; Rani & Radhab, 2021). The composition of SEDDS allows the alteration of the lipid arrangement of the SC. Natural oils, used as vehicles, are solvents to lipophilic drugs, allowing administration of the lipophilic molecules in a solution (Van Staden et al., 2020a).

Although the mechanism of spontaneous emulsification of SEDDS after topical administration is not clear, the scientific evidence of the therapeutic efficacy confirms the SEDDS as potential carriers for increased bioavailability of poorly soluble drugs administered topically, including herbal derivatives. Compared to conventional systems and nanocarriers such as nanoemulsions and liposomes, SEDDS have the advantages of high drug loading capacity, drug targeting, as well evident lymphatic uptake. Uptake of drugs into the lymphatic pathway after dermal administration may be an advantage in the treatment of diseases aggravated by lymphatic spread, for example, human immunodeficiency virus (HIV), metastatic cancers, and endogenous extrapulmonary tuberculosis (Van Staden et al., 2020b).

Herbal extracts are formed for compounds mostly with low solubility and permeability, as they contain lipophilic phytoconstituents, such as terpenoids, and steroids, among others, in addition to phytoconstituents of greater polarity such as polyphenols and glycosides. SEDDS can increase the solubility, permeability, bioavailability, and consequently, the biological activity of herbal extracts and phytoconstituents (Teja et al., 2022).

Self-emulsifying systems loaded with curcumin were prepared by mixing different excipients (oils, surfactants, and co-solvents). The formulations had a size from 32.4 to 80.0 nm and zeta potential of –1.56 to –4.8. Antileishmanial and antimicrobial activities against *Escherichia coli*, *Pseudomonas aeruginosa*, *Staphylococcus aureus*, and *Klebsiella pneumoniae* were evaluated. IC_{50} values against Leishmania ranged from 0.19 to 0.37 μg/ml and minimum inhibitory concentration (MICs) values were 48–62 μg/ml. The systems showed high spreadability and permeability on the skin, enhancing the biological activity of curcumin (Singh et al., 2013a, b, 2015; Kesharwani et al., 2011; Upadhyaya et al., 2009). Curcumin-loaded SEDDS can provide an effective therapy against cutaneous leishmaniasis (CL) co-infected with secondary bacteria at lower doses compared to free curcumin (Khan et al., 2019; Vyas et al., 2010; Kesharwani et al., 2015, 2018; Mishra et al., 2019; Singh et al., 2016).

Chrysin, a bioactive phytoconstituent, has a wide range of pharmacological spectra showing anti-inflammatory, antioxidant, anti-aging, anti-cancer, and cardioprotective properties. However, chrysin is poorly soluble in water and has low bioavailability. The incorporation of chrysin into self-nanoemulsifying DDSs increased percutaneous absorption measured as flux, apparent permeability coefficient, steady-state diffusion coefficient, and drug deposition when evaluated in an *ex vivo* permeation study through the abdominal mouse skin. *In vitro* cytotoxicity on A375 and SK-MEL-2 cell lines showed a significantly improved therapeutic effect, thus ensuring dose reduction (Nagaraja et al., 2021).

It is important to highlight that plant extracts have been successfully incorporated into SEDDS for oral administration, such as propolis ethanolic extract (Wang et al., 2021), *Moringa oleífera* (Sermkaew & Plyduang, 2020), *Garcinia kola* (Mukubwa et al., 2020), *Annona muricata* (Sulkhan et al., 2019), *Citrus aurantium* (Nazari-Vanani et al., 2018), *Eugenia polyantha* (Prihapsara et al., 2018), *Eugenia Polyantha* (Prihapsara et al., 2018), *Zingiber officinale* (Wijayanti et al., 2019; Ogino et al., 2018), *Physalis peruviana* (Cardona et al., 2021), *Cannabis* (Monton et al., 2022), *Passiflora ligularis* (Echeverry et al., 2021), and *Sonchus oleraceus* (Chen et al., 2020) with therapeutic application as antimicrobial, antioxidant, antimalarial, anticancer, hypoglycemic activity, and hepatoprotective effect. Therefore, self-emulsifying systems are promising carriers for topical and transdermal delivery of herbal extracts to be scientifically studied and commercially exploited.

10.6 POLYMERIC NANOPARTICLES

Polymeric nanoparticles are the term used for particles smaller than 100 nm, which, in their composition, contain some drug, whether encapsulated by a polymer or dispersed in a polymeric matrix (Figure 10.3). Nanoparticles intrinsically carry, due to their small dimensions and the use of biocompatible polymers, some desired advantages for drug delivery. The possibility of a controlled release, combined with drug vectoring and reduction of the administered dose, results in greater bioavailability (Zielińska et al., 2020).

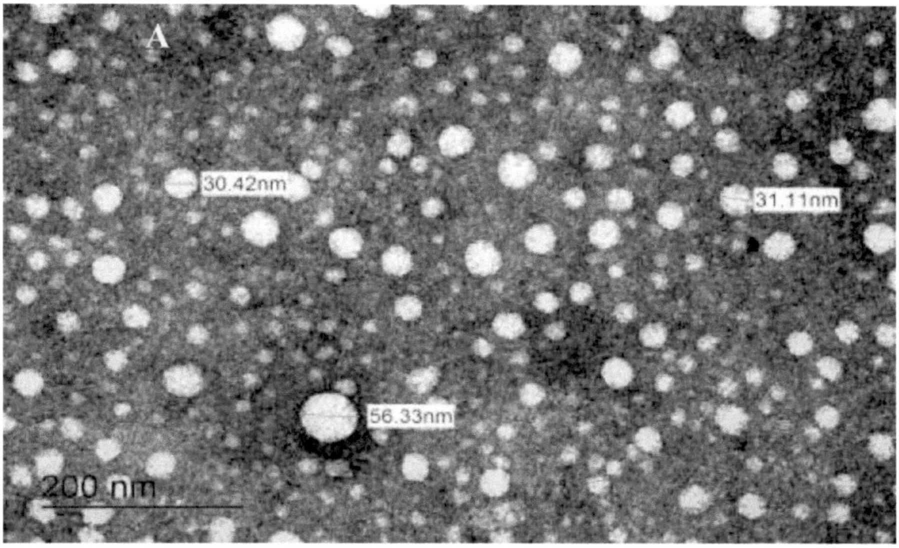

FIGURE 10.3 Morphology of the chitosan nanoparticles containing extract of *Rapanea ferruginea* stem bark extracts by TEM. Magnification of 30,000x (A); and 50,000x (B).

Source: Authorized for publication by De Carli (2017).

Polymeric nanoparticulate systems have been developed for administration by different routes of administration such as oral, topical, transdermal, parenteral, pulmonary, ocular, nasal, and vaginal (Cheng et al., 2015). The advantages of polymeric micro- and nano-particles are the increase in the chemical and physical stability of the active ingredients, greater availability and maintenance of the active ingredient in the target tissue, greater solubility of hydrophobic active ingredients, reduction of side effects and toxicity, as well as the number of doses and frequency of administration, which provides greater comfort for the patient (Faria-Tischer & Tischer, 2012).

The safety in the use of polymeric nanoparticles is derived from their origin (precursors) and composition, which currently follows trends in green chemistry. Therefore, biocompatible, biodegradable, non-toxic ingredients, with isolated phytoconstituents, herbal extracts, and even metallic ions (Ag and Au) are widely used for therapeutic purposes. In this context, natural polymers such as peptides and polysaccharides have been used as coating material (Naikoo et al., 2021).

The various possibilities and combinations of polymer and isolated active substances, drugs, and herbal extracts, can be found as a nanocapsule, in which the active ingredient is protected/stored internally in a sphere of polymeric material, or the active ingredient can be dispersed in the matrix of a polymeric sphere, forming a nanosphere. In metallic nanoparticles, the similar morphology of the nanospheres occurs through the stabilization of the surface charge of the metallic ion used, usually from the metallic salt, where the polymer, in solution, acts as a stabilizing agent, causing the ion to remain in nanometer size and does not aggregate with the others to form macromolecules. To obtain polymeric nanoparticles, it is essential to fully understand the system, the physicochemical characteristics of the polymer to be used as well as the drug (Zielińska et al., 2020).

Due to the advantages provided by nanometric systems, the incorporation of herbal extracts has gained space and is being evaluated comparatively with systems with isolated actives, seeking to take advantage of the complexity and synergism of the molecules present in the extracts (Silva et al., 2015; Abdel-Mottaleb et al., 2012). Nanoparticles containing extracts can exert anti-inflammatory, antimicrobial, antitumor action in a sustained way with the use of some polymer that controls its release, increasing the stability and bioavailability of the extract, with low or no toxicity through the choice of biocompatible polymers and non-toxic, such as poly(lactic acid-co-glycolic acid) (PLGA), chitosan (QTS), α or β-cyclodextrin, caprolactone, sodium alginate among others (Sanna et al., 2015; Servat-Medina et al., 2015).

Chitosan nanoparticles containing anti-inflammatory extract from the bark of *Rapanea ferruginea* were developed using chitosan cross-linked with tripolyphosphate by the simple coacervation method (De Carli, 2017). The diameter of the nanoparticles was dependent on both the extract:polymer and TPP ratio in the matrix, being between 50 and 270 nm and with a zeta potential between –38 and –50 mV. The nanoparticles had a spherical shape and were not agglomerated. The morphology of chitosan nanoparticles containing *R. ferruginea* extract can be seen in Figure 10.3.

10.7 CONCLUSION

Herbal extracts are complex mixtures of molecules with different solubility and permeability. They stand out for their synergistic effect, therapeutic potential, and low toxicity. On the other hand, the complexity of the mixture makes it difficult to improve its biopharmaceutical properties. Nanometric systems are DDSs capable of carrying extracts. Topical administration challenges for the treatment of skin diseases are solved with extract incorporation in the lipid nanoparticles, polymeric nanoparticles, and nanoemulsion systems (nanoemulsion, SEDDS, and nanoemulgels). These nanosystems increase the permeability of phytoconstituents in the skin and improve the efficacy and Safetire producibility, allowing the development of new drugs for relevant diseases such as viral infections, microbial infections, inflammatory, and painful processes, and skin cancer. New medicines developed based on nanotechnology have the potential to improve pharmacological action and overcome the problems related to these constituents, being relevant therapeutic alternatives to synthetic drugs. The technology involved is easy to scale up and the excipients are common in the pharmaceutical field, which makes it possible to produce new medicines from natural products. Scientific studies with these products have grown in recent years, but research about dose standardization and understanding of the release mechanism and biological activity of extracts and phytoconstituents are necessary, highlighting the importance of studies in this area.

KEYWORDS

- **herbal extracts**
- **lipid nanoparticles**
- **nanoemulsion**
- **nanostructure**
- **phytochemicals**
- **self-emulsifying systems**
- **skin disease**

REFERENCES

Abdel-Mottaleb, M. M. A., Moulari, B., Beduneau, A., Pellequer, Y., & Lamprecht, A., (2012). Nanoparticles enhance therapeutic outcome in inflamed skin therapy. *Eur J Pharm Biopharms.*, *82*(1), 151–157.

Agrawal, U., Gupta, M., & Vyas, S. P., (2015). Capsaicin delivery into the skin with lipidic nanoparticles for the treatment of psoriasis. *Artif. Cells Nanomed Biotechnol.*, *43*, 33–39.

Algahtani, M. S., Ahmad, M. Z., & Ahmad, J., (2020). Nanoemulgel for improved topical delivery of retinyl palmitate: Formulation design and stability evaluation. *Nanomaterials, 10*, 848.

Aman, R. M., Hashim, I. I. A., & Meshali, M. M., (2020). Novel clove essential oil nanoemulgel tailored by Taguchi's model and scaffold-based nanofibers: Phytopharmaceuticals with promising potential as cyclooxygenase-2 inhibitors in external inflammation. *Int. J. Nanomedicine, 15*, 2171–2195.

Ansari, S. H., Islam, F., & Sameem, M., (2012). Influence of nanotechnology on herbal drugs: A review. *J. Adv PharmTechnol Res., 3*(3), 142–146.

Assali, M., & Zaid, A. N., (2022). Features, applications, and sustainability of lipid nanoparticles in cosmeceuticals. *Saudi Pharm J., 30*(1), 53–65.

Baig, M. S., Keservani, R. K., Ahmad, M. F., & Baig, M. E., (2018). Smart delivery of nanobiomaterials in drug delivery. In: *Nanobiomaterials* (pp. 241–287). Apple Academic Press. ISBN: 9781771885911.

Barata, L., (2005). Empirismo e ciência: Fonte de novos *fitomedicamentos. Rev Ciência Cult., 57*(4), 4-5.

Bashir, M., Junaid, A. J., Asif, M., Khan, S., Irfan, M., Ibrahim, A. I., Asghar, S., et al., (2021). Nanoemulgel, an innovative carrier for diflunisal topical delivery with profound anti-inflammatory effect: *In vitro* and *in vivo* evaluation. *Int. J. Nanomedicine*, (16), 1457–1472.

Behera, J., Keservani, R. K., Yadav, A., Tripathi, M., & Chadoker, A., (2010). Methoxsalen loaded chitosan coated microemulsion for effective treatment of psoriasis. *International Journal of Drug Delivery, 2*(2).

Bidone, J., Argenta, D. F., Kratz, J., Pettenuzzo, L. F., Horn, A. P., Koester, L. S., Bassani, V. L., et al., (2015). Antiherpes activity and skin/mucosa distribution of flavonoids from *Achyrocline satureioides* extract incorporated into topical nanoemulsions. *BioMed Res Int.* Article ID 238010.

Bidone, J., Zorzi, G. K., Carvalho, E. L.S., Simões, C. M. O., Koester, L. S., Bassani, V. L., & Teixeira, H. F., (2014). Incorporation of *Achyrocline satureioides* (Lam.) DC extracts into topical nanoemulsions obtained by means of spontaneous emulsification procedure. *Ind. Crops Products., 62*, 421–429.

Buranajaree, S., Donsing, P., Jeenapongsa, R., & Viyoch, J., (2011). Depigmenting action of a nanoemulsion containing heartwood extract of *Artocarpus incisus* on UVB-induced hyperpigmentation in C57BL/6 mice. *J. Cosmetic. Sci., 62*(1), 1-14.

Burger, C., Shahzad, Y., Brümmer, A., Gerber, M., & Du Plessis, J., (2017). Traversing the skin barrier with nano-emulsions. *Curr Drug Deliv., 14*(4), 458–472.

Caesar, L. K., & Cech, N. B., (2019). Synergy and antagonism in natural product extracts: When 1 + 1 does not equal 2. *Nat. Prod Rep., 36*(6), 869–888.

Cápek, I., (2004). Degradation of kinetically-stable o/w emulsions. *Adv. Colloid Interface Sci., 107*, 125–155.

Chaiittianan, R., & Sripanidkulchai, B., (2014). Development of a nanoemulsion of *Phyllanthus emblica* L. branch extract. *Drug Dev. Ind. Pharm., 40*(12), 1597–1606.

Chen, B. H., & Inbaraj, B. S., (2019). Nanoemulsion and nanoliposome based strategies for improving anthocyanin stability and bioavailability. *Nutrients, 11*(5), 1052.

Cheng, C. J., Tietjen, G. T., Saucier-Sawyer, J. K., & Saltzman, W. M., (2015). A holistic approach to targeting disease with polymeric nanoparticles. *Nature Rev Drug Discov.*, 1–9.

Chime, S. A., Kenechukwu, F. C., & Attama, A. A., (2014). *Nanoemulsions – Advances in Formulation, Characterization and Applications in Drug Delivery.* Croatia: Intech Books.

Christofori, M. R. R., Nastiti, T. P., Abd, E., Grice, J. E., Benson, H. A. E., & Roberts, M. S., (2017). Topical nano and microemulsions for skin delivery. *Pharmaceutics*, *9*(4), 37.

Cragg, G. M., & Newman, D. J., (2013). Natural products: A continuing source of novel drug leads. *Biochim Biophys Acta*, *1830*(6), 3670–3695.

Dal Mas, J., Zermiani, T., Thiesen, L. C., Silveira, J. L. M., Silva, K. A. B. S., Souza, M. M., Malheiros, A., et al., (2016). Nanoemulsion as a carrier to improve the topical anti-inflammatory activity of stem bark extract of *Rapanea ferruginea*. *Int. J. Nanomedicine*, *11*, 4495–4507.

De Carli, R. B. G., (2017). *Desenvolvimento e Avaliação Biológica de Sistemas Micro e Nanoparticulados Contendo Extrato das Cascas de RAPANEA Ferruginea Mez.* (Primulaceae). Universidade do Vale do Itajaí, Itajaí.

Dionysio, M. E. D., (2019). *Nanoemulgel Como Carreador Dermocosmético Para Aplicação do Extrato Glicólico das Cascas de Rapanea Ferruginea com Potencial Antioxidante e Anti-inflamatório.* Universidade do Vale do Itajaí, Itajaí.

Eid, A. M., & Hawash, M., (2021). Biological evaluation of safrole oil and safrole oil nanoemulgel as antioxidant, antidiabetic, antibacterial, antifungal and anticâncer. *BMC Complement Med. Ther.*, *21*, 159.

Eid, A. M., Issa, L., Al-kharouf, O., Jaber, R., & Hreash, F., (2021). Development of *Coriandrum sativum* oil nanoemulgel and evaluation of its antimicrobial and anticancer activity. *BioMed Res Int.*, Article ID 5247816.

Faria-Tischer, P. C. S., & Tischer, C. A., (2012). Nanobiotechnology: Platform technology for biomaterials and biological applications the nanostructures. *Biochem Biotechnol Reports*. *1*(1), 32–53.

Forouz, F., Dabbaghi, M., Namjoshi, S., Mohammed, Y., Roberts, M. S., & Grice, J. E., (2020). Development of an oil-in-water self-emulsifying microemulsion for cutaneous delivery of rose Bengal: Investigation of anti-melanoma properties. *Pharmaceutics*, *12*(947), 947.

Gad, H. A., El-Rahman, F. A. A., & Hamdy, G. M., (2019). Chamomile oil loaded solid lipid nanoparticles: A naturally formulated remedy to enhance the wound healing. *J. Drug Deliv. Sci. Technol.*, *50*, 329–338.

Geetha, T., Kapila, M., Prakash, O., Deol, P. K., Kakkar, V., & Kaur, I. P., (2015). Sesamol-loaded solid lipid nanoparticles for treatment of skin cancer. *J. Drug Target, 2*, 159–169.

Jarouliya, U., Kesharwani, R. K., & Kesharwani, R. K., (2018). Advances of nanotechnology in cancer therapy. In: *Nanobiomaterials* (pp. 291–328). Apple Academic Press. ISBN: 9781771885911.

Jyothi, V. G. S. S., Ghouse, S. M., Khatri, D. K., Nanduri, S., Singh, B. S., & Madan, J., (2022). Lipid nanoparticles in topical dermal drug delivery: Does chemistry of lipid persuade skin penetration. *J Drug Deliv Sci Technol.*, *69*, 103176.

Kaur, G., Bedi, P. M. S., & Narang, J. K., (2017). Topical nanoemulgel: A novel pathway for investigating alopecia. *J. Nanomedicine Nanotechnol.*, *8*, 6.

Keservani, R. K., & Gautam, S. P., (2020). Formulation and evaluation of baclofen liposome vesicles using lecithin. *ARS Pharmaceutica, 61*(3), 175–180.

Keservani, R. K., Bandopadhyay, S., Bandyopadhyay, N., & Sharma, A. K., (2020a). Design and fabrication of transdermal/skin drug-delivery system. In: *Drug Delivery Systems* (pp. 131–178). Academic Press.

Keservani, R. K., Sharma, A. K., & Kesharwani, R. K., (2016). *Novel Approaches for Drug Delivery*. IGI Global. ISBN13, 9781522507543.

Keservani, R. K., Sharma, A. K., & Kesharwani, R. K., (2017). *Drug Delivery Approaches and Nanosystems, Two-Volume Set*. CRC Press. ISBN:9781771885850.

Keservani, R. K., Sharma, A. K., & Kesharwani, R. K., (2018). Nanoparticulate nanocarriers in drug delivery. In: *Nanobiomaterials* (pp. 3–22). Apple Academic Press. ISBN: 9781771885911.

Keservani, R. K., Sharma, A. K., & Kesharwani, R. K., (2019). *Nanocarriers for Brain Targeting: Principles and Applications.* CRC Press. ISBN:9781771887304.

Kesharwani, R. K., & Misra, K., (2011). Prediction of binding site for curcuminoids at human topoisomerase II α protein; an in silico approach. *Current Science*, 1060–1065.

Kesharwani, R. K., Singh, D. B., Singh, D. V., & Misra, K., (2018). Computational study of curcumin analogues by targeting DNA topoisomerase II: A structure-based drug designing approach. *Network Modeling Analysis in Health Informatics and Bioinformatics, 7*(1), 1–7.

Kesharwani, R. K., Srivastava, V., Singh, P., Rizvi, S. I., Adeppa, K., & Misra, K., (2015). A novel approach for overcoming drug resistance in breast cancer chemotherapy by targeting new synthetic curcumin analogues against aldehyde dehydrogenase 1 (ALDH1A1) and glycogen synthase kinase-3 β (GSK-3β). *Applied Biochemistry and Biotechnology, 176*(7), 1996–2017.

Khan, M., Khan, M., Ali, M., Shah, W., Shah, A., & Yasinzai, M. Y., (2019). Curcumin-loaded self-emulsifying drug delivery system (cu-SEDDS): A promising approach for the control of primary pathogen and secondary bacterial infections in cutaneous leishmaniasis. *Appl. Microbiol. Biotechnol., 103*(18), 7481–7490.

Khezri, K., Farahpour, M. R., & Mounesi, R. S., (2019). Accelerated infected wound healing by topical application of encapsulated Rosemary essential oil into nanostructured lipid carriers. *Artif. Cells Nanomed Biotechnol.*, *47*, 980–988.

Lacatusu, I., Badea, N., Badea, G., Mihaila, M., Ott, C., Stan, R., & Meghea, A., (2019). Advanced bioactive lipid nanocarriers loaded with natural and synthetic anti-inflammatory actives. *Mater. Sci. Eng.,200*, 113–126.

Leelapornpisid, P., Kiattisin, K., Jantrawut, P., & Phrutivorapongkul, A., (2014). Nanoemulsion loaded with marigold flower extract (*Tagetes erecta* Linn) in gel preparations as anti-wrinkles cosmeceutical. *Int. J. Pharm. PharmSci.*, *6*(2), 231–236.

Lewińska, A., Domżał-Kędzia, M., Jaromin, A., & Łukaszewicz, M., (2020). Nanoemulsion stabilized by safe surfactin from *Bacillus subtilis* as a multifunctional, custom-designed smart delivery system. *Pharmaceutics, 12,* 953.

Mahdi, E. S., Noor, A. M., Sakeena, M. H., Abdullah, G. Z., Abdulkarim, M. F., & Sattar, M. A., (2011). Formulation and *in vitro* release evaluation of newly synthesized palm kernel oil esters-based nanoemulsion delivery system for 30% ethanolic dried extract derived from local *Phyllanthus urinaria* for skin antiaging. *Int. J. Nanomedicine*, *6*, 2499–2512.

Malay, N. J., Chandresh, P. P., & Bhupendra, G. P., (2018). Nanoemulgel innovative approach for topical gel-based formulation. *Res. Rev. Health Care Open Acc. J.*, *1*(2), 18–23.

Mandal, S. C., Mandal, V., & Kumar, A., (2015). History and background on the use of natural products obtained from plants as therapeutic agents. In: *Essentials of Botanical Extraction: Principles and Applications* (pp. 7–17). New York: Academic Press, cap. 2.

Mehnert, W., & Mader, K., (2001). Solid lipid nanoparticles: Production, characterization, and applications. *Adv. Drug Deliv. Rev.*, *47*, 165–196.

Micale, N., Citarella, A., Molonia, M. S., Speciale, A., Cimino, F., Saija, A., & Cristani, M., (2020). Hydrogels for the delivery of plant-derived (poly)phenols. *Molecules*, *25*, 3254.

Mikušová, V., Ferková, J., Žigrayová, D., Krchˇ nák, D., & Mikuš, P., (2022). Comparative study of polysaccharide-based hydrogels: Rheological and texture properties and ibuprofen release. *Gels.*, *8*, 168.

Miranda, M., Cruz, M. T., Vitorino, C., & Cabral, C., (2019). Nanostructuring lipid carriers using *Ridolfia segetum* (L.) Moris essential oil. *Materials Sci. Eng. C.*, 103.

Mishra, H., Kesharwani, R. K., Singh, D. B., Tripathi, S., Dubey, S. K., &Misra, K., (2019). Computational simulation of inhibitory effects of curcumin, retinoic acid, and their conjugates on GSK-3 beta. *Network Modeling Analysis in Health Informatics and Bioinformatics, 8*(1), 3.

Muller, R. H., Shegokar, R., & Keck, C. M., (2011). 20 years of lipid nanoparticles (SLN and NLC): Present state of development and industrial applications. *Curr. Drug. Discov. Technol., 8*, 207–227.

Nagaraja, S., Basavarajappa, G. M., Attimarad, M., & Pund, S., (2021). Topical nanoemulgel for the treatment of skin cancer: Proof of-technology. *Pharmaceutics., 13*, 902.

Naikoo, G. A., Mustaqeem, M., Hassan, I. U., Awan, T., Arshad, F., Salim, H., & Qurashi, A., (2021). Bioinspired and green synthesis of nanoparticles from plant extracts with antiviral and antimicrobial properties: A critical review. *J. Saudi Chem. Soc., 25*(9), 17.

Namdar, M., Eatemadi, A., Soleimaninejad, M., & Hammed, A. T., (2017). A brief review on the application of nanoparticle enclosed herbal medicine for the treatment of infective endocarditis. *Biomed Pharmacother., 87*, 321–331.

Newman, D. J., & Cragg, G. M., (2020). Natural products as sources of new drugs over the nearly four decades from 01/1981 to 09/2019). *World Disease Weekly*, 150.

Pandey, R., Bhairam, M., Shukla, S. S., & Gidwani, B., (2021). Colloidal and vesicular delivery system for herbal bioactive constituents. *Daru, 29*(2), 415–438.

Pham, D. T. T., Tran, P. H. L., & Tran, T. T. D., (2019). Development of solid dispersion lipid nanoparticles for improving skin delivery. *Saudi Pharm. J., 27*, 1019–1024.

Pivetta, T. P., Simões, S., Araújo, M. M., Carvalho, T., Arruda, C., & Marcato, P. D., (2018). Development of nanoparticles from natural lipids for topical delivery of thymol: Investigation of its anti-inflammatory properties. *Colloids Surf. B Biointerfaces, 164*, 281–290.

Prameelarani, A., Desavathu, M., & Reddy, L. S., (2020). A state of the art review on self-emulsifying drug delivery system. *Int. J. Pharm. Sci. Res., 11*(9), 4244–4260.

Puglia, C., Offerta, A., Tirendi, G. G., Tarico, M. S., Curreri, S., Bonina, F., & Perrotta, R. E., (2016). Design of solid lipid nanoparticles for caffeine topical administration. *Drug Deliv., 23*, 36–40.

Qadir, A., Aqil, M., Ali, A., Warsi, M. H., Mujeeb, M., Ahmad, F. J., Ahmad, S., & Beg, S., (2019). Nanostructured lipidic carriers for dual drug delivery in the management of psoriasis: Systematic optimization, dermatokinetic and preclinical evaluation. *J. Drug Deliv. Sci., Technol., 57*, 101775.

Rai, V. K., Mishra, N., Yadav, K. S., & Yadav, N. P., (2018). Nanoemulsion as pharmaceutical carrier for dermal and transdermal drug delivery: Formulation development, stability issues, basic considerations, and applications. *J. Control Release, 270*, 203.

Raina, H., Soni, G., Jauhari, N., Sharm, N., & Bharadvaja, N., (2014). Phytochemical importance of medicinal plants as potential sources of anticancer agents. *Turk. J. Botany, 38*, 1027–1035.

Rane, B. R., Bharath, M. S., Patil, R. R., Keservani, R. K., & Jain, A. S., (2020b). Novel approaches in nutraceuticals. In: Rajesh, K. K., Raj, K. K., & Anil, K. S., (eds.), *Enhancing the Therapeutic Efficacy of Herbal Formulations through Novel Drug Delivery Systems* (pp. 241–266). IGI Global International Publisher, Pennsylvania, USA, Chapter 11. ISBN13: 9781799844532.

Rane, B. R., Bharath, M. S., Patil, R. R., Keservani, R. K., & Jain, A. S., (2020a). Novel approaches in herbal formulation. In: Rajesh, K. K., Raj, K. K., & Anil, K. S., (eds.), *Enhancing the Therapeutic Efficacy of Herbal Formulations through Novel Drug Delivery Systems* (pp. 43–68). IGI Global International Publisher, Pennsylvania, USA, Chapter 2. ISBN13: 9781799844532.

Rane, B. R., Tadavi, S. A., & Keservani, R. K., (2020c). "Naturopathy." In: Anil, K. S., Raj, K. K., & Surya, P. G., (eds.), *Herbal Product Development* (pp. 321–347). Apple Academic Press, CRC Press, Taylor & Francis Group, Chapter 12. ISBN: 9781771888776.

Rani, E. R., & Radhab, G. V., (2021). Insights into novel excipients of self-emulsifying drug delivery systems and their significance: An updated review. *Crit. Rev. Ther. Drug Carrier Syst., 38*(2), 27–74.

Rao, V., Vani, D. B. S., & Padmalatha, K., (2021). Topical nanoemulgel: A novel approach for wound healing efficacy. *J. Chem. Pharm Res., 13*(9), 01–09.

Rizg, W. Y., Hosny, K. M., Mahmoud, S. S., Kammoun, A. K., Alamoudi, A. J., Tayeb, H. H., Bukhary, H. A., et al., (2022). Repurposing lovastatin cytotoxicity against the tongue carcinoma HSC3 cell line using a eucalyptus oil-based nanoemulgel carrier. *Gels, 8*, 176.

Rocha, A. C. F., (2017). *Desenvolvimento de Nanoemulsão Contendo Extrato Das Folhas de Aleurites moluccanus L. willd (Euphorbiaceae) Com Atividade Anti-inflamatória Tópica.* Universidade do Vale do Itajaí, Itajaí.

Rocha, A. C. F., (2022). *Sistema Autoemulsificável Para Transporte Nariz-cérebro de Ácido Mirsinoico: Desenvolvimento e Avaliação da Atividade tipo Antidepressiva in Vivo.* Tese de doutorado. Universidade do Vale do Itajaí, Itajaí.

Rocha, P. B. R., Souza, B. S., Andrade, L. M., Anjos, J. L. V., Mendanha, S. A., Alonso, Neves, R., et al., (2019). Enhanced asiaticoside skin permeation by *Centella asiatica*-loaded lipid nanoparticles: Effects of extract type and study of stratum corneum lipid dynamics. *J. Drug Deliv Sci Technol., 50*, 305–312.

Rodenak-Kladniew, B., German, A. I., Bravo, M. G., Durán, N., & Castro, G. R., (2017). Design, characterization, and *in vitro* evaluation of linalool-loaded solid lipid nanoparticles as potent tool in cancer therapy. *Colloids Surf. B., 154*, 123–132.

Sanna, V., Lubinu, G., Madau, P., Pala, N., Nurra, S., Mariani, A., & Sechi, M., (2015). Polymeric nanoparticles encapsulating white tea extract for nutraceutical application. *J. Agricult. Food Chem., 63*(7), 2026–2032.

Saraf, A. S., (2010). Applications of novel drug delivery system for herbal formulations. *Fitoterapia, 81*, 680–689.

Servat-Medina, L., González-Gómez, A., Reyes-Ortega, F., Sousa, I. M. O., Queiroz, N. C. A., Zago, P. M. W., Jorge, M. P., et al., (2015). Chitosan–tripolyphosphate nanoparticles as *Arrabidaea chica* standardized extract carrier: Synthesis, characterization, biocompatibility, and antiulcerogenic activity. *Int J Nanomedicine, 9*(10), 3897–3910.

Shah, P., Bhalodia, D., & Shelat, P., (2010). Nanoemulsion: A Pharmaceutical review. *Sys. Rev. Pharm., 1*, 24–32.

Sharma, A. K., Keservani, R. K., & Gautam, S. P., (2020). *Herbal Product Development.* Apple Academic Press, CRC Press, Taylor & Francis Group. ISBN: 9781771888776.

Sharma, A. K., Keservani, R. K., & Keseharwani, R. K., (2018). *Nanobiomaterials: Applications in Drug Delivery.* CRC Press. ISBN:9781771885911.

Sharma, S., Sathasivam, T., Rawat, P., Pushpamalar, J., & Langford, P., (2021). Lycopene-loaded nanostructured lipid carrier from carboxymethyl oil palm empty fruit bunch cellulose for topical administration. *Carbohyd. Polym. Technol. Appl.,* 100049.

Silva, A. C., Amaral, M. H., Lobo, J. M., & Lopes, C. M., (2015). Lipid nanoparticles for the delivery of biopharmaceuticals. *Curr. Pharm. Biotechnol., 16,* 291–302.

Silva, C. O., Rijo, P., Molpeceres, J., Figueiredo, I. V., Ascensão, L., Fernandes, A. S., Roberto, A., & Reis, C. P., (2015). Polymeric nanoparticles modified with fatty acids encapsulating betamethasone for anti-inflammatory treatment. *Int. J. Pharmaceutics, 493*(1, 2), 271–284.

Singh, D. B., Gupta, M. K., Kesharwani, R. K., & Misra, K., (2013a). Comparative docking and ADMET study of some curcumin derivatives and herbal congeners targeting β-amyloid. *Network Modeling Analysis in Health Informatics and Bioinformatics, 2*(1), 13–27.

Singh, D. V., Agarwal, S., Kesharwani, R. K., & Misra, K., (2013b). 3D QSAR and pharmacophore study of curcuminoids and curcumin analogs: Interaction with thioredoxin reductase. *Interdisciplinary Sciences: Computational Life Sciences, 5*(4), 286–295.

Singh, P., Kesharwani, R. K., Misra, K., & Rizvi, S. I., (2015). The modulation of erythrocyte Na+/K+-ATPase activity by curcumin. *Journal of Advanced Research, 6*(6), 1023–1030.

Singh, P., Kesharwani, R. K., Misra, K., & Rizvi, S. I., (2016). Modulation of erythrocyte plasma membrane redox system activity by curcumin. *Biochemistry Research International,* ArticleID 702039.

Soliman, W. E., Shehata, T. M., Mohamed, M. E., Younis, N. S., & Elsewedy, H. S., (2021). Enhancement of curcumin anti-inflammatory effect via formulation into myrrh oil-based nanoemulgel. *Polymers, 13,* 577.

Souto, E. B., Zielinska, A., Souto, S. B., Durazzo, A., Lucarini, M., Santini, A., Silva, A. M., et al., (2020). (+)-limonene 1,2-epoxide-loaded SLNs: Evaluation of drug release, antioxidant activity, and cytotoxicity in an HaCaT cell line. *Int. J. Mol. Sci., 21*(4), 1449.

Sultan, M. H., Javed, S., Madkhali, O. A., Alam, M. I., Almoshari, Y., Bakkari, M. A., Sivadasan, D., et al., (2022). Development and optimization of methylcellulose-based nanoemulgel loaded *Withnigella sativa* oil for oral health management: Quadratic model approach. *Molecules, 27,* 1796.

Sungpud, C., Panpipat, W., Chaijan, M., & Sae, Y. A., (2020). Techno-biofunctionality of mangostin extract-loaded virgin coconut oil nanoemulsion and nanoemulgel. *PLoS One, 15*(1), 1–22.

Tadros, T., Izquierdo, P., Esquena, J., & Solans, C., (2004). Formation and stability of nano-emultions. *Adv. Colloid Interf. Sci., 108, 109,* 303–318.

Teaima, T. H., Badawi, N. M., Attia, D. A., El-Nabarawi, M. A., Elmazar, M. M., & Mousa, S. A., (2022). Efficacy of pomegranate extract loaded solid lipid nanoparticles transdermal emulgel against Ehrlich ascites carcinoma. *Nanotechnol. Biol. Med., 39,* 102466.

Teja, P. K., Teja, P. K., Mithiya, J., Kate, A. S., Bairwa, K., & Chauthe, S. K., (2022). Herbal nanomedicines: Recent advancements, challenges, opportunities, and regulatory overview. *Phytomedicine, 96,* 153890.

Ting, T. C., Rahim, N. F. A., Zaudin, N. A. C., Abdullah, N. H., Mohamad, M., Shoparwe, N. F., Ramle, S. F. M., et al., (2020). Development and characterization of nanoemulgel containing *Piper betle* essential oil as active ingredient. *IOP Conf. Series: Earth and Environmental Science,* 596.

Toscano, R. J. M., (2011). *Plantas Medicinais.* Lisboa: Academia das Ciências de Lisboa.

Upadhyaya, J., Kesharwani, R. K., & Misra, K., (2009). Metabolism, pharmacokinetics, and bioavailability of ascorbic acid; synergistic effect with tocopherols and curcumin. *J. Comput. Intell. Bioinform., 2*(1), 77–84.

Van, S. D., Du Plessis, J., & Viljoen, J., (2020a). Development of a self-emulsifying drug delivery system for optimized topical delivery of clofazimine. *Pharmaceutics, 12*(6), 1-24.

Van, S. D., Du Plessis, J., & Viljoen, J., (2020b). Development of topical/transdermal self-emulsifying drug delivery systems, not as simple as expected. *Scientia Pharm., 88*(2), 1–24.

Vyas, N., Keservani, R. K., Nayak, A., Jain, S., & Singhal, M., (2010). Effect of *Tamarindus indica* and *Curcuma longa* on stress induced alopecia. *Pharmacology Online, 1*, 377–384.

Waghule, T., Gorantla, S., Rapalli, V. K., Shah, P., Dubey, S. K., Saha, R. N., & Singhvi, G., (2020). Emerging trends in topical delivery of curcumin through lipid nanocarriers: Effectiveness in skin disorders. *AAPS PharmSciTech, 21*(7).

Wissing, S., Lippacher, A., & Muller, R., (2001). Investigations on the occlusive properties of solid lipid nanoparticles (SLN). *J. Cosmet. Sci., 52*, 313–324.

Wu, Y., Li, Y. H., Gao, X. H., & Chen, H. D., (2013). The application of nanoemulsion in dermatology: An overview. The application of nanoemulsion in dermatology: An overview. *J. Drug Target., 21*(4), 321–327.

Zhai, Y., & Zhai, G., (2014). Advances in lipid-based colloid systems as drug carrier for topic delivery. *J. Control Release, 193*, 90–99.

Zhang, L., Song, J., Kong, L., Yuan, T., Li, W., & Zhang, W., (2020). The strategies and techniques of drug discovery from natural products. *Pharmacol. Ther.*, 216.

Zhang, Y., Li, Z., Zhang, K., Yang, G., Wang, Z., Zhao, J., Hu, R., & Feng, N., (2016). Ethyl oleate-containing nanostructured lipid carriers improve oral bioavailability of trans-ferulic acid as compared with conventional solid lipid nanoparticles. *Int. J. Pharm., 511*, 57–64.

Zielińska, A., Carreiró, F., Oliveira, A. M., Neves, A., Pires, B., Venkatesh, D. N., Durazzo, A., et al., (2020). Polymeric nanoparticles: Production, characterization, toxicology, and ecotoxicology. *Molecules, 25*(16), 3731.

Zielinska, A., Ferreira, N. R., Durazzo, A., Lucarini, M., Cicero, N., Mamouni, S. E., Silva, A. M., et al., (2019). Development and optimization of alpha-pinene-loaded solid lipid nanoparticles (SLN) using experimental factorial design and dispersion analysis. *Molecules, 24*(15), 2683.

Zielinska, A., Ferreira, N. R., Feliczak-Guzik, A., Nowak, I., & Souto, E. B., (2020). Loading, release profile and accelerated stability assessment of monoterpenes-loaded solid lipid nanoparticles (SLN), *Pharm Dev Technol., 25*, 832–844.

Zielinska, A., Martins-Gomes, C., Ferreira, N. R., Silva, A. M., Nowak, I., & Souto, E. B., (2018). Anti-inflammatory and anti-cancer activity of citral: Optimization of citral-loaded solid lipid nanoparticles (SLN) using experimental factorial design and LUMiSizer(R). *Int. J. Pharm., 553*, 428–440.

CHAPTER 11

Medicinal Plant in Skin Topical Treatment Based on Nanotechnology

BUI THANH TUNG, NGO THI HUE, TRAN VIET LINH, NGUYEN VIET LONG, NGUYEN THUY NGOC, and NGUYEN ĐUC THUAN

VNU University of Medicine and Pharmacy, Vietnam National University, Ha Noi, Vietnam

ABSTRACT

The skin is the large organ that covers and protects the body. Therefore, it is continuously exposed to agents and oxygen species reactions in the environment and causes lots of skin diseases such as acne, skin infections, psoriasis, fungal skin diseases, atopic dermatitis (AD), and skin cancer. They affect the quality of human life, so since ancient times, people have known to use herbal plants to treat them. Some medicinal plants are known for their good biological activities, which are widely used in the treatment of skin diseases like *Aloe vera*, *Curcuma longa*, *Melaleuca alternifolia*, *Panax ginseng*, *Berberis aristata*, *Rheum officinale*, etc. However, the traditional methods using medicinal plants show a limited ability to dissolve and penetrate the skin. To exploit and maximize the benefits of medicinal plants, recent research is directed towards the preparation of medicinal plant products in the form of nanoparticles. In this review, we summarize several studies on this method, thereby giving an overview of it. The results show that the application of nanotechnology in the treatment of skin diseases brings good results and opens a new perspective in the further development of nano-compounds from medicinal plants.

Novel Nanocarriers forSkin Diseases: Advances and Applications.
Raj K. Keservani and Júlia Scherer Santos (Eds.)

11.1 INTRODUCTION

Plant knowledge and use as herbal remedies have occurred in various populations, beginning with man's learning to select plants for nourishment and to treat maladies and diseases (Patra et al., 2018). Natural products have remarkable properties such as exceptional chemical diversity, chemical, and biological properties with macromolecular specificity, and lower toxicity (Rout et al., 2018).

Topical drug delivery has inherent advantages over other routes of administration. However, the presence of the SC limits drug diffusion to small, lipophilic molecules. Fortunately, the advancement of nanotechnology opens up new avenues for addressing this issue (Cui et al., 2020). The use of large-sized materials in drug delivery presents significant challenges, including *in vivo* instability, poor bioavailability and solubility, poor absorption in the body, issues with target-specific delivery and tonic effectiveness, and potential adverse drug effects (Jahangirian et al., 2017).

Nanocarriers such as liposomes, polymeric nanoparticles, gold nanoparticles (AuNPs), and framework nucleic acids have been used to transport drugs across the skin barrier to the epidermis and dermis layers due to their unique size and surface chemistry (Chang et al., 2021). Various nanotechnology methods, such as nanoemulsions, liposomes, solid lipid nanoparticles (SLNs), smaller-sized nanoparticles, hydrogels, and dendrimers, play active roles in beauty enhancement (Karthivashan et al., 2018). Liposomes, niosomes, nanoemulsions, microemulsions, SLNs, nanostructured lipid carriers (NLCs), and nanospheres are examples of novel nanocarriers that have replaced traditional delivery systems. These novel nanocarriers have advantages such as improved skin penetration, controlled, and sustained drug release, increased stability, site-specific targeting, and high entrapment efficiency (Kaul et al., 2018).

Nanoparticles used as drug delivery vehicles are typically 100 nm in at least one dimension and are composed of various biodegradable materials such as natural or synthetic polymers, lipids, or metals (Pudlarz & Szemraj, 2018). In particular, nano-drug delivery systems (DDSs) anchor bioactive molecules to the applied area, sustain drug release, and explicitly improve drug therapeutic efficacies, making a fine figure in the field of skin regeneration (Patra et al., 2018). Nanoparticles can be used to improve the uptake of poorly soluble drugs at the site of disease, drug targeting to a specific site, and drug bioavailability (Pudlarz & Szemraj, 2018). Nanosystems enable profitable skin penetration and a consistent ingredient release profile, resulting in improved technological performance (Santos et al., 2019). Nanotechnology, which has a better protective and skin-health-improving efficiency, can cure most difficulties (Ganesan & Choi, 2016).

Skin, which is the largest organ in the human body, accounts for 16% of body weight and an adult's skin area is up to 1.8–2.0 m^2. The skin has the function of protecting the body from harmful effects from the surrounding environment and allowing interaction with the surrounding environment. The main function of the skin is to maintain the internal environment of the body, allowing the organism to protect and reproduce DNA correctly. Therefore, the skin is an organ that often suffers from disease problems (Dąbrowska et al., 2018). Some common skin diseases are presented below:

1. **Acne Vulgaris:** It is a skin condition where small pimples appear when the hair follicles on the skin become clogged with oil or dead skin cells. It can cause red spots and pimples anywhere on the body, especially on the face, shoulders, back, neck, chest, and upper arms. Therefore, the patient feels a substantial cutaneous and significant psychological influence (Knutsen-Larson et al., 2012; Williams et al., 2012).

2. **Atopic Dermatitis (AD):** Commonly known as eczema, is a common chronic, relapsing skin disease characterized by pruritus, and presenting at any age (Sohn et al., 2011). The incidence of AD is approximately 15% to 20% of children and 1% to 3% of adults worldwide. Risk factors for developing topic dermatitis include a genetic defect in the gene encoding filaggrin (FLG) and a family history of the atopic disease (Avena-Woods, 2017). AD patients are at higher risk for skin infections because of bacterial and viral superinfections ex: *Staphylococcus aureus* skin infections, eczema herpeticum, eczema vaccinatum, and eczema coxsackium (Ong & Leung, 2016).

3. **Bacterial and Viral Infections:** These are common diseases in patients with multiple trauma, diabetes, immunocompromised, obese, or malnourished patients. Bacterial dermatitis: *Staphylococcus*, *Streptococcus*, *Methicillin-resistant Staphylococcus aureus* (MRSA), etc., can cause a lot of diseases such as MRSA skin infection, cellulitis, boils, impetigo, leprosy, etc. It can be treated early with antibiotics, but severe infections and antibiotic resistance should be limited. Viral dermatitis: *Herpes simplex virus* (type 1,2), *Poxvirus*, *Papillomavirus*, etc., can cause a lot of diseases such as

hand, foot, and mouth disease, shingles, warts, chickenpox, measles, etc. But some viruses need treatment, or they will leave scars on the skin (Solanki, 2011).

4. **Dermatophytosis:** It is a common disease in tropical monsoon climate countries with an infection rate of about 27.3% and the highest in children. The disease has many common ways of transmission such as infection from fungal spores present in the air and the surrounding environment, infected animals transmitting to humans, sick people infecting healthy people, etc. So, disease prevention and treatment are difficult. Some fungi cause fungal infections of the skin such as *Piedra hortai*, *Pityrosporum ovale*, *Candida albicans*, *Epidermophyton*, *Microsporum*, and *Trichophyton* spp. Common fungal skin diseases are Tinea capitis, Tinea corporis, Tinea pedis, Tinea cruris, Tinea unguium, Pityriasis versicolor, and Mucocutaneous candidiasis (Gupta et al., 2017).
5. **Psoriasis:** It is a common, chronic papulosquamous skin disease occurring worldwide, and presenting at any age (Griffiths et al., 2021). According to the World Psoriasis Day consortium, about 2–3% of the world's population suffers from this disease (Lowes et al., 2014). Risk factors for developing psoriasis include genetic and exogenous factors (trauma, prolonged stress, sunburn, surgery, skin infections) (Kamiya et al., 2019). Several clinical phenotypes of psoriasis include psoriasis vulgaris (account for 90% of cases), psoriasis pustular, psoriasis scalp (Griffiths & Barker, 2007).
6. **Skin Cancer:** It is a common disease nowadays is a pre-eminent public health threat, the incidence is increasing yearly. Three separate forms of skin cancer are basal cell carcinoma (BCC), squamous cell carcinoma (SCC), and melanoma. BCC which is commonly known as "freckles," is the most common skin cancer (Jarouliya et al., 2018), representing about 70% of all types. The best way to prevent illness is sunscreen. SCC is a malignant tumor of the skin due to atypical proliferation of spinous cells, of an invasive character, which can produce metastases. The expressive lesions are nodules or plaques, reddish, and thick, which bleed at the slightest trauma. Clinically, melanoma is usually asymptomatic, but the itching and bleeding may be the first manifestation of melanoma (Gordon, 2013; Linares et al., 2015; Souto et al., 2021).

11.2 MEDICINAL PLANTS

Medicinal plants are found to be an important role in the treatment of skin disorders (De Wet et al., 2013). Most of the biologically active constituents of plants extracts, which are highly soluble in water, but have low absorption, because they are unable to cross the lipid membranes of the cells, have excessively high molecular size, or are poorly absorbed, leading to loss of bioavailability and efficacy. Recently, the wide proposal to combine medicinal plants with nanotechnology because nanostructured systems may be ready to potentiate the action of plant extracts, reducing the required dose and side effects, and improving activity. Nanosystems (Keservani et al., 2017) can deliver the active constituent at a sufficient concentration during the entire treatment period, direct it to the specified of action (Bonifacio et al., 2014). Below, we are going to summarize several medicinal plants such as *Aloe vera*, *Centella asiatica*, *Ocimum sanctum*, e.g., that are used with nanotechnology in dermatology treatments.

11.2.1 ALOE VERA

Aloe vera is perennial, tropical, drought-resistant, a succulent plant belonging to the Liliaceae. It is used for a variety of medicinal purposes. It is about 60–100 cm tall, has 12–16 leaves usually, and weighs up to 2–3 kilograms on maturity (Parthasarathy et al., 2016). It has 75 potentially active constituents and also the entire goodness of aloe lies in its leaf, which may be divided into three parts: the thick protective outer layer; the skinny yellowish middle layer; and also, the fleshy inner layer (Tyler, 1993).

Aloe vera gel contains about 200 active ingredients like minerals, lipids, vitamins, proteins, polysaccharides, and amino acids. So, it is used to make topical medications for skin conditions, such as burns, wounds, rashes, psoriasis, cold sores, or dry skin (Hekmatpou et al., 2019). Regarding the biological effects of *Aloe vera*, it can prevent injury to the epithelium and promote the healing of injured tissues. It also has antibacterial, antifungal, and increases blood flow to wounded areas. It stimulates fibroblasts, the skin cells responsible for wound healing, and the production of collagen, the protein that controls the aging process of the skin and wrinkling (Parthasarathy et al., 2016).

Recently, the strong development of nanotechnology has brought effective new prospects for aloe vera in medical applications. The usage of *Aloe vera* in the form of hydrogels, nanoparticles, nanocomposites, nanofibers, and bio-inspired sponges has extended its well-established application spectrum in the fields of wound healing, in topical therapy of psoriasis and drug delivery (Balaji et al., 2015; Fereig et al., 2020). The metal nanoparticles in *Aloe vera* extract have the ability to treat fungal skin diseases, antibacterial, and wound-healing effects well than *Aloe vera* gel (Burange et al., 2021). The study of antifungal properties of green synthesized silver nanoparticles (AgNPs) from *Aloe vera* leaf extract against two pathogenic fungus *Rhizopus* sp. and *Aspergillus* sp. are carried out by Shreya Medda et al. The results show that AgNPs have great potential in controlling pathogenic fungi on the skin (Parthasarathy et al., 2016). AgNPs have also been shown to have the ability to combat serious infections caused by *MRSA*, *S. aureus*, *P. aeruginosa*, and *E. coli* (Ibrahim et al., 2020). Mariam et al. also reported a study of zinc oxide (ZnO) nanoparticles obtained from *Aloe vera* hot extract (ZnO-AH). It showed *S. aureus*, *S. pyogenes*, *P. aeruginosa*, *E. coli*, and *S. typhi* and fungal strains are *A. niger*, *A. flavus*, *A. fumigatous*, *Rhizopus indicus*, and *Mucor indicus* are inhibited (Parthasarathy et al., 2016). Moreover, nanoparticles extracted from *Aloe vera* also show other benefits such as being cheap, easy to use, and environmentally friendly. Another research has shown that nanotechnology-based *Aloe vera* products are highly effective in treating skin diseases and skincare. This method can solve the limitations of phytocompounds such as low solubility and permeability, whitening effect, and low stability (Ganesan & Choi, 2016). Currently, scientists are continuing to study the application of nanotechnology to further exploit the effects of *Aloe vera* in skin topical treatment.

11.2.2 BERBERIS ARISTATA

Berberis aristata is an Indian medicinal plant that has been widely employed in traditional medicines for skin diseases and it belongs to the family Berberidaceae. Many studies indicate that Rasaut, a decoction of *Berberis aristata*, was commonly accustomed treat skin disorders (Qadir et al., 2021). *Berberis aristata* contains mainly alkaloids like berberine (BRB), oxyberberine, aromoline, berbamine, a protoberberine alkaloid karachine and so on. Among the several compounds, BRB, which is a benzylisoquinoline alkaloid, main constitute having various pharmacological actions, occurs as an active constituent in numerous medicinal plants, and has an array of pharmacological properties (Chander et al., 2017). Novel *B. aristata* extracts (roots, ethanolic 70%,) loaded nanovesicular transferosomal gel are prepared. These prepared nanovesicles have a bearing on skin disorders specifically psoriasis (Nimisha et al., 2017). *Berberis aristata* extract loaded transferosomes were prepared using soy phosphatidylcholine and edge activators (Tween 80, Span 80, and sodium deoxycholate) by a modified lipid film hydration technique using a rotary evaporator and evaluated for various parameters (Jain et al., 2003). The quantification and standardization of extract are disbursed using its alkaloid content as BRB as a biomarker (Elsayed et al., 2006). Transferosomes were further added to Carbopol 934P for gel formation and subsequently evaluated for their physicochemical properties. Their efficacy against inflammation, IMQ-induced (Imiquimod-induced) psoriasis, and skin sensitivity were compared with conventional formulation (commercial formulation-Angle Gloss, Phytolab Pvt. Ltd.). The first irritation index was found to be less than 0.4 inferring its safe use for topical formulation. The histopathological report showed that psoriasis-induced animals treated with topical application of extract loaded transferosomal gel showed a marked reduction in thickness of the epidermis, length of rete ridges as compared to traditional gel formulation. The remarkable enhancement within the *in vitro* release efficiency of *Berberis aristata* extract loaded transferosomal gel improved anti-inflammatory activity. It is supposed that *Berberis aristata* extracts loaded transferosomal gel can function as a potential antipsoriatic formulation and anti-inflammatory (Nimisha et al., 2017).

11.2.3 CENTELLA ASIATICA

Centella asiatica is a valued traditional medicinal plant used in medicine to treat various diseases. It is a tropical medicinal plant from the Apiaceae family native to India, Sri Lanka, China, South Africa, Madagascar, Indonesia, Vietnam (Chandrika & Kumara, 2015). *Centella asiatica* is used in the treatment of skin conditions such as eczema, excoriations, burns, psoriasis, scleroderma as well as small wounds and hypertrophic wounds (Bylka et al., 2014). The most important active compounds extracted from *Centella asiatica* are ursane type pentacyclic triterpenoids known as centelloids, chiefly: asiaticoside, madecasosside, asiatic acid, and madecassic acid (Hashim et al., 2011). Besides, *Centella asiatica* also contains other components, including flavonoids, phenolic acids, triterpenic steroids, amino acids, and vitamins, which have important effects on antioxidant, anti-inflammatory, antimicrobial, and anticarcinogenic activity (Ratz-Łyko et al., 2016). Numerous *in vitro, in vivo*, and clinical studies have demonstrated the role of *Centella asiatica* extracts and their individual compounds in the process of healing wounds, psoriasis, and scleroderma lesions by acid (Bylka et al., 2014). Additionally, several studies have demonstrated the therapeutic potential of *Centella asiatica* in the treatment of acne, burns, and AD but further intensive clinical trials are required to confirm its efficacy as a therapeutic agent for treating skin diseases (Park, 2021).

Recently, Lee Yonghyeon et al. have discovered the anti-inflammatory and immunomodulatory effects of the *Centella asiatica* ethanol extract on AD which is a chronic inflammatory skin disease caused mainly by a chronic inflammatory skin disease immune dysregulation (Lee et al., 2020). Because of *Centella asiatica's* medicinal importance, the synthesis of nanoparticles from this plant is one of the important applications in the field of nanobiotechnology. One of the important applications of nanotechnology in improving the extraction of *Centella asiatica* is the synthesis of high payload nanosuspension. High-payload nanocrystal suspensions, which could improve the loading capacity of the preparation and the skin absorption of active compounds such as Asiatic acid, and madecassic acid; could improve skin delivery of *Centella asiatica* without any skin irritation or need for surfactants (Kim et al., 2021). Besides, extracts of *Centella asiatica* were encapsulated by the gelatin nano-encapsulation process to enhance skin protection (Kwon et al., 2012) and *Centella asiatica* mediated facile green synthesis of nano-ZnO (Pavan Kumar et al., 2021) and AgNPs (Roy, 2017).

11.2.4 CURCUMA LONGA

Curcuma longa is a rhizomatous perennial plant of Zingiberaceae, a ginger family. The active compound is curcuminoid that has antioxidant, anti-inflammatory, antimicrobial, and anticancer activity (Suryawati & Jawi). It has a good effect on the skin, so it is used to treat AD. However, its extract is limited in terms of release and penetration through the skin. Therefore, researchers have combined nanotechnology and *Curcuma longa* in the topical treatment of skin diseases (Kesharwani et al., 2011; Vyas et al., 2010; Kesharwani et al., 2015, 2018). Typically, research by Cristina et al. prepared SLNs of *Curcuma longa* by the hot melt emulsion method (Zamarioli et al., 2015). Another study with AgNPs from *Curcuma longa* also showed significant antibacterial activity against pathogens causing skin infections (Maghimaa & Alharbi, 2020). They performed experiments with *S. aureus*,

P. aeruginosa, *S. pyogenes*, and *C. albicans* and showed that their growth was significantly inhibited. In a recent report on ZnO nano- and *Curcuma longa* nano, Zeeshan Ahmad Bhutta et al. concluded that the application of nano-ZnO/CUR composite ointment will heal third-degree burn wounds rapidly as compared to solus alone application (Nimisha et al., 2017). *Curcuma longa's* lipid-based nanocarrier systems have shown potential in treating skin diseases, overcome the problems associated with conventional topical dosage forms. The nano-size, which is lipophilic in nature, with elastic properties and clogging effect of lipid nanocarriers provide high drug delivery, skin hydration, stability, enhanced penetration through the stratum corneum (SC), and release and slow curcumin in the targeted skin layers (Rapalli et al., 2020). Nanoparticles, lipid-based nanocarriers have become predominant for topical drug delivery against superficial fungal infections (Nene et al., 2021). Synthetic nanoparticles are friendly and do not pollute the environment (Maghimaa & Alharbi, 2020). From these benefits, the beneficial compounds in turmeric are actively being discovered by scientists to combine with nanotechnology in the treatment of skin diseases, especially curcumin. Green synthesis of AgNPs from *Curcuma longa* and coating on the cotton fabrics for antimicrobial applications and wound healing activity (Maghimaa & Alharbi, 2020).

11.2.5 GARCINIA MANGOSTANA

Garcinia mangostana L. (Clusiaceae) is a tropical tree endemic to Southeast Asia known as mangosteen. Mangosteen seeds and pericarps have long been used in traditional medicinal practices in the region, and beverages containing mangosteen pulp and pericarps are offered as nutritional supplements all over the world. Isoprenylated xanthones, a class of secondary metabolites with diverse biological properties such as antioxidant, anti-proliferative, pro-apoptotic, antinociceptive, hypoglycemic, neuroprotective, and anti-obesity, are the principal phytochemicals found in the species (Ovalle-Magallanes et al., 2017). A topical application of a very stable oil-in-water nanoemulsion containing mangosteens derived from the pericarp of *Garcinia mangostana* is a potential technique for protecting mangosteens and improving their penetration through the skins. The nanoemulsion made with xanthan gum as the thickening agent and blended at a temperature of 40°C showed the highest quantity of mangosteen entering into the skin, with the maximum flux occurring after one hour of application, according to the *in vitro* percutaneous penetration test. These findings suggest that VCO (virgin coconut oil) nanoemulsions made with a low-energy emulsification method and xanthan gum as a thickening agent could be used to distribute mangosteen extract topically (Krisanti et al., 2021). In young adults, acne vulgaris is the most common inflammatory sebaceous gland condition. In the treatment of acne, resistant strains of *Propionibacterium acnes* are becoming more common. The study aimed to compare the efficacy of 0.5% topical mangosteen extract in nanoparticle-loaded gel (including alpha-mangostin) to 1% clindamycin gel in treating mild to moderate acne vulgaris. After a 12-week treatment with mangosteen fruit rind extract, comedones, and inflammatory lesions were reduced by 66.86% and 67.05%, respectively ($p<0.001$). The mangosteen fruit rind extract could be a phytopharmaceutical therapy for the treatment of mild and moderate acne vulgaris, similar to 1% clindamycin gel, but without the severe side effects (Lueangarun et al., 2019). *Garcinia mangostana* peel extract was used to reduce gold ions in an aqueous solution, resulting in AuNPs. Additionally, the antibacterial activity and free radical scavenging activity of 1,1-diphenyl-2-picrylhydrazyl (DPPH) were investigated utilizing various microorganisms. The data analysis (pathological alterations) revealed that the AuNPs were not harmful. *Garcinia mangostana* peel extract and AuNPs made by this extract were combined to form a lotion that was used to treat wounds. As a consequence, compared to controls, AuNPs had a significant role in wound healing advancement, which could be attributable to their anti-inflammatory, antibacterial, and antioxidant properties. Therefore, AuNPs have the potential to be used as promising agents in the creation of novel medications (Jassim et al., 2021).

11.2.6 *MELALEUCA ALTERNIFOLIA*

More than 40 plant-derived OTC pharmaceuticals, dietary supplements, cosmetics, herbal medicines, and functional foods containing complex mixtures (e.g., *Melaleuca alternifolia* essential oi, Glycyrrhiza glabra extract, l, and Pistacia lentiscus resin), pure compounds (e.g., berberine, benzoic acid, salicylic acid, eucalyptol, & thymol) as well as their derivatives and complexes (e.g., bismuth subsalicylate and zinc pyrithione) have been identified (Kokoska et al., 2019). *Melaleuca alternifolia* essential oil (MEO) has generally been utilized because of its recuperating and antimicrobial activity. Develop, characterize, and assess the *in vivo* pharmacological activity of MEO-containing bicontinuous microemulsions (BME). Diagram construction, a formulation consisting of Kolliphor® HS 15 (31.05%), Span® 80 (3.45%), isopropyl myristate (34.5%), and distilled water (31%) was selected & MEO was incorporated in the proportion of 3.45% (v/v) (de Assis et al., 2020). *In vivo* studies suggest that BME loaded with MEO may aid in the healing of skin wounds and have antibacterial activity against Gram-positive and Gram-negative bacteria (Gnatta et al., 2021). *In vivo* wounds, the healing potential of three chitosan-based topical preparations loaded with either tea tree essential oil, rosemary essential oil, or a combination of both oils is investigated in the study. GC/MS analysis of *Melaleuca alternifolia* and *R. officinale* essential oils revealed richness in oxygenated monoterpenes, representing 51.06% and 69.61% of the total oil composition, respectively. When compared to either group treated with individual essential oils or the untreated group, topical application of a chitosan-based formulation loaded with a mixture of tea tree and rosemary oils resulted in a significant increase in wound contraction percentage (Labib et al., 2019). A randomized controlled trial had used in this study to investigate the effects of a tea tree (*Melaleuca alternifolia*) oil disinfectant on hand disinfection and skin condition. The study found that tea tree oil could be introduced into nursing practice as a new hand hygiene product to help prevent and reduce healthcare-associated infections (Youn et al., 2021).

11.2.7 OCIMUM SANCTUM

Ocimum sanctum L. (Tulsi), known as the Queen of Herbs, is one of the most revered and cherished of the many healing and health-giving herbs. *Ocimum sanctum* L. is a tropical plant native throughout the world tropics and is widespread as a cultivated plant (Pattanayak et al., 2010). *Ocimum sanctum* L. is supposed to promote general health, prevent disease, longevity, and deal with the demands of daily life. Tulsi is also said to improve the appearance of the skin, the sweetness of the voice, and the development of attractiveness, intelligence, stamina, and a calm emotional disposition (Cohen, 2014). The leaf extract of Tulsi is used to be efficient in terms of reaction time and stability of the synthesized AgNPs. For six months after manufacture, this nanoparticulate solution has exceptional stability. The antibacterial activity of AgNPs against *E. coli* and *Staphylococcus aureus* had investigated, and it had discovered that Tulsi extract stabilized AgNPs had significant potential for usage as an antimicrobial agent in the medical field, as well as the food and cosmetic industries (Ramteke et al., 2013).

When compared to marketed silver nitrate gel (0.2% w/w), the improved AgNPs gel (0.025% w/w) demonstrated a virtually comparable zone of inhibition against all harmful microorganisms. In partial-thickness burns, the AgNPs gel encouraged faster-wound healing. As a result, biosynthesized silver nano-gel is a promising topical antibacterial alternative in antibiotic-resistant strains for infection treatment and wound healing. That is one of the first studies on AgNP optimization utilizing *O. sanctum* leaf extracts and their efficiency on wound healing potential in rats (Sood & Chopra, 2018). *Ocimum sanctum* is also a natural source of anti-aging compounds for the skin, such as antioxidants, anti-inflammatories, hyaluronic acid inhibition, and collagen fiber degradation inhibition. As a result, the ethanolic extract of *O. sanctum* is an appealing cosmetic active component for anti-aging products. NLC was chosen as the best method because it improves the dermal administration of RA and has a significant skin retention rate of 27 ± 1.8 ($p < 0.05$). After 24 hours, RA was released from NLC in a consistent pattern, with a release amount of 1.29 ± 0.15%. NLC did not irritate the skin and did not penetrate it. Therefore, NLC with *Ocimum sanctum* extract was an appealing dermal delivery strategy for RA that was safe and effective. In the future, it might be used as a topical anti-aging medication, according to the researchers (Chaiyana et al., 2020).

11.2.8 PANAX GINSENG

Panax ginseng's anti-melanogenesis effect, skin-protective effect, and cellular mechanism, particularly *P. ginseng* calyx (Pg-C-EE). Pg-C-EE inhibited melanin synthesis and secretion by inhibiting activator protein-1 regulatory enzymes such as p38, ERKs (extracellular signal-regulated kinases), and cyclic adenosine monophosphate response element-binding protein. Pg-C-EE also inhibited ROS production induced by H_2O_2 and UVB. Pg-C-EE treatment increased cell viability while lowering the expression of matrix metalloproteinases (MMPs), mitogen-activated protein kinases, and hyaluronidases. As a result, Pg-C-EE had the potential to be used as a skin-improving agent with moisture retention and whitening properties (Han et al., 2018). BIOGF1K, a *Panax ginseng* fraction, has anti-melanogenic, anti-inflammatory, and anti-photoaging properties that could be useful in treating skin conditions, particularly AD (Lorz, Kim, & Cho, 2020). BIOGF1K inhibited the AD response by decreasing histamine and β-hexosaminidase release IL-4, IL-5, and IL-13 secretion levels in RBL-2H3 cells and IL-4 and

IL-13 secretion levels in HMC-1 cells. Furthermore, BIOGF1K inhibited MAPK pathway activation in RBL-2H3 and HMC-1 cells (Lorz, Kim, & Cho, 2020). Lower eczema area and severity index, transepidermal water loss (TEWL), immunoglobulin E (IgE) levels, and higher sleep quality are all favorable effects of *P. ginseng* in AD patients. As a result, *P. ginseng* and its ginsenosides are unquestionably a nontoxic effective way to treat AD (Lorz, Kim, Kim et al., 2020). Besides, those found in *P. ginseng* have been shown in a large number of preclinical studies to promote hair growth (Choi, 2018).

11.2.9 PODOPHYLLUM PELTATUM

Podophyllum peltatum is a long-standing medicinal plant in the family Berberidaceae native to eastern North America (Maleš et al., 2019). For centuries, Native American tribes used the *Podophyllum peltatum* to treat ulcers, furuncles, warts, laxatives, parasitic worm infections, and snake bites (Colantonio & Rivers, 2017). Podophyllin resin is the crude alcohol extract of the plant's root and consists of four different components: podophyllotoxin, 4-demethylpodophyllotoxin, a-peltatin, and b-peltatin. Podophyllotoxin is the most biologically active component and has a lot of medical applications (Schwartz & Norton, 2002). The mechanism of action of podophyllotoxin prevents cell proliferation through the inhibition of the polymerization of tubulin into microtubules and inhibits the release of cytokines like IL-1 and TNFα (Colantonio & Rivers, 2017). For a long time, numerous studies have demonstrated the use of podophyllotoxin in the treatment of condyloma acuminatum, psoriasis vulgaris, skin cancer (Singh et al., 2018). Podophyllotoxin has been used in the treatment of warts for many years, most lesions disappeared within four days after one application of podophyllotoxin, which was demonstrated in a clinical trial in 200 patients with warts. Today podophyllotoxin is still used to treat warts because of its medicinal value (Singh et al., 2018). Podophyllotoxin is a candidate for the treatment of psoriasis vulgaris because it inhibits the release of cytokines, about 75% of patients improved after 2 weeks of daily podophyllotoxin treatment (Singh et al., 2018). Podophyllotoxin can inhibit the proliferation of tumors. However, podophyllotoxin has not been clinically used as an antineoplastic agent, because of its high toxicity. Instead of this, less toxic derivatives of podophyllotoxin have been researched and developed an antineoplastic effect. A study has demonstrated the effectiveness of topical podophyllotoxin in treating

BCC, where 32 patients had 96% of basal cell lesions clinically cleared with 2–6 sessions using podophyllin resin (Singh et al., 2018). The application of nanotechnology in products containing podophyllotoxin helps to enhance the effectiveness of treatment as well as reduce adverse effects (Colantonio & Rivers, 2017). Nanoparticles have a significant role in retaining the drug at the site of action and by modifying the release profile, which has more effective treatments for skin chemotherapy and psoriasis (Souto et al., 2021).

11.2.10 RHEUM OFFICINALE BAILL.

Rheum officinale Baill. (Chinese rhubarb) is one of the most popular Chinese herbal medicines that are widely and traditionally used for wound healing, including topical skin wounds (Clementi & Misiti, 2010). The main chemical compositions of rhubarb include anthraquinones, anthrones, stilbenes, tannins, polysaccharides (Cao et al., 2017). It has pharmacological activities such as cathartic, antimicrobial, anti-inflammatory, and antioxidative with its major active ingredient being emodin (1,3,8-trihydroxy-6-methyl-anthraquinone), an anthraquinone (Tang et al., 2007). The nanofibers of emodin in polyvinylpyrrolidone were harmless, bioactive, anti-allergenic, and dissolved at a fast rate compared to the pure compound. Detailed analysis of the blended nanofibrous membrane by scanning electron microscopy, differential scanning calorimetry and X-ray diffraction revealed that emodin was well distributed within the ultrafine fibers in the type of amorphous nano-solid dispersions (Dai et al., 2012). Re-epithelialization occurred at the wounded area, the medicated nanofibrous material is non-toxic, non-allergenic, and highly biocompatible to the wound surface and its application can accelerate wound healing (Dai et al., 2012). To extend the composition of collagen in human cells to 100%, emodin was incorporated in cellulose acetate nanostructure fibers (Panichpakdee et al., 2016). The study provides evidence that the *Rheum officinale*'s compounds loaded nanofibrous membrane is more effective as a healing accelerator and the loaded drug retained its biological functionality. It is supposed that using electrospinning in combining nanotechnology with *Rheum officinale* may be a good method to incorporate and release drugs in nanofibrous materials, which have great potential in strategies to develop promising material and DDS for novel therapeutic applications, such as biomedical wound dressings for the acceleration healing of acute full-thickness skin wounds (Schneider et al., 2009).

11.3 BIOACTIVE COMPOUNDS FOR SKIN DISEASES

Nanotechnology shows potential as a powerful method for increasing the bioactivity of bioactive substances. Nanomaterials with very small dimensions have a variety of applications due to their unique size and physical qualities, which provide a variety of distinguishing traits. Scientists are eventually exploring these advantages are to overcome the physical and chemical limitations of biological molecules generated from natural sources (Majumdar et al., 2020). The study focuses on substances that protect the skin from oxidative and UV-induced damage, as well as dryness and elasticity loss: vitamins A, C, and E; copper; alkaloids; carotenoids; and polyphenols (Michalak et al., 2021).

11.3.1 ASTAXANTHIN

Carotenoids are organic pigments that occur naturally mainly in plants and play an important role in the human body. Currently, there are about 800 types of carotenoids, and it is classified into two main groups: xanthophylls and carotenes (Michalak et al., 2021). Carotenoids prevent aging, stimulate fibroblasts to produce collagen and elastin, inhibit MMP activity, and exhibit anti-inflammatory and UV-filtering effects. In addition, carotenoids provide health benefits, such as enhancing resistance to infections, and preventing damage to DNA and other genetic material (Michalak et al., 2021). Astaxanthin which belongs to the group of xanthophylls-oxygenated carotenoids derives from aquatic animals, such as lobsters, crabs, salmon, trout, crustaceans, microalgae *Phaffia rhodozyma*, *Chlorella vulgaris*, *Haematococcus pluvialis*, etc. (Davinelli et al., 2018). Numerous studies have demonstrated diverse biological activities of astaxanthin *in vitro* and *in vivo* (Ng et al., 2021). Astaxanthin has been shown to have anti-inflammatory, immune-modulating, and DNA repair properties, which has been recommended to use skincare and tackle skin damage (Singh et al., 2020). Astaxanthin is a carotenoid widely used to decrease the fine lines, wrinkles, and age spots as an anti-aging agent (Singh et al., 2020). Some studies have demonstrated the effectiveness of astaxanthin in improving the moisture content of the skin and decreasing the TEWL, so it may be utilized to tackle the problem of dry skin, secondary to seasonal stress (Singh et al., 2020). Astaxanthin has been found to decrease UV-induced skin changes and thus prevent UV damage, so it may be used as a food supplement to tackle UV-induced dermatological effects (Ito et al., 2018; Singh et al., 2020). Besides, the antioxidant effect of astaxanthin can neutralize the elevated free radical molecules, thus reducing the potential attack of these harmful components on skin cells (Singh et al., 2020). Because of the immense effects of astaxanthin, an effective delivery system is needed that targets astaxanthin to the skin in therapeutic quantities. Self-nano-emulsifying drug delivery systems (SNEDDS) have successfully been developed and studied to increase the skin penetration of astaxanthin and target its antioxidant and anti-inflammatory potential to the epidermis and dermis (Ponto et al., 2021). SNEDDS has been demonstrated to be an effective formulation for enhanced skin delivery of the highly lipophilic astaxanthin to the deeper skin tissues that constitute the target site for therapeutic antioxidant and anti-inflammatory activity (Ponto et al., 2021).

11.3.2 BERBERINE

Berberine (BRB) (5,6-dihydro-9,10-dimethoxybenzo[g]-1,3-benzodioxolo [5,6-a] quinolinium) is an isoquinoline alkaloid with promising pharmacological effects (Neag et al., 2018). It is found in some plants such as barberry (*Berberis*), meadow rue (*Thalictrum*), celandine (*Chelidonium*), goldenseal (*Hydrastis canadensis* L.), and *Phellodendron amurense* (Germán-Acacio et al., 2020). Plants that contain BRB, have been traditionally used in different parts of the world for the treatment of skin diseases, inflammatory disorders, wound healing, reducing fevers, affections of eyes, tumors treatment, digestive, and respiratory diseases, and microbial pathologies (Neag et al., 2018). In the study, combining BRB in nanotechnology like novel berberine nano-hydrogel (BNH) was demonstrated to improve and promote wound healing of diabetics. BNH would create a relatively closed environment for wound healing and serve as a carrier for sustained release of BRB, that effectively maintain a high BRB concentration and a moist environment at the site of skin lesions over a long period of time (Zhang et al., 2020). Additionally, another study report showed topical BRB-loaded hyalurosomes can apply in vitiligo treatment. BRB-hyalurosomes are hyaluronan-immobilized phospholipid nanovesicles that showed promising *in vitro* physicochemical properties and they showed significant improvement of the biochemical markers and enhancement in the biological activity confirming its intrinsic activity. BRB-hyalurosomes is considered a novel nanodermatological tool that paves the way for its clinical application for vitiligo treatment (Elhalmoushy et al., 2022).

11.3.3 CATECHINS

Catechins are a type of polyphenol chemical found in a variety of medicinal plants and offer numerous advantages, including the ability to prevent or reduce skin damage (Bae et al., 2020). The bioactive compounds found in natural green tea readily lose functional groups when exposed to environmental conditions, lowering their stability and limiting their use in cosmeceutical products. Nanodelivery techniques increase the bioavailability of these compounds in cosmeceutical products, by enhancing their usage in the novel development of green tea-based cosmeceuticals (Ganesan & Choi, 2016).

In another study, scientists used topical application to improve skin permeability and the whitening effect of catechin-loaded transfersomes (TRAs). The study aimed to create catechin-loaded TRAs that would increase medication permeability when applied topically to the skin to protect it from UV-induced photodamage. The *in vitro* skin permeation test stated that the catechin-loaded TRAs enhanced the skin permeability by 85% compared to the catechin aqueous solution. As a result, topical injection of catechin-loaded TRAs could be explored as a therapy option for UV-induced oxidative skin damage (Hsieh et al., 2021).

The delivery of bioactive molecules through the skin is challenging given the complex structure of its outer layer (Keservani et al., 2020a). The scientists look at the possibilities of encapsulating natural substances in nanocarriers with permeation enhancers that can change the fluidity of the lipids in the SC. This method should make cutaneous or transdermal release easier. For antioxidant topical administration, bile salts had added to lipid liquid crystalline nanoparticles (NPs) composed of monoolein. Under the same experimental settings and with the same antioxidant, the effects of two alternative lipid formulations without bile salts were examined. In comparison to formulations without bile salts, the formulation with bile salts performed the best, allowing for improved catechin penetration in the various skin layers (Fornasier et al., 2021).

11.3.4 COPPER

Copper is an essential mineral that is involved in a variety of physiological and metabolic processes, including angiogenesis, skin formation, and the expression and stability of extracellular skin proteins, as well as having antibacterial characteristics. Copper is an appealing material for improving skin health because it combines these two features (Salvo & Sandoval, 2022). Copper nano-form has a wide range of applications, raising the risk of environmental contamination. Bioaccumulation and toxicity of copper nanoparticles (CuNPs) have been established in plants and animals, whereas released nanoparticles undergo numerous transformation processes in the environment. This toxicity is assumed to be a combined effect of intracellular particles and the release of dissolved copper ions. CuNPs' antibacterial properties make them excellent components for use in biomedicine, and they've lately been studied for use as drug delivery agents in cancer therapy (Ameh & Sayes, 2019).

Recently, nanomaterials such as CuNPs have sparked a lot of interest in wound healing research. The potential therapeutic effect of various CuNPs concentrations (1 μM, 10 μM, 100 μM, 1 mM, and 10 mM) and sizes (20 nm, 40 nm, and 80 nm) in wound healing investigated by the authors. The results show that CuNP (80 nm/1 μM) is a potential NP for wound healing applications without adverse side effects (Alizadeh et al., 2019). Another study by Mohammed S. Saddik's aimed to create and test phenytoin (PHT)-loaded copper nanoparticles (PHT-loaded CuNPs) for wound healing. CuNPs biosynthesized using the licorice aqueous extract. The prepared CuNPs were loaded with PHT by characterized, adsorption, and evaluated for wound-healing efficiency. Both plain and PHT-loaded CuNPs were monodisperse and had a cubic and hexagonal shape, according to the findings. When compared to control rats, PHT-loaded CuNPs accelerated epidermal regeneration and encouraged granulation and tissue development. Finally, PHT-loaded CuNPs appear to be a viable platform for wound healing that is both effective and quick (Saddik et al., 2020). Copper peptides are small copper peptides with a long history of use in skincare products and a good safety record. GHK-Cu (glycyl-L-histidyl-L-lysine), a short copper-binding peptide found in human plasma, is the most researched copper peptide. GHK-Cu has a list of health benefits, including enhancing wound contraction and increasing growth factor synthesis and antioxidant enzyme activity. Furthermore, copper peptides, which have DNA-repair characteristics, are gaining interest as potent gene modulators capable of reversing the expression of various genes implicated in biochemical processes linked to cancer growth and progression (Pickart & Margolina, 2018).

11.3.5 CURCUMIN

Curcumin is a polyphenol and yellow pigment extracted from the rhizome of *Curcuma longa* (turmeric) (Carvalho et al., 2016). Curcumin is known for a lot of benefits such as anti-inflammatory, antibacterial, and wound-healing activities for centuries ago. It seems to be more advantageous in providing a localized effect in skin diseases such as inflammatory skin diseases, psoriasis, AD, wound care, skin aging, skin cancer, skin infections (Vollono et al., 2019). Although it has great potential, its ability to be soluble in water that makes the flexibility penetrate poor skin and degradation has limited its application. According to Nutraceutical Bioavailability Classification Scheme (NuBACS), Curcumin has poor bioaccessibility, because of its low solubility in water and low stability (McClements et al., 2015). To improve this limitation, a combination of nano-formulas with Curcumin is usually recommended to point out to boost Curcumin bioavailability and therapeutic potential. Lipid-based nanocarrier systems including liposomes (Keservani & Gautam, 2020), niosomes (Keservani & Gautam, 2022), SLNs (Keservani et al., 2017a), NLCs (Keservani et al., 2018), lyotropic liquid crystal nanoparticles, lipospheres, and lipid nanocapsules have found potential as carriers to beat the problems related to conventional topical dosage forms (Nene et al., 2021). The report of Laura Vollono et al. reported the results of the evaluation of the use of Curcumin in nanoformulations and also showed good results of this method (Vollono et al., 2019). The incorporation of Curcumin in nanocarriers may achieve faster wound healing at a lower dose compared to free molecules (Liakopoulou et al., 2021). Studies show that Curcumin in nano-form is simpler within the topical treatment of the skin, which may optimize the pharmacokinetic profile and increase the bioavailability of the free compound Curcumin.

11.3.6 GALLIC ACID

Gallic acid (3,4,5-trihydroxybenzoic acid), a phenolic compound, is a ubiquitous secondary metabolite found both as a free state and as a constituent of tannins, namely, Gallotannin (Fitzpatric & Woldemariam, 2017) Gallic acid and its derivatives are present in nearly every part of the plant, such as bark, wood, leaf, fruit, root, and seed, with appreciable concentrations in grapes seed, rose flowers, sumac, oak, and witch hazel (Goldberg & Rokem, 2009). It exhibits powerful antioxidant, anti-inflammatory, antimicrobial, and anti-cancer activities. The most intriguing benefit has been reported to be on the skin. So, gallic acid and its derivatives have been extensively used as an adjuvant in a number of therapeutic formulations, as a substitute for hydrocortisone in children with AD and other skin conditions (hyperpigmentation, wound healing), and as a cosmetic ingredient (Khan et al., 2018). Synthesized, environmentally friendly gallic acid-coated gold nanoparticles (GA–AuNPs) have been evaluated as an anti-aging antioxidant for the skin (Eren Böncü et al., 2021). Additionally, the present data showed that GA–AuNPs have a superior ability to inhibit high glucose-mediated matrix metalloproteinase-1-elicited (MM-1) type I collagen degradation in dermal fibroblast cells (Choi et al., 2020). Anti-skin-aging treatments for their antioxidant properties and inhibition of MMP-1 *in vitro* assays and for anti-wrinkle properties as shown *in vivo* skin tests (Shin et al., 2020). The studies showed that GA–AuNPs are valuable as an active ingredient in anti-aging products, particularly for high glucose-induced skin aging (Ng et al., 2021).

11.3.7 VITAMIN A

Vitamin A is a fat-soluble vitamin that has a lot of effects on the skin. Vitamin A from animal sources is mainly acquired in the form of retinyl esters (palmitate, propionate, and acetate) such as liver, fish liver oils, dairy products, butter, cheese, egg yolk, meat products, certain saltwater fish, etc. Vitamin A has derived from plants that contain provitamin A (β-carotene) (Michalak et al., 2021). Derivatives of vitamin A, called retinoids, include both natural and many synthetic retinol derivatives with activity similar to that of vitamin A. Vitamin A and derivatives of vitamins stimulate the synthesis of epidermal proteins; stimulate proliferation of epidermal cells, and regulates exfoliation of keratinocytes; stimulate fibroblasts to synthesize collagen and elastin, protects collagen against MMP-induced degradation; take part in angiogenesis in the dermis; influence skin thickness; influence melanin degradation and skin color; protect the skin against UV radiation; reduce sebum and limit the development of Propionibacterium acnes (Michalak et al., 2021). Vitamin A and all of its derivatives applied systemically or topically, have a significant influence on skin health. Retinoids have a lot of research on their anti-aging effects. Retinoids slow down the aging processes and improve the aging condition of the skin (Michalak et al., 2021).

Vitamin A plays an important role in skin immunity. If Vitamin A is deficient, it will lead to impaired immune response and increased susceptibility to skin infections and inflammatory skin disease (Roche & Harris-Tryon, 2021). Besides, Retinoic acid and its derivatives have therapeutic potential for a variety of serious dermatological disorders including some malignant conditions (Szymański et al., 2020). Today, the application of nanotechnology is widely applied in the delivery of drugs to tissues. In order to improve their pharmacological properties and circulating half-life, while minimizing their off-target uptake, various retinoid delivery systems have been recently developed (Bensa et al., 2021). Overcoming retinoids using fenretinide-loaded liposomes, which have raised interest within the scientific community thanks, among others, to their beneficial effects in cancer (Bensa et al., 2021). Because the topical application of tretinoin is followed by a high incidence of side effects, one method to overcome the problem is loading tretinoin into lipid nanoparticles (Nasrollahi et al., 2017). A new drug delivery system (DDS) improves total retinoic acid therapy (atRA) for external treatments of damaged skin. Inorganic-coated atRA nanoparticles have many pharmacological improvements and have many good clinical applications (Yamaguchi et al., 2005).

11.3.8 VITAMIN C

Vitamin C (L-ascorbic acid) is a highly water-soluble, sugar-like alpha-ketolactone produced from D-glucose. Vitamin C has a crucial role in the metabolism of essential substances and maintaining human physiological activities. Benefits of Vitamin C include photoprotection from UV A & B, neocollagenesis, inhibition of melanogenesis, and improvement of a spread of inflammatory skin disorders (Stamford, 2012). A human cannot synthesize vitamin C on their own but can only get and absorb it through food. Vitamin C is most abundantly stored in the skin and is responsible for the biosynthesis of collagen, which has an anti-wrinkle effect. It also configures the symbolic barrier and strengthens the cells, preventing water loss and protecting the skin (Carita et al., 2020; Michalak et al., 2021). However, this vitamin is unstable and loses effectiveness with poorly formulated strategies. Nanotechnology has been effectively used to promote the stability and therapeutic activity of various drug molecules (Keservani et al., 2019). With this context, the objective of the work was set to formulate a topical delivery system of vitamin C nanoparticles incorporated into the polymeric gel. In the study of human albumin serum (HAS) contains vitamin C within the treatment of wounds, the results showed that the wound healing speed was increased after treatment with 20 HAS nanoparticles loaded Vitamin C (Shojania et al., 2019). Another study on the treatment of skin and soft tissue infections shows that *S.*

aureus shows that Polyelectrolyte-Vitamin C Nanoparticulates incorporate a strong anti-autopsy activity 5 times compared to Vancomycin (George et al., 2017). Additionally, vitamin C is combined with a NLC to treat acne (Jain et al., 2016). These activities suggest the important role of Vitamin C nanoparticles in the treatment of skin.

11.3.9 VITAMIN E

Plants are the only ones that can synthesize vitamin E and all forms supplied to the human body through food (Khadangi & Azzi, 2019). Vitamin E is essential for maintaining skin health and has been used in dermatology for over 50 years. The most likely physiologic function of epidermal vitamin E is to contribute to the skin's antioxidant defenses and protect the epidermis and dermis from oxidative stress caused by environmental factors. In humans, vitamin E is the most important lipid-soluble antioxidant (Michalak et al., 2021). Because of its antioxidant and anti-inflammatory bioactivities, vitamin E has great potential as an adjunctive treatment for AD (Teo et al., 2021). The modified vesicles based on ethanol and either vitamin E or PEGylated castor oil derivatives demonstrated the highest transdermal fluxes, as confirmed by confocal laser microscopy tracking to the dermis (Abdel-Messih et al., 2019). Dermatitis was alleviated using a combination of microwave and nanotechnology, which promotes vitamin E delivery and translates to a positive dermatitis treatment outcome that warrants further investigation (Harun et al., 2021).

11.4 CONCLUSION

Medicinal plants have an excellent value in the treatment of topical skin diseases. When combining them with nanotechnology, nanoparticles help release drugs slowly and have little degradation, so they have detached a replacement resolution in topical skin treatment. Studies have shown that this method can improve the constraints of stability and low permeability when only using medicinal herbs. Therefore, the development of medicinal plant analogs supported by nanotechnology with better bioavailability or alternative formulations is urgently needed. Research on this field is continuously developing and applied more and more in dermatology problems.

KEYWORDS

- **astaxanthin**
- **bioactive compounds**
- **herbal plants**
- **medicinal plants**
- **nanotechnology**
- **skin diseases**

REFERENCES

Abdel-Messih, H. A., Ishak, R. A. H., Geneidi, A. S., & Mansour, S., (2019). Tailoring novel soft nano-vesicles 'flexosomes' for enhanced transdermal drug delivery: Optimization, characterization, and comprehensive *ex vivo – in vivo* evaluation. *International Journal of Pharmaceutics, 560,* 101–115. https://doi.org/https://doi.org/10.1016/j.ijpharm.2019.01.072.

Alizadeh, S., Seyedalipour, B., Shafieyan, S., Kheime, A., Mohammadi, P., & Aghdami, N., (2019). Copper nanoparticles promote rapid wound healing in acute full thickness defect via acceleration of skin cell migration, proliferation, and neovascularization. *Biochemical and Biophysical Research Communications, 517*(4), 684–690.

Ameh, T., & Sayes, C. M., (2019). The potential exposure and hazards of copper nanoparticles: A review. *Environmental Toxicology and Pharmacology, 71,* 103220.

Avena-Woods, C., (2017). Overview of atopic dermatitis. *The American Journal of Managed Care, 23*(8 Suppl), S115–S123.

Bae, J., Kim, N., Shin, Y., Kim, S. Y., & Kim, Y. J., (2020). Activity of catechins and their applications. *Biomedical Dermatology, 4*(1), 1–10.

Balaji, A., Vellayappan, M. V., John, A. A., Subramanian, A. P., Jaganathan, S. K., SelvaKumar, M., & Yusof, M., (2015). Biomaterials based nano-applications of aloe vera and its perspective: A review. *RSC Advances, 5*(105), 86199-86213.

Bensa, V., Calarco, E., Giusto, E., Perri, P., Corrias, M. V., Ponzoni, M., & Pastorino, F., (2021). Retinoids delivery systems in cancer: Liposomal fenretinide for neuroectodermal-derived tumors. *Pharmaceuticals, 14*(9), 854.

Bonifacio, B. V., Da Silva, P. B., Dos Santos, R. M. A., Negri, K. M. S., Bauab, T. M., & Chorilli, M., (2014). Nanotechnology-based drug delivery systems and herbal medicines: A review. *International Journal of Nanomedicine, 9,* 1.

Burange, P. J., Tawar, M. G., Bairagi, R. A., Malviya, V. R., Sahu, V. K., Shewatkar, S. N., & Mamurkar, R. R., (2021). Synthesis of silver nanoparticles by using Aloe vera and Thuja orientalis leaves extract and their biological activity: A comprehensive review. *Bulletin of the National Research Centre, 45*(1), 1–13.

Bylka, W., Znajdek-Awiżeń, P., Studzińska-Sroka, E., Dańczak-Pazdrowska, A., & Brzezińska, M., (2014). Centella asiatica in dermatology: An overview. *Phytotherapy Research, 28*(8), 1117–1124.

Cao, Y. J., Pu, Z. J., Tang, Y. P., Shen, J., Chen, Y. Y., Kang, A., & Duan, J. A., (2017). Advances in bio-active constituents, pharmacology, and clinical applications of rhubarb. *Chinese Medicine, 12*(1), 1–12.

Carita, C., Fonseca-Santos, B., Shultz, J. D., Michniak-Kohn, B., Chorilli, M., & Leonardi, G. R., (2020). Vitamin C: One compound, several uses. Advances for delivery, efficiency, and stability. *Nanomedicine: Nanotechnology, Biology and Medicine, 24*, 102117.

Carvalho, A. C., Gomes, A. C., Pereira-Wilson, C., & Lima, C. F., (2016). Mechanisms of action of curcumin on aging: Nutritional and pharmacological applications. In: *Molecular Basis of Nutrition and Aging* (pp. 491–511). Elsevier.

Chaiyana, W., Anuchapreeda, S., Somwongin, S., Marsup, P., Lee, K. H., Lin, W. C., & Lue, S. C., (2020). Dermal delivery enhancement of natural anti-ageing compounds from *Ocimum sanctum* Linn. extract by nanostructured lipid carriers. *Pharmaceutics, 12*(4), 309.

Chander, V., Aswal, J., Dobhal, R., & Uniyal, D., (2017). A review on pharmacological potential of berberine; an active component of Himalayan *Berberis aristata. J. Phytopharmacol, 6*(1), 53–58.

Chandrika, U. G., & Kumara, P. A. P., (2015). Gotu kola (*Centella asiatica*): Nutritional properties and plausible health benefits. *Advances in Food and Nutrition Research, 76*, 125–157.

Chang, H., Chew, S. W., Zheng, M., Lio, D. C. S., Wiraja, C., Mei, Y., & Shi, P., (2021). Cryomicroneedles for transdermal cell delivery. *Nature Biomedical Engineering, 5*(9), 1008–1018.

Choi, B. Y., (2018). Hair-growth potential of ginseng and its major metabolites: A review on its molecular mechanisms. *International Journal of Molecular Sciences, 19*(9). https://doi.org/10.3390/ijms19092703.

Choi, H. J., Alam, M. B., Baek, M. E., Kwon, Y. G., Lim, J. Y., & Lee, S. H., (2020). Protection against UVB-induced photoaging by *Nypa fruticans* via inhibition of MAPK/AP-1/MMP-1 signaling. *Oxidative Medicine and Cellular Longevity, 2020.*

Clementi, E. M., & Misiti, F., (2010). Potential health benefits of rhubarb. In: *Bioactive Foods in Promoting Health* (pp. 407–423). Elsevier.

Cohen, M. M., (2014). Tulsi-*Ocimum* sanctum: A herb for all reasons. *Journal of Ayurveda and Integrative Medicine*, *5*(4), 251.

Colantonio, S., & Rivers, J. K., (2017). Botanicals with dermatologic properties derived from first nations healing: Part 2—Plants and algae. *Journal of Cutaneous Medicine and Surgery*, *21*(4), 299–307.

Cui, M., Wiraja, C., Chew, S. W. T., & Xu, C., (2020). Nanodelivery systems for topical management of skin disorders. *Molecular Pharmaceutics*, *18*(2), 491–505.

Dąbrowska, A., Spano, F., Derler, S., Adlhart, C., Spencer, N. D., & Rossi, R. M., (2018). The relationship between skin function, barrier properties, and body-dependent factors. *Skin Research and Technology*, *24*(2), 165–174.

Dai, X. Y., Nie, W., Wang, Y. C., Shen, Y., Li, Y., & Gan, S. J., (2012). Electrospun emodin polyvinylpyrrolidone blended nanofibrous membrane: A novel medicated biomaterial for drug delivery and accelerated wound healing. *Journal of Materials Science: Materials in Medicine*, *23*(11), 2709–2716.

Davinelli, S., Nielsen, M. E., & Scapagnini, G., (2018). Astaxanthin in skin health, repair, and disease: A comprehensive review. *Nutrients, 10*(4), 522.

De Assis, K. M. A., Da Silva, L. J. M., De Melo, D. F., Borges, J. C., Santana, L. M. B., Dos Reis, M. M. L., & Dos Santos, S. G., (2020). Bicontinuous microemulsions containing *Melaleuca alternifolia* essential oil as a therapeutic agent for cutaneous wound healing. *Drug Delivery and Translational Research, 10*(6), 1748–1763.

De Wet, H., Nciki, S., & Van, V. S. F., (2013). Medicinal plants used for the treatment of various skin disorders by a rural community in northern Maputaland, South Africa. *J. Ethnobiol. Ethnomed., 9*, 51. https://doi.org/10.1186/1746-4269-9-51.

Elhalmoushy, P. M., Elsheikh, M. A., Matar, N. A., El-Hadidy, W. F., Kamel, M. A., Omran, G. A., & Elnaggar, Y. S., (2022). Novel berberine-loaded hyalurosomes as a promising nanodermatological treatment for vitiligo: Biochemical, biological and gene expression studies. *International Journal of Pharmaceutics*, 121523.

Elsayed, M. M., Abdallah, O. Y., Naggar, V. F., & Khalafallah, N. M., (2006). Deformable liposomes and ethosomes: Mechanism of enhanced skin delivery. *International Journal of Pharmaceutics, 322*(1, 2), 60–66.

Eren, B. T., Yücel, Ç., Şeker, K. G., & Takır, E., (2021). Gallic acid-loaded microemulsion and microemulsion gel: Development, characterization, and evaluation of antioxidant effectiveness. *Indian Journal of Natural Products and Resources (IJNPR)[Formerly Natural Product Radiance (NPR)], 12*(1), 128–135.

Fereig, S. A., El-Zaafarany, G. M., Arafa, M. G., & Abdel-Mottaleb, M. M., (2020). Tackling the various classes of nano-therapeutics employed in topical therapy of psoriasis. *Drug Delivery, 27*(1), 662–680.

Fornasier, M., Pireddu, R., Del Giudice, A., Sinico, C., Nylander, T., Schillǃ╚n, K., & Murgia, S., (2021). Tuning lipid structure by bile salts: Hexosomes for topical administration of catechin. *Colloids and Surfaces B: Biointerfaces, 199*, 111564.

Ganesan, P., & Choi, D. K., (2016). Current application of phytocompound-based nanocosmeceuticals for beauty and skin therapy. *International Journal of Nanomedicine, 11*, 1987.

George, L., Bavya, M. C., Rohan, K. V., & Srivastava, R., (2017). A therapeutic polyelectrolyte ق│ôvitamin C nanoparticulate system in polyvinyl alcoholق│ôalginate hydrogel: An approach to treat skin and soft tissue infections caused by *Staphylococcus aureus*. *Colloids and Surfaces B: Biointerfaces, 160*, 315–324.

Germán-Acacio, J. M., Meza-Sánchez, D. E., & Morales-Morales, D., (2020). Therapeutically relevant natural products as AMPK activators in the treatment of diabetes. In: *Studies in Natural Products Chemistry* (Vol. 66, pp. 57–90). Elsevier.

Gnatta, J. R., De Brito, P. V., Padoveze, M. C., Graziano, K. U., Turrini, R. N. T., & Da Silva, M. J. P., (2021). Melaleuca alternifolia essential oil soap: A potential alternative for hand hygiene. *European Journal of Clinical Microbiology & Infectious Diseases, 40*(7), 1517–1520. https://doi.org/10.1007/s10096-021-04190-w.

Gordon, R., (2013). Skin cancer: An overview of epidemiology and risk factors. *Seminars in Oncology Nursing.*

Griffiths, C. E. M., Armstrong, A. W., Gudjonsson, J. E., & Barker, J., (2021). Psoriasis. *Lancet, 397*(10281), 1301–1315. https://doi.org/10.1016/s0140-6736(20)32549-6.

Griffiths, C. E., & Barker, J. N., (2007). Pathogenesis and clinical features of psoriasis. *The Lancet, 370*(9583), 263–271.

Gupta, A. K., MacLeod, M. A., Foley, K. A., Gupta, G., & Friedlander, S. F., (2017). Fungal skin infections. *Pediatrics in Review*, *38*(1), 8–22.

Han, S. Y., Kim, J., Kim, E., Kim, S. H., Seo, D. B., Kim, J. H., & Cho, J. Y., (2018). AKT-targeted anti-inflammatory activity of panax ginseng calyx ethanolic extract. *Journal of Ginseng Research*, *42*(4), 496–503. https://doi.org/https://doi.org/10.1016/j.jgr.2017.06.003.

Harun, M. S., Wong, T. W., & Fong, C. W., (2021). Advancing skin delivery of α-tocopherol and γ-tocotrienol for dermatitis treatment via nanotechnology and microwave technology. *International Journal of Pharmaceutics*, *593*, 120099. https://doi.org/https://doi.org/10.1016/j.ijpharm.2020.120099.

Hashim, P., Sidek, H., Helan, M. H. M., Sabery, A., Palanisamy, U. D., & Ilham, M., (2011). Triterpene composition and bioactivities of *Centella asiatica*. *Molecules*, *16*(2), 1310–1322.

Hekmatpou, D., Mehrabi, F., Rahzani, K., & Aminiyan, A., (2019). The effect of Aloe vera clinical trials on prevention and healing of skin wound: A systematic review. *Iranian Journal of Medical Sciences*, *44*(1), 1.

Hsieh, W. C., Fang, C. W., Suhail, M., Vu, Q. L., Chuang, C. H., & Wu, P. C., (2021). Improved skin permeability and whitening effect of catechin-loaded transfersomes through topical delivery. *International Journal of Pharmaceutics*, *607*, 121030.

Ibrahim, O., Abed, A., & Yahea, N., (2020). Evaluation of biological silver nanoparticles using aloe vera gel extract as antibacterial agent in-vitro and in-activity of greenly synthesized vivo. *Iraqi J. of Agric. Sci*, *51*(6), 1706–1715.

Ito, N., Seki, S., & Ueda, F., (2018). The protective role of astaxanthin for UV-induced skin deterioration in healthy people—A randomized, double-blind, placebo-controlled trial. *Nutrients*, *10*(7), 817.

Jahangirian, H., Lemraski, E. G., Webster, T. J., Rafiee-Moghaddam, R., & Abdollahi, Y., (2017). A review of drug delivery systems based on nanotechnology and green chemistry: Green nanomedicine. *International Journal of Nanomedicine*, *12*, 2957.

Jain, A., Garg, N. K., Jain, A., Kesharwani, P., Jain, A. K., Nirbhavane, P., & Tyagi, R. K., (2016). A synergistic approach of adapalene-loaded nanostructured lipid carriers, and vitamin C co-administration for treating acne. *Drug Development and Industrial Pharmacy*, *42*(6), 897–905.

Jain, S., Jain, P., Umamaheshwari, R., & Jain, N., (2003). Transfersomes—A novel vesicular carrier for enhanced transdermal delivery: Development, characterization, and performance evaluation. *Drug Development and Industrial Pharmacy*, *29*(9), 1013–1026.

Jarouliya, U., Kesharwani, R. K., & Kesharwani, R. K., (2018). Advances of nanotechnology in cancer therapy. In: *Nanobiomaterials* (pp. 291–328). Apple Academic Press. ISBN: 9781771885911.

Jassim, A. M. N., Shafy, G. M., Mohammed, M. T., Farhan, S. A., & Noori, O. M., (2021). Antioxidant, anti-inflammatory and wound healing of biosynthetic gold nanoparticles using mangosteen (*G. Mangostona*). *Iraqi Journal of Industrial Research*, *8*(2), 59–74.

Kamiya, K., Kishimoto, M., Sugai, J., Komine, M., & Ohtsuki, M., (2019). Risk factors for the development of psoriasis. *International Journal of Molecular Sciences*, *20*(18), 4347.

Karthivashan, G., Ganesan, P., Park, S. Y., Kim, J. S., & Choi, D. K., (2018). Therapeutic strategies and nano-drug delivery applications in management of ageing Alzheimer's disease. *Drug Delivery*, *25*(1), 307–320.

Kaul, S., Gulati, N., Verma, D., Mukherjee, S., & Nagaich, U., (2018). Role of nanotechnology in cosmeceuticals: A review of recent advances. *Journal of Pharmaceutics*, *2018*.

Keservani, R. K., & Gautam, S. P., (2020). Formulation and evaluation of baclofen liposome vesicles using lecithin. *ARS Pharmaceutica, 61*(3), 175–180.

Keservani, R. K., & Gautam, S. P., (2022). Skeletal muscle relaxant activity of different formulation of span 60 niosome. *ARS Pharmaceutica, 63*(91), 32–44.

Keservani, R. K., Bandopadhyay, S., Bandyopadhyay, N., & Sharma, A. K., (2020a). Design and fabrication of transdermal/skin drug-delivery system. In: *Drug Delivery Systems* (pp. 131–178). Academic Press.

Keservani, R. K., Kesharwani, R. K., & Sharma, A. K., (2017a). Introduction to nanotechnology in drug delivery. In: *Drug Delivery Approaches and Nanosystems* (pp. 1–19). Apple Academic Press. ISBN: 9781771885836.

Keservani, R. K., Sharma, A. K., & Kesharwani, R. K., (2017). *Drug Delivery Approaches and Nanosystems, Two-Volume Set*. CRC Press. ISBN:9781771885850.

Keservani, R. K., Sharma, A. K., & Kesharwani, R. K., (2018). Nanoparticulate nanocarriers in drug delivery. In: *Nanobiomaterials* (pp. 3–22). Apple Academic Press. ISBN: 9781771885911.

Keservani, R. K., Sharma, A. K., & Kesharwani, R. K., (2019). *Nanocarriers for Brain Targeting: Principles and Applications*. CRC Press. ISBN:9781771887304.

Keservani, R. K., Sharma, A. K., & Ramteke, S., (2010). Novel vesicular approach for topical delivery of baclofen via niosomes. *Lat. Am. J. Pharm., 29*, 1364–1370.

Kesharwani, R. K., & Misra, K., (2011). Prediction of binding site for curcuminoids at human topoisomerase II α protein; an in silico approach. *Current Science*, 1060–1065.

Kesharwani, R. K., Singh, D. B., Singh, D. V., & Misra, K., (2018). Computational study of curcumin analogues by targeting DNA topoisomerase II: A structure-based drug designing approach. *Network Modeling Analysis in Health Informatics and Bioinformatics, 7*(1), 1–7.

Kesharwani, R. K., Srivastava, V., Singh, P., Rizvi, S. I., Adeppa, K., & Misra, K., (2015). A novel approach for overcoming drug resistance in breast cancer chemotherapy by targeting new synthetic curcumin analogues against aldehyde dehydrogenase 1 (ALDH1A1) and glycogen synthase kinase-3 β (GSK-3β). *Applied Biochemistry and Biotechnology, 176*(7), 1996–2017.

Khadangi, F., & Azzi, A., (2019). Vitamin E–the next 100 years. *IUBMB Life*, *71*(4), 411–415.

Khan, B. A., Mahmood, T., Menaa, F., Shahzad, Y., Yousaf, A. M., Hussain, T., & Ray, S. D., (2018). New perspectives on the efficacy of gallic acid in cosmetics & nanocosmeceuticals. *Current Pharmaceutical Design*, *24*(43), 5181–5187.

Kim, E. A., Park, J. S., Kim, M. S., Jeong, M. Y., Park, H. J., Choi, J. H., & Kang, M. J., (2021). High-payload nanosuspension of *Centella asiatica* extract for improved skin delivery with no irritation. *International Journal of Nanomedicine*, *16*, 7417.

Knutsen-Larson, S., Dawson, A. L., Dunnick, C. A., & Dellavalle, R. P., (2012). Acne vulgaris: Pathogenesis, treatment, and needs assessment. *Dermatologic Clinics*, *30*(1), 99–106.

Kokoska, L., Kloucek, P., Leuner, O., & Novy, P., (2019). Plant-derived products as antibacterial and antifungal agents in human health care. *Current Medicinal Chemistry*, *26*(29), 5501–5541.

Krisanti, E. A., Kirana, D. P., & Mulia, K., (2021). Nanoemulsions containing *Garcinia mangostana* L. pericarp extract for topical applications: Development, characterization, and *in vitro* percutaneous penetration assay. *PloS One*, *16*(12), e0261792.

Kwon, M. C., Choi, W. Y., Seo, Y. C., Kim, J. S., Yoon, C. S., Lim, H. W., & Lee, H. Y., (2012). Enhancement of the skin-protective activities of *Centella asiatica* L. urban by a nano-encapsulation process. *Journal of Biotechnology*, *157*(1), 100–106.

Labib, R. M., Ayoub, I. M., Michel, H. E., Mehanny, M., Kamil, V., Hany, M., & Mohamed, A., (2019). Appraisal on the wound healing potential of *Melaleuca alternifolia* and *Rosmarinus officinalis* L. essential oil-loaded chitosan topical preparations. *PloS One*, *14*(9), e0219561. https://doi.org/10.1371/journal.pone.0219561.

Lee, Y., Choi, H. K., N'deh, K. P. U., Choi, Y. J., Fan, M., Kim, E. K., & An, J. H., (2020). Inhibitory effect of *Centella asiatica* extract on DNCB-induced atopic dermatitis in HaCaT cells and BALB/c mice. *Nutrients*, *12*(2), 411.

Liakopoulou, A., Mourelatou, E., & Hatziantoniou, S., (2021). Exploitation of traditional healing properties, using the nanotechnology's advantages: The case of curcumin. *Toxicology Reports*, *8*, 1143–1155.

Linares, M. A., Zakaria, A., & Nizran, P., (2015). Skin cancer. *Primary Care: Clinics in Office Practice*, *42*(4), 645–659.

Lorz, L. R., Kim, D., Kim, M. Y., & Cho, J. Y., (2020). Panax ginseng–derived fraction BIOGF1K reduces atopic dermatitis responses via suppression of mitogen-activated protein kinase signaling pathway. *Journal of Ginseng Research*, *44*(3), 453–460. https://doi.org/https://doi.org/10.1016/j.jgr.2019.02.003.

Lorz, L. R., Kim, M. Y., & Cho, J. Y., (2020). Medicinal potential of panax ginseng and its ginsenosides in atopic dermatitis treatment. *Journal of Ginseng Research*, *44*(1), 8-13.

Lowes, M. A., Suarez-Farinas, M., & Krueger, J. G., (2014). Immunology of psoriasis. *Annual Review of Immunology*, *32*, 227–255.

Lueangarun, S., Sriviriyakul, K., Tempark, T., Managit, C., & Sithisarn, P., (2019). Clinical efficacy of 0.5% topical mangosteen extract in nanoparticle loaded gel in treatment of mild-to-moderate acne vulgaris: A 12-week, split-face, double-blinded, randomized, controlled trial. *Journal of Cosmetic Dermatology*, *18*(5), 1395–1403.

Maghimaa, M., & Alharbi, S. A., (2020). Green synthesis of silver nanoparticles from *Curcuma longa* L. and coating on the cotton fabrics for antimicrobial applications and wound healing activity. *Journal of Photochemistry and Photobiology B: Biology*, *204*, 111806.

Majumdar, M., Shivalkar, S., Pal, A., Verma, M. L., Sahoo, A. K., & Roy, D. N., (2020). Nanotechnology for enhanced bioactivity of bioactive compounds. In: *Biotechnological Production of Bioactive Compounds* (pp. 433–466). Elsevier.

Maleš, Ž., Ledić, D. D., Duka, I., & Žužul, K., (2019). Application of medicinal plants in several dermatovenerological entities. *Acta Pharmaceutica*, *69*(4), 525–531.

McClements, D. J., Li, F., & Xiao, H., (2015). The nutraceutical bioavailability classification scheme: Classifying nutraceuticals according to factors limiting their oral bioavailability. *Annual Review of Food Science and Technology*, *6*, 299–327.

Michalak, M., Pierzak, M., Kręcisz, B., & Suliga, E., (2021). Bioactive compounds for skin health: A review. *Nutrients*, *13*(1), 203.

Nasrollahi, S. A., Hassanzade, H., Moradi, A., Sabouri, M., Samadi, A., & Firooz, A., (2017). Safety assessment of tretinoin loaded nano emulsion and nanostructured lipid carriers: A non-invasive trial on human volunteers. *Current Drug Delivery*, *14*(4), 575–580.

Neag, M. A., Mocan, A., Echeverría, J., Pop, R. M., Bocsan, C. I., Crişan, G., & Buzoianu, A. D., (2018). Berberine: Botanical occurrence, traditional uses, extraction methods, and relevance in cardiovascular, metabolic, hepatic, and renal disorders. *Frontiers in Pharmacology*, *9*, 557.

Nene, S., Shah, S., Rangaraj, N., Mehra, N. K., Singh, P. K., & Srivastava, S., (2021). Lipid based nanocarriers: A novel paradigm for topical antifungal therapy. *Journal of Drug Delivery Science and Technology*, *62*, 102397.

Ng, Q. X., De Deyn, M. L. Z. Q., Loke, W., Foo, N. X., Chan, H. W., & Yeo, W. S., (2021). Effects of astaxanthin supplementation on skin health: A systematic review of clinical studies. *Journal of Dietary Supplements, 18*(2), 169–182.

Nimisha, D. A. R., Fatima, Z., & Neema, C. D. K., (2017). Antipsoriatic and anti-inflammatory studies of *Berberis aristata* extract loaded nanovesicular gels. *Pharmacognosy Magazine, 13*(Suppl 3), S587.

Ong, P. Y., & Leung, D. Y., (2016). Bacterial and viral infections in atopic dermatitis: A comprehensive review. *Clinical Reviews in Allergy & Immunology, 51*(3), 329–337.

Ovalle-Magallanes, B., Eugenio-Pérez, D., & Pedraza-Chaverri, J., (2017). Medicinal properties of mangosteen (*Garcinia mangostana* L.): A comprehensive update. *Food and Chemical Toxicology, 109*, 102–122.

Panichpakdee, J., Pavasant, P., & Supaphol, P., (2016). Electrospun cellulose acetate fiber mats containing emodin with potential for use as wound dressing. *Chiang Mai. J. Sci, 43*(1), 1249–1259.

Park, K. S., (2021). Pharmacological effects of *Centella asiatica* on skin diseases: Evidence and possible mechanisms. *Evidence-Based Complementary and Alternative Medicine, 2021*.

Parthasarathy, G., Saroja, M., Venkatachalam, M., Gowthaman, P., & Evanjelene, V., (2016). Synthesis of nano particles from aloe vera extract–review paper. *Int. J. Intercult. Relat., 2*, 1570–1575.

Patra, J. K., Das, G., Fraceto, L. F., Campos, E. V. R., Rodriguez-Torres, M. D. P., Acosta-Torres, L. S., & Sharma, S., (2018). Nano based drug delivery systems: Recent developments and future prospects. *Journal of Nanobiotechnology, 16*(1), 1-33.

Pattanayak, P., Behera, P., Das, D., & Panda, S. K., (2010). *Ocimum sanctum* Linn. A reservoir plant for therapeutic applications: An overview. *Pharmacognosy Reviews, 4*(7), 95.

Pavan, K. M. A., Suresh, D., & Sneharani, A. H., (2021). *Centella asiatica* mediated facile green synthesis of nano zinc oxide and its photo-catalytic and biological properties. *Inorganic Chemistry Communications, 133*, 108865. https://doi.org/https://doi.org/10.1016/j.inoche.2021.108865.

Pickart, L., & Margolina, A., (2018). Skin regenerative and anti-cancer actions of copper peptides. *Cosmetics, 5*(2), 29.

Ponto, T., Latter, G., Luna, G., Leite-Silva, V. R., Wright, A., & Benson, H. A., (2021). Novel self-nano-emulsifying drug delivery systems containing astaxanthin for topical skin delivery. *Pharmaceutics, 13*(5), 649.

Pudlarz, A., & Szemraj, J., (2018). Nanoparticles as carriers of proteins, peptides, and other therapeutic molecules. *Open Life Sciences, 13*(1), 285–298.

Qadir, A., Jahan, S., Aqil, M., Warsi, M. H., Alhakamy, N. A., Alfaleh, M. A., & Ali, A., (2021). Phytochemical-based nano-pharmacotherapeutics for management of burn wound healing. *Gels, 7*(4), 209.

Ramteke, C., Chakrabarti, T., Sarangi, B. K., & Pandey, R. A., (2013). Synthesis of silver nanoparticles from the aqueous extract of leaves of *Ocimum sanctum* for enhanced antibacterial activity. *Journal of Chemistry, 2013*.

Rapalli, V. K., Kaul, V., Waghule, T., Gorantla, S., Sharma, S., Roy, A., & Singhvi, G., (2020). Curcumin loaded nanostructured lipid carriers for enhanced skin retained topical delivery: Optimization, scale-up, in-vitro characterization and assessment of ex-vivo skin deposition. *European Journal of Pharmaceutical Sciences, 152*, 105438.

Ratz-Łyko, A., Arct, J., & Pytkowska, K., (2016). Moisturizing and anti-inflammatory properties of cosmetic formulations containing *Centella asiatica* extract. *Indian Journal of Pharmaceutical Sciences*, *78*(1), 27.

Roche, F. C., & Harris-Tryon, T. A., (2021). Illuminating the role of vitamin A in skin innate immunity and the skin microbiome: A narrative review. *Nutrients*, *13*(2), 302.

Rout, G. K., Shin, H. S., Gouda, S., Sahoo, S., Das, G., Fraceto, L. F., & Patra, J. K., (2018). Current advances in nanocarriers for biomedical research and their applications. *Artificial Cells, Nanomedicine, and Biotechnology*, *46*(sup2), 1053–1062.

Roy, A., & Bharadvaja, A., (2017). Centella Asiatica: A Pharmaceutically Important Medicinal Plant, Current Trends in Biomedical Engineering & Biosciences, Juniper Publishers Inc., *5*(3), 47–51.

Saddik, M. S., Alsharif, F. M., El-Mokhtar, M. A., Al-Hakkani, M. F., El-Mahdy, M. M., Farghaly, H. S., & Abou-Taleb, H. A., (2020). Biosynthesis, characterization, and wound-healing activity of phenytoin-loaded copper nanoparticles. *AAPS PharmSciTech*, *21*(5), 1–12.

Salvo, J., & Sandoval, C., (2022). Role of copper nanoparticles in wound healing for chronic wounds: Literature review. *Burns & Trauma*, *10*.

Santos, A. C., Morais, F., Simões, A., Pereira, I., Sequeira, J. A., Pereira-Silva, M., & Ribeiro, A., (2019). Nanotechnology for the development of new cosmetic formulations. *Expert Opinion on Drug Delivery*, *16*(4), 313–330.

Schneider, A., Wang, X., Kaplan, D., Garlick, J., & Egles, C., (2009). Biofunctionalized electrospun silk mats as a topical bioactive dressing for accelerated wound healing. *Acta Biomaterialia*, *5*(7), 2570–2578.

Schwartz, J., & Norton, S. A., (2002). Useful plants of dermatology. VI. The mayapple (*Podophyllum*). *Journal of the American Academy of Dermatology*, *47*(5), 774–775.

Shin, S., Cho, S. H., Park, D., & Jung, E., (2020). Anti-skin aging properties of protocatechuic acid *in vitro* and *in vivo*. *Journal of Cosmetic Dermatology*, *19*(4), 977–984.

Shojania, H. R., Momeni-Moghaddam, M., Hossini, S. E., Armin, M., & Omrani, B. J., (2019). MicroRNA 155 downregulation by vitamin c-loaded human serum albumin nanoparticles during cutaneous wound healing in mice. *The International Journal of Lower Extremity Wounds*, *18*(2), 143–152.

Singh, D., Fisher, J., Shagalov, D., Varma, A., & Siegel, D. M., (2018). Dangerous plants in dermatology: Legal and controlled. *Clinics in Dermatology*, *36*(3), 399–419.

Singh, K. N., Patil, S., & Barkate, H., (2020). Protective effects of astaxanthin on skin: Recent scientific evidence, possible mechanisms, and potential indications. *Journal of Cosmetic Dermatology*, *19*(1), 22–27.

Sohn, A., Frankel, A., Patel, R. V., & Goldenberg, G., (2011). Eczema. *Mt Sinai J Med*, *78*(5), 730–739. https://doi.org/10.1002/msj.20289.

Solanki, R., (2011). Treatment of skin diseases through medicinal plants in different regions of the world. *Int. J. Biomed. Res.*, *2*(1), 73.

Sood, R., & Chopra, D. S., (2018). Optimization of reaction conditions to fabricate *Ocimum sanctum* synthesized silver nanoparticles and its application to nano-gel systems for burn wounds. *Materials Science and Engineering: C.*, *92*, 575–589.

Souto, E. B., De Souza, A. L., Dos Santos, F. K., Sanchez-Lopez, E., Cano, A., Zielińska, A., & Chorilli, M., (2021). Lipid nanocarriers for hyperproliferative skin diseases. *Cancers*, *13*(22), 5619.

Stamford, N. P. J., (2012). Stability, transdermal penetration, and cutaneous effects of ascorbic acid and its derivatives. *Journal of Cosmetic Dermatology*, *11*(4), 310–317.

Suryawati, N., & Jawi, I. M. (2020). *Potential Development of Turmeric Extract Nanoparticles as a Topical Anti-Inflammatory Agent. 9*(3), 10–21.

Szymański, Ł., Skopek, R., Palusińska, M., Schenk, T., Stengel, S., Lewicki, S., & Zelent, A., (2020). Retinoic acid and its derivatives in skin. *Cells*, *9*(12), 2660.

Tang, T., Yin, L., Yang, J., & Shan, G., (2007). Emodin, an anthraquinone derivative from *Rheum officinale* Baill, enhances cutaneous wound healing in rats. *European Journal of Pharmacology*, *567*(3), 177–185.

Teo, C. W. L., Tay, S. H. Y., Tey, H. L., Ung, Y. W., & Yap, W. N., (2021). Vitamin E in atopic dermatitis: From preclinical to clinical studies. *Dermatology*, *237*(4), 553–564. https://doi.org/10.1159/000510653.

Tyler, V. E., (1993). *A Sensible Guide to the Use of Herbs and Related Remedies*. Haworth Press, Incorporated.

Vollono, L., Falconi, M., Gaziano, R., Iacovelli, F., Dika, E., Terracciano, C., & Campione, E., (2019). Potential of curcumin in skin disorders. *Nutrients*, *11*(9), 2169.

Vyas, N., Keservani, R. K., Nayak, A., Jain, S., & Singhal, M., (2010). Effect of *Tamarindus indica* and *Curcuma longa* on stress induced alopecia. *Pharmacology Online, 1*, 377–384.

Williams, H. C., Dellavalle, R. P., & Garner, S., (2012). Acne vulgaris. *Lancet*, *379*(9813), 361–372. https://doi.org/10.1016/s0140-6736(11)60321-8.

Yamaguchi, Y., Nagasawa, T., Nakamura, N., Takenaga, M., Mizoguchi, M., Kawai, S. I., & Igarashi, R., (2005). Successful treatment of photo-damaged skin of nano-scale atRA particles using a novel transdermal delivery. *Journal of Controlled Release*, *104*(1), 29–40.

Youn, B. H., Kim, Y. S., Yoo, S., & Hur, M. H., (2021). Antimicrobial and hand hygiene effects of tea tree essential oil disinfectant: A randomized control trial. *International Journal of Clinical Practice*, *75*(8), e14206.

Zamarioli, C. M., Martins, R. M., Carvalho, E. C., & Freitas, L. A., (2015). Nanoparticles containing curcuminoids (*Curcuma longa*): Development of topical delivery formulation. *Revista Brasileira de Farmacognosia*, *25*, 53–60.

Zhang, P., He, L., Zhang, J., Mei, X., Zhang, Y., Tian, H., & Chen, Z., (2020). Preparation of novel berberine nano-colloids for improving wound healing of diabetic rats by acting Sirt1/NF-κB pathway. *Colloids and Surfaces B: Biointerfaces*, *187*, 110647.

CHAPTER 12

Biodegradable Nanoparticles to Skin Diseases

EKNATH D. AHIRE,[1] RAJ K. KESERVANI,[2] and SANJAY J. KSHIRSAGAR[1]

[1]*Department of Pharmaceutics, MET's Institute of Pharmacy, Bhujbal Knowledge City, Affiliated to Savitribai Phule Pune University, Adgaon, Nashik, Maharashtra, India*

[2]*Faculty of B. Pharmacy, CSM Group of Institutions, Prayagraj, Uttar Pradesh, India*

ABSTRACT

Biodegradable polymeric substances are perfect carrier structures for distinct biomedical applications. Features like controlled and sustained delivery, stepped forward drug pharmacokinetics, decreased facet results and secure degradation make the usage of those substances very attractive in lots of clinical fields, with dermatology included. A variety of research have proven that particle-primarily based totally formulations can enhance the pores and skin penetration of topically implemented drugs. However, for a successful translation of these promising consequences right into a scientific application, a greater rational technique is wanted to recall the distinct homes of diseased pores and skin and the destiny of those polymeric substances after topical application. Higher expertise of such mechanisms has the capacity to enhance the efficacy of service-primarily based totally dermal therapy. Such expertise could permit the knowledgeable desire of the kind of biodegradable service relying at the pores and skin situation to be treated, the kind of drug to be loaded, and the favored launch kinetics. Furthermore, higher manipulate of polymer degradation and launch homes according with the pores and skin surroundings could enhance the protection and selectivity of drug launch.

Novel Nanocarriers forSkin Diseases: Advances and Applications.
Raj K. Keservani and Júlia Scherer Santos (Eds.)

This overview objectives at summarizing the modern-day expertise on how polymeric shipping structures have interaction with healthful and diseased pores and skin, giving a top-level view of the demanding situations that distinct pathological pores and skin situations pose to the improvement of more secure and greater particular dermal therapies.

12.1 INTRODUCTION

Nanotechnology gives a sizeable opportunity to enhance shipping, bioavailability, and concentration on of medicine and cosmetics to pores and skin. Considering the coolest accessibility of pores and skin, the opportunity to deal with pores and skin problems via way of topical treatment plans may be very appealing (Keservani et al., 2019). This approach of management will increase affected person compliance, reduce aspect effects, avoid the hepatic first by skip metabolism, hereby improving the quantity of drug on the site of action, and will assist in lessening the dose required to reap healing effects (Saranya & Radha, 2014). Supramolecular drug delivery systems (DDS) implemented topically to diseased pores and skin need to gather and launch the drug on the site of action. In diseased pores and skin, due to impaired stratum corneum (SC) and/or activated immune system, the penetration of macromolecules and particulate substances is regularly altered with recognize to wholesome pores and skin. Thus, to keep away from viable aspect effects, the use and improvement of biodegradable and biocompatible nanomaterials is necessary. In medicine, the time period biodegradable describes materials recent advances in the area of nanotechnology has allowed the production of elaborated nanometer-sized debris for diverse biomedical programs (Hans & Lowman, 2002). A huge spectrum of debris, extending from diverse lipid nanostructures inclusive of liposomes and strong lipid nanoparticles to metal, nanocrystalline, and polymer debris have already been examined as drug shipping structures in special animal fashions with notable results, promising an in-depth commercialization inside the coming years. Controlled drug launch to pores and skin and pores and skin appendages, concentrated on hair follicle-unique mobile populations, transcutaneous vaccination, and transdermal gene remedy are just a few of those new programs. Carrier structures of the brand new era take benefit of progressed pores and skin penetration properties, depot impact with sustained drug launch and of floor functionalization (e.g., the binding to unique ligands) permitting unique cell and subcellular concentrated on. Drug career via skin by microparticles and nanocarriers may want to revolutionize the remedy of numerous pores and skin problems. However, the toxicological and environmental protection of micro-and nanoparticles needs to be evaluated by the use of unique toxicological research previous toa much wider implementation of the brand-new technology (Zhang et al., 2013; Kayser et al., 2005).

These assessment ambitions to provide a top-level view of the maximum investigated programs of transcutaneously implemented particle-primarily based totally formulations withinside the fields of cosmetics and dermatology. The time period particle derives from the Latin phrase particular, because of this that a small part. A particle is consequently described as a small item that behaves as an entire unit. Particles at the nanometer scale are normally defined as nanoparticles (Berthet et al., 2017; Shinde et al., 2012). Currently, there's no global standard definition concerning their dimensions, even though the British Standards Institution (BSI) set a 100 nm because the top restriction and 1 nm because of the decrease restriction. Particles with size over this restriction are taken into consideration microparticles. An extraordinary type of substances inclusive of polymers, lipids, metals, and ceramics had been used so far, and loads of shapes had been engineered to create particulate pills or drug shipping structures (DDS). There are some opportunities to categorize and list nanoparticle types (Couvreur, 2013; Kumari, Yadav, & Yadav, 2010).

Particles may be divided into natural and inorganic, or they may be categorized in keeping with their form, size, floor fee, and physicochemical properties. Nevertheless, from the factor of view of particle interactions with organic surfaces and limitations like pores and skin, it is able to be beneficial to differentiate between gentle and inflexible debris (Badilli et al., 2018; Desai & Shah, 2013). In general, gentle debris is the product of natural substances (e.g., lipids, proteins, polymers) and may briefly adjust their form via way of pressure or touch with surfaces, even as stable particles are the product of inorganic substances and aren't deformable (Badri et al., 2014).

12.2 TYPES OF BIODEGRADABLE MATERIALS IN NANOPARTICULATE DRUG DELIVERY SYSTEM (DDS)

Liposomes were the first delivery systems to be studied and promoted for dermatological and esthetic uses. After that, nanostructured lipid carriers (NLC) and SLNs were created (Keservani et al., 2017a, 2020a; Sharma et al., 2018), which may be stronger, have larger pores, and have skin penetration. More and more polymeric carriers have been looked into in recent years for topical drug delivery. Benefits of using biodegradable polymers over lipid-based suppliers (Locatelli & Franchini, 2012). Each hydrophobic and hydrophilic capsule may be encapsulated or adsorbed, they may be functionalized, but most importantly, their physicochemical properties may be properly tuned to ensure a controlled release of the encapsulated medicine. They may be stored over months. Different types of polymer-based fully DDS have been tested for medication delivery. In tissue engineering, polymeric fibers are used as scaffolds for tissue rebuilding and wound healing. Collagen, hyaluronic acid, and poly(-caprolactone) (PCL) are a few polymers that are utilized to construct organic matrixes (Mobaraki et al., 2020). They might be packed with angiogenic or growth-promoting agents to encourage tissue renewal or antimicrobials to prevent wound infection. Hydrogels are made up of hydrophilic molecules, or "gelling agents," that can form a three-dimensional community by chemically or physically cross-linking with one another and soaking up excessive amounts of water (Pathak et al., 2019). Alginate, chitosan, dextran, as well as synthetic materials like poly(ethylene glycol) (PEG) and poly(lactic acid-glycolic acid) (PLGA) or a blend of both can be used to make hydrogels. They have been extensively researched for drug delivery in medicine and may be loaded with several capsules, particularly hydrophilic ones. Organogels are networks of gelling agents that can contain oil or natural solvents (Bala & Kumar, 2004). Polymers like poly(ethylene) and PEG, in addition to copolymers of methacrylic acid and methyl methacrylate (MMA), are generally used. These polymers are non-biodegradable however are taken into consideration biocompatible; due to their lipophilic nature, they could comprise hydrophobic capsules and feature higher pores and skin penetration (Brannon-Peppas, 1995; Gou et al., 2008). Additionally, hydrogels have been employed as a delivery system for wound healing and to disseminate nanocarriers, enhancing their dispersion at the skin's pores and skin's surface. Organogels and hydrogels on a nanoscale are called nanogels. It is possible to construct nanogels stimulus-responsive by using the right linkers (e.g., temperature, pH, light). Thus, the release of encapsulated capsules may be controlled by taking use of the specific characteristics of sick skin and pores or even by employing an external trigger (Hans & Lowman, 2002; George, Shah, & Shrivastav, 2019).

12.3 MECHANISM OF ACTION AFTER DERMAL APPLICATION

12.3.1 INTERFERENCE WITH STRATUM CORNEUM (SC)

The protein-rich cells that make up the SC are encased in a lipid extracellular matrix. The bricks and mortar concept has been used to describe this organization. Additionally, intercellular protein networks called corneodesmosomes help attach corneocytes to one another. Macromolecules and supramolecular carriers interact with this extremely complex barrier in diverse ways depending on their make-up, size, and form (Abd-Allah et al., 2020; Puglia et al., 2008). According to a theory, polymeric particles may interact differently with the extracellular lipids of the SC than lipid-based totally debris because they are more hydrophilic and have a tendency to blend with skin lipid layers. Although the lipids of the SC do not fuse with the additions of polymeric businesses, the interaction with the SC can also extrude their three-dimensional structure, which can lead to adsorption, instability, or agglomeration (Bolzinger et al., 2011). Additionally, the SC is covered in sebum, which is rich in lipids and proteins and interacts with the polymeric materials to destabilize them or alter how they interact with various skin additives. Numerous different commensal microbe species can interact with installed materials because they are found at the skin's surface, in its furrows, and on its appendages. The SC's surface has a pH between 4.2 and 5.6. The stability of particles' colloidal systems can be impacted by a pH this acidic (Patzelt & Lademann, 2020). The rate of hydrolysis and the activity of pH-sensitive enzymes are both accelerated by the acidic pH, which may hasten the destruction of polymeric particles. Finally, because the SC is a continually developing structure, it is possible to differentiate a looser element close to a more compact region (stratum compactum) due to desquamation processes (stratum disjuncture). By shedding the topmost layers, items accumulated in the stratum disjuncture are quickly eliminated, and the SC can serve as a repository for particulate materials that penetrate deeper (Rancan, 2016; Korting & Schäfer-Korting, 2010).

12.3.2 HAIR FOLLICLE ROUTE

The pilosebaceous unit's hair follicle canal serves as a reservoir for material with a diameter of micron, submicron, and nanometer. It took some time before the hair follicle was recognized as a potential skin penetration gateway. Although hair follicle orifices make up only 0.1% of the skin's surface, it was once believed that sebum prevented materials from penetrating the hair follicle canal. The significance of the transfollicular pathway, particularly for the preferential penetration of particulate elements, was only partially established by studies over the course of the following decade. For days before they can be removed, particles that collect inside the hair follicle are protected from SC turnover (Lohanin et al., 2014; Patzelt & Lademann, 2020). The interaction surface of the hair follicle infundibulum has been calculated to be roughly 0.068 cm^2 for empty or complete follicles, respectively. The size of the hair follicle orifices levels between 17,270 m in terminal hair follicles and 8,637 m in vellus hair follicles (Patzelt & Lademann, 2015). As a result, the hair follicle infundibulum constitutes not just a reservoir but also a sizable surface area where interaction between accumulated material and skin systems might take place. The hair follicle serves as a shunt for extremely quick substance penetration. In individuals with open hair follicles, the compounds used in the experiment attained equal blood values when the hair follicle orifices were selectively closed (Knorr et al., 2009; Fang et al., 2014). This is likely due to the fact that the SC barrier is thinner inside the deep infundibulum, where molecules can diffuse more unexpectedly than at the skin's surface where the SC has several more layers (Chenthamara et al., 2019). Additionally, the drug is released by the one's suppliers gathered inside the hair follicle canal, resulting in an excessive local concentration of the drug that acts as a riding pressure for its diffusion to the potential pores and skin. The removal of the contents of the hair follicles (sebum, cell debris, and ultimately germs) makes it easier for topically applied particle materials to penetrate the skin (Rancan et al., 2013).

12.3.3 TRANSLOCATION THROUGHOUT THE STRATUM CORNEUM (SC)

It is generally accepted that most effective lipophilic molecules with a molecular weight under 500 Dalton can bypass the skin barrier, while the penetration of hydrophilic molecules, macromolecules, and nanoparticles is significantly hindered, even though the discussion regarding the translocation of particulate material throughout the SC isn't yet closed (Rancan et al., 2009). There is no evidence to support the translocation of all debris across the intact SC of healthy skin, despite the fact that liposomes, potent lipid nanoparticles, and polymeric DDS have been shown to improve the skin penetration of loaded material. Instead, it appears that some of the lipid-based total particles' constituent parts dissolve into the lipids of the SC, increasing its permeability (Knorr et al., 2019). Most of the studies cited in this text observed the released fluorochrome (or medication) in the case of polymer-based carriers, but only a few studies attempted to determine the fate of the carrier following topical application, hence in formation at penetration through the SC are negative (Nohynek et al., 2008). By using transmission electron microscopy (TEM), these biocompatible carriers have in fact been found inside the acceptor liquid of the Franz diffusion cell. The lipid matrix and corneodesmosomes may be damaged by heating epidermal sheets at 60°C, therefore those effects only apply to partial thickness skin (Gwinn & Vallyathan, 2006; Patzelt & Lademann, 2020).

12.3.4 MATERIAL DIFFUSION ACROSS DISTURB SKIN BARRIERS

The specific characteristics of skin that is ill should be taken into account when growing DDS for skin illnesses. In contrast to how particle carriers in healthy skin penetrate the SC and the hair follicle canals, releasing the loaded medications there, carrier structures in ill skin, where the integrity of the SC is compromised, may breach the SC barrier and enter the dermis and epidermis (Badri et al., 2014). There have been a number of methods developed to avoid the SC, such as disturbing it using sticky tapes and abrasion, altering it with permeabilizing chemicals, or using microneedles. Most of the methods had been tested for transcutaneous medication delivery or immunization procedures (Gul et al., 2018). The penetration of particles through diseased animal or human skin was only lightly studied in studies. In actuality, the majority of animal researchers focus on the efficacy and diffusion of the released medications rather than the fate of the utilized carrier materials. The majority of writers discovered that diseased skin had much higher drug permeability than healthy skin. These effects are shown by the tissue swelling and the rapid intercellular fluid within the dermis, which may control the tight junction structure (Ghasemiyeh & Mohammadi-Samani, 2020). There was, however, no concrete proof of nanoparticle transfer. In general, researchers who examine the use of mechanical or ultraviolet (UV) irradiation to jolt the immune system and disturb the SC have confirmed that topically applied nanoparticles can be found inside the possible skin layers. Once particles have crossed the SC, they may also reach the subcutaneous lymph nodes through passive transport after the lymph outflow or by being picked up by pores and skin antigen-offering cells. These results highlight the need for a similar understanding of the interactions and outcome of the carrier system following topical administration to sick skin (Desai et al., 2010; Hasanovic, 2010).

12.3.5 CELLULAR UPTAKE

A carrier system or medicine can diffuse across the extracellular space or be absorbed through dermis and epidermis cells once it has successfully penetrated the skin barrier and reached the practicable epidermis layers

(Choi et al., 2014). Small amphiphilic particles can pass across the cell membrane, while macromolecules including proteins and nucleic acids, as well as nano- and submicron-sized materials, can only be ingested by means of cells through the energy-based endocytosis mechanism. The most useful positive cell types can often swallow particles longer than 200 nm (Suh et al., 1998). For instance, we found that the nimblest dendritic cells absorbed each particle when dendritic cells and T-cells were co-cultured and treated with fluorescently categorized bacteria and polystyrene particles (200 nm). The Langerhans cells in the dermis are cells that are skilled in absorbing particles that penetrate through a compromised skin barrier (Jung et al., 2000). Additionally, keratinocytes, which make up 90% of the dermis' cells, have the ability to internalize chemicals that have pierced the skin. However, *in vitro* studies using newly removed epidermal cells showed that keratinocytes are substantially less prone than Langerhans cells to ingest particles depending on the article length (Panyam & Labhasetwar, 2003). Cells including fibroblasts, mast cells, and T-cells are in contact with penetrated material in the dermis. The most likely cells to ingest them are dendritic cells and macrophages, though. Once ingested, the carrier systems can degrade inside the lysosomes' acidic and hydrolytic environment, releasing the medicine that was loaded. Although the same activities can be harmful for positively loaded molecules like proteins or nucleic acids, hydrolysis, and enzymatic degradation can be used as a mechanism for medication release. It is necessary to establish endosomal break-out to prevent degradation. On the other hand, it is desirable to absorb antigen-loaded carriers by the use of antigen-imparting cells and their intracellular breakdown for vaccination purposes (Benfer & Kissel, 2012; Fenton et al., 2018).

12.4 BIOMATERIAL DEGRADATION AND DRUG RELEASE

Depending on the nature of the polymer, polymeric biomaterials can be destroyed after applied to the skin's surface utilizing chemical and/or enzymatic reactions. Proteases, esterases, glycosidases, and phosphatases are examples of hydrolytic enzymes that can facilitate the water-mediated breaking of a variety of chemical bonds (Jo et al., 2009; Langer et al., 1990). The release of the loaded medicine frequently exhibits non-linear kinetics, and the breakdown of polymer particles is typically a difficult process. Additionally, the polymer's breakdown may damage the loaded pharmaceuticals or otherwise interfere with the drug's release, either inhibiting or speeding it. A biodegradable polymer should ideally break down into non-toxic byproducts and disintegrate under controlled conditions. By doing this, the drug's selectivity and efficacy are improved in addition to the protection it offers. For instance, the drug-carrier bond may be hydrolyzed by adding linkers that can be broken down by enzymes that are mostly found inside the target cell or the diseased tissue (Commandeur et al., 2006). These methods are prompted through skin parameters like temperature, pH, and protein concentration (Pritchard & Kaplan, 2011). Additionally, including degrading enzymes inside the polymer matrix is viable. When and where the service degrades and the drug is released depends on the type of polymer, the nature of interactions between the drug and polymer, and the drug's affinity for skin additives (Liow et al., 2016). After entering the SC, after entering the epidermis and dermis, or best after cell absorption, polymers may simply be hydrolyzed. A loaded medicine may also be released by other methods, such as conformational alterations of the particles (destabilization, swelling, or shrinkage). When applied topically, medications that have been adsorbed at the carrier surface can be released either through affinity-driven diffusion or an alternative method involving skin additives such proteins. It appears that the carriers' physicochemical characteristics are critical for drug release and diffusion (Prestwich & Luo, 2001; Deshayes & Kasko, 2013).

12.5 CONCLUSION

The effectiveness and advantages of biodegradable polymeric materials as carriers or delivery systems in dermatology have been supported by numerous studies. These compounds are safe and offer ways to improve carrier systems specifically designed for each individual dermatological illness. Future research must be aware of more specific information about the interactions between polymeric provider structures and the skin environment in order to achieve this goal. Drug permeation and efficacy assessments must be supplemented with precise studies on supplier skin penetration, uptake through the skin cells, degradation mechanism, drug release, as well as toxicological aspects. Additionally, it is crucial that these studies be conducted using skin and pore models of the specific clinical disorders that need to be treated. To improve the selectivity and specificity of drug administration, it will be possible to modify polymeric materials by examining how delivery systems interact with damaged skin barriers or activated immune systems. The vast capacity of those biodegradable and flexible materials is demonstrated by the fact that new polymer-based carrier systems are being developed and by the great range in their dermatological programs that is always expanding.

ACKNOWLEDGMENTS

We, thank the MET, Institute of Pharmacy, BKC, affiliated under Savitribai Phule Pune University, Nashik, for their constant support and providing all facilities to complete this work. We are also thankful to the Ministry of Tribal Affairs Government of India for providing financial assistance in the form of a fellowship (Award No.: 202021-NFST-MAH-01235).

KEYWORDS

- **biodegradable nanoparticles**
- **biomaterial degradation**
- **dermal application**
- **hair follicles**
- **material diffusion**
- **nanocarriers**
- **skin barriers**
- **skin penetration**

REFERENCES

Abd-Allah, H., Abdel-Aziz, R. T., & Nasr, M., (2020). Chitosan nanoparticles making their way to clinical practice: A feasibility study on their topical use for acne treatment. *International Journal of Biological Macromolecules, 156,* 262–270.

Badilli, U., Gumustas, M., Uslu, B., & Ozkan, S. A., (2018). Lipid-based nanoparticles for dermal drug delivery. In: *Organic Materials as Smart Nanocarriers for Drug Delivery* (pp. 369–413). William Andrew Publishing.

Badri, W., Eddabra, R., Fessi, H., & Elaissari, A., (2014). Biodegradable polymer-based nanoparticles: Dermal and transdermal drug delivery. *Journal of Colloid Science and Biotechnology*, *3*(2), 141–149.

Bala, I., Hariharan, S., & Kumar, M. R., (2004). PLGA nanoparticles in drug delivery: The state of the art. *Critical Reviews™ in Therapeutic Drug Carrier Systems*, *21*(5).

Benfer, M., & Kissel, T., (2012). Cellular uptake mechanism and knockdown activity of siRNA-loaded biodegradable DEAPA-PVA-g-PLGA nanoparticles. *European Journal of Pharmaceutics and Biopharmaceutics, 80*(2), 247–256.

Berthet, M., Gauthier, Y., Lacroix, C., Verrier, B., & Monge, C., (2017). Nanoparticle-based dressing: The future of wound treatment? *Trends in Biotechnology, 35*(8), 770–784.

Bolzinger, M. A., Briançon, S., & Chevalier, Y., (2011). Nanoparticles through the skin: Managing conflicting results of inorganic and organic particles in cosmetics and pharmaceutics. *Wiley Interdisciplinary Reviews: Nanomedicine and Nanobiotechnology, 3*(5), 463–478.

Brannon-Peppas, L., (1995). Recent advances on the use of biodegradable microparticles and nanoparticles in controlled drug delivery. *International Journal of Pharmaceutics, 116*(1), 1–9.

Chenthamara, D., Subramaniam, S., Ramakrishnan, S. G., Krishnaswamy, S., Essa, M. M., Lin, F. H., & Qoronfleh, M. W., (2019). Therapeutic efficacy of nanoparticles and routes of administration. *Biomaterials Research, 23*(1), 1–29.

Choi, J. S., Cao, J., Naeem, M., Noh, J., Hasan, N., Choi, H. K., & Yoo, J. W., (2014). Size-controlled biodegradable nanoparticles: Preparation and size-dependent cellular uptake and tumor cell growth inhibition. *Colloids and Surfaces B: Biointerfaces, 122,* 545–551.

Commandeur, S., Van, B. H. M., & Van, D. G. W. J., (2006). Polymers, drug release, and drug-eluting stents. *Journal of Interventional Cardiology, 19*(6), 500–506.

Couvreur, P., (2013). Nanoparticles in drug delivery: Past, present, and future. *Advanced Drug Delivery Reviews, 65*(1), 21–23.

Desai, D., & Shah, D., (2013). Implication of nanoparticles for controlled drug delivery system. *International Journal of Pharmaceutical Sciences and Research, 4*(7), 2478.

Desai, P., Patlolla, R. R., & Singh, M., (2010). Interaction of nanoparticles and cell-penetrating peptides with skin for transdermal drug delivery. *Molecular Membrane Biology, 27*(7), 247–259.

Deshayes, S., & Kasko, A. M., (2013). Polymeric biomaterials with engineered degradation. *Journal of Polymer Science Part A: Polymer Chemistry, 51*(17), 3531–3566.

Fang, C. L., Aljuffali, I. A., Li, Y. C., & Fang, J. Y., (2014). Delivery and targeting of nanoparticles into hair follicles. *Therapeutic Delivery, 5*(9), 991–1006.

Fenton, O. S., Olafson, K. N., Pillai, P. S., Mitchell, M. J., & Langer, R., (2018). Advances in biomaterials for drug delivery. *Advanced Materials, 30*(29), 1705328.

George, A., Shah, P. A., & Shrivastav, P. S., (2019). Natural biodegradable polymers-based nano-formulations for drug delivery: A review. *International Journal of Pharmaceutics, 561,* 244–264.

Ghasemiyeh, P., & Mohammadi-Samani, S., (2020). Potential of nanoparticles as permeation enhancers and targeted delivery options for skin: Advantages and disadvantages. *Drug Design, Development and Therapy, 14,* 3271.

Gou, M., Li, X., Dai, M., Gong, C., Wang, X., Xie, Y., Deng, H., et al., (2008). A novel injectable local hydrophobic drug delivery system: Biodegradable nanoparticles in thermo-sensitive hydrogel. *International Journal of Pharmaceutics, 359*(1, 2), 228–233.

Gul, R., Ahmed, N., Ullah, N., Khan, M. I., Elaissari, A., & Rehman, A., (2018). Biodegradable ingredient-based emulgel loaded with ketoprofen nanoparticles. *AAPS Pharmscitech, 19*(4), 1869–1881.

Gwinn, M. R., & Vallyathan, V., (2006). Nanoparticles: Health effects—Pros and cons. *Environmental Health Perspectives, 114*(12), 1818–1825.

Hans, M. L., & Lowman, A. M., (2002). Biodegradable nanoparticles for drug delivery and targeting. *Current Opinion in Solid State and Materials Science*, *6*(4), 319–327.

Hasanovic, A., (2010). *Nanoparticles of Biodegradable Polymers and DPPC Liposomes for Skin Diffusion Studies and Physicochemical Stabilization of the Incorporated Model Drugs.*

Jo, Y. S., Gantz, J., Hubbell, J. A., & Lutolf, M. P., (2009). Tailoring hydrogel degradation and drug release via neighboring amino acid-controlled ester hydrolysis. *Soft Matter*, *5*(2), 440–446.

Jung, T., Kamm, W., Breitenbach, A., Kaiserling, E., Xiao, J. X., & Kissel, T., (2000). Biodegradable nanoparticles for oral delivery of peptides: Is there a role for polymers to affect mucosal uptake? *European Journal of Pharmaceutics and Biopharmaceutics*, *50*(1), 147–160.

Kayser, O., Lemke, A., & Hernandez-Trejo, N., (2005). The impact of nanobiotechnology on the development of new drug delivery systems. *Current Pharmaceutical Biotechnology*, *6*(1), 3–5.

Keservani, R. K., Bandopadhyay, S., Bandyopadhyay, N., & Sharma, A. K., (2020a). Design and fabrication of transdermal/skin drug-delivery system. In: *Drug Delivery Systems* (pp. 131–178). Academic Press.

Keservani, R. K., Kesharwani, R. K., & Sharma, A. K., (2017a). Introduction to nanotechnology in drug delivery. In: *Drug Delivery Approaches and Nanosystems* (pp. 1–19). Apple Academic Press. ISBN: 9781771885836.

Keservani, R. K., Sharma, A. K., & Kesharwani, R. K., (2019). *Nanocarriers for Brain Targeting: Principles and Applications*. CRC Press. ISBN:9781771887304.

Knorr, F., Lademann, J., Patzelt, A., Sterry, W., Blume-Peytavi, U., & Vogt, A., (2009). Follicular transport route–research progress and future perspectives. *European Journal of Pharmaceutics and Biopharmaceutics*, *71*(2), 173–180.

Knorr, F., Patzelt, A., Meinke, M. C., Vogt, A., Blume-Peytavi, U., Rühl, E., & Lademann, J., (2019). Interactions of nanoparticles with skin. In: *Biological Responses to Nanoscale Particles* (pp. 329–339). Springer, Cham.

Korting, H. C., & Schäfer-Korting, M., (2010). Carriers in the topical treatment of skin disease. *Drug Delivery*, 435–468.

Kumari, A., Yadav, S. K., & Yadav, S. C., (2010). Biodegradable polymeric nanoparticles-based drug delivery systems. *Colloids and Surfaces B: Biointerfaces*, *75*(1), 1–18.

Langer, R., Cima, L. G., Tamada, J. A., & Wintermantel, E., (1990). Future directions in biomaterials. *Biomaterials*, *11*(9), 738–745.

Liow, S. S., Dou, Q., Kai, D., Karim, A. A., Zhang, K., Xu, F., & Loh, X. J., (2016). Thermogels: In situ gelling biomaterial. *ACS Biomaterials Science & Engineering*, *2*(3), 295–316.

Locatelli, E., & Comes, F. M., (2012). Biodegradable PLGA-b-PEG polymeric nanoparticles: Synthesis, properties, and nanomedical applications as drug delivery system. *Journal of Nanoparticle Research*, *14*(12), 1–17.

Lohani, A., Verma, A., Joshi, H., Yadav, N., & Karki, N., (2014). Nanotechnology-based cosmeceuticals. *International Scholarly Research Notices*, *2014*.

Mobaraki, M., Soltani, M., Zare, H. S., Zoudani, E. L, Daliri, R., Aghamirsalim, M., & Raahemifar, K., (2020). Biodegradable nanoparticle for cornea drug delivery: Focus review. *Pharmaceutics*, *12*(12), 1232.

Nohynek, G. J., Dufour, E. K., & Roberts, M. S., (2008). Nanotechnology, cosmetics, and the skin: Is there a health risk? *Skin Pharmacology and Physiology*, *21*(3), 136–149.

Panyam, J., & Labhasetwar, V., (2003). Biodegradable nanoparticles for drug and gene delivery to cells and tissue. *Advanced Drug Delivery Reviews, 55*(3), 329–347.

Pathak, C., Vaidya, F. U., & Pandey, S. M., (2019). Mechanism for development of nanobased drug delivery system. *Applications of Targeted Nano Drugs and Delivery Systems*, 35–67.

Patzelt, A., & Lademann, J., (2015). The increasing importance of the hair follicle route in dermal and transdermal drug delivery. In: *Percutaneous Penetration Enhancers Chemical Methods in Penetration Enhancement* (pp. 43–53). Springer, Berlin, Heidelberg.

Patzelt, A., & Lademann, J., (2020). Recent advances in follicular drug delivery of nanoparticles. *Expert Opinion on Drug Delivery, 17*(1), 49–60.

Prestwich, G. D., & Luo, Y., (2001). Novel biomaterials for drug delivery. *Expert Opinion on Therapeutic Patents, 11*(9), 1395–1410.

Pritchard, E. M., & Kaplan, D. L., (2011). Silk fibroin biomaterials for controlled release drug delivery. *Expert Opinion on Drug Delivery, 8*(6), 797–811.

Puglia, C., Blasi, P., Rizza, L., Schoubben, A., Bonina, F., Rossi, C., & Ricci, M., (2008). Lipid nanoparticles for prolonged topical delivery: An *in vitro* and *in vivo* investigation. *International Journal of Pharmaceutics, 357*(1, 2), 295–304.

Rancan, F., (2016). Biodegradable, biocompatible, and bioconjugate materials as delivery agents in dermatology: Safe drug delivery to skin. In: *Nanoscience in Dermatology* (pp. 73–87). Academic Press.

Rancan, F., Afraz, Z., Combadiere, B., Blume-Peytavi, U., & Vogt, A., (2013). Hair follicle targeting with nanoparticles. In: *Nanotechnology in Dermatology* (pp. 95–107). Springer, New York, NY.

Rancan, F., Papakostas, D., Hadam, S., Hackbarth, S., Delair, T., Primard, C., Verrier, B., et al., (2009). Investigation of polylactic acid (PLA) nanoparticles as drug delivery systems for local dermatotherapy. *Pharmaceutical Research, 26*(8), 2027–2036.

Saranya, S., & Radha, K. V., (2014). Review of nanobiopolymers for controlled drug delivery. *Polymer-Plastics Technology and Engineering, 53*(15), 1636–1646.

Sharma, A. K., Keservani, R. K., & Keseharwani, R. K., (2018). *Nanobiomaterials: Applications in Drug Delivery*. CRC Press. ISBN:9781771885911.

Shinde, N. C., Keskar, N. J., & Argade, P. D., (2012). Nanoparticles: Advances in drug delivery systems. *Res. J. Pharm. Biol. Chem. Sci, 3*(1), 922–929.

Suh, H., Jeong, B., Liu, F., & Kim, S. W., (1998). Cellular uptake study of biodegradable nanoparticles in vascular smooth muscle cells. *Pharmaceutical Research, 15*(9), 1495.

Zhang, Z., Tsai, P. C., Ramezanli, T., & Michniak-Kohn, B. B., (2013). Polymeric nanoparticles-based topical delivery systems for the treatment of dermatological diseases. *Wiley Interdisciplinary Reviews: Nanomedicine and Nanobiotechnology, 5*(3), 205–218.

CHAPTER 13

Skin Topical Treatment Based on Nanotechnology

MEENAKSHI PANCHAL[1] and R. S. RAGHUWANSHI[2]

[1]*Department of Pharmaceutics, Corporate Institute of Pharmacy, Bhopal, Madhya Pradesh, India*

[2]*Department of Pharmaceutical Chemistry, Corporate Institute of Pharmacy, Bhopal, Madhya Pradesh, India*

ABSTRACT

The role of numerous functions of the human being skin is well identified. It works as an immune and sensory system that protects the human body from unsafe ecological impacts such as physical threats, mechanical, and chemical, reduces UV radiation effects, prevents moisture loss, and helps thermoregulation. Nano-systems support numerous rewards, attending to the opportunity of controlled active ingredient release, superior skin permeation, and lower skin irritation. However, a novel nano-technological outlook for acne treatment and care can provide new side effects, but also environmental nano-pollution. Nanotechnology-based formulations are little acknowledged about the toxicology, for that reason, as outlook, additional studies should be conducted to ensure the consumers' health and environmental safety.

13.1 INTRODUCTION

13.1.1 SKIN

The largest part of the body is the skin which is made of water, fat minerals, and proteins. The role of skin as a safeguard for your body from microorganisms and normalizes body temperature. Also, feel the sensation of cold

Novel Nanocarriers forSkin Diseases: Advances and Applications.
Raj K. Keservani and Júlia Scherer Santos (Eds.)

and hot with the help of nerves in the skin. Your skin, along with your hair, nails, oil glands, and sweat glands are included in the integumentary system (Antonio et al., 2014).

Human skin is composed by three following layers (Paiva-Santos et al., 2021):

- epidermis (top layer);
- dermis (middle layer); and
- hypodermis (bottom or fatty layer).

13.1.1.1 EPIDERMIS (TOP LAYER OF SKIN)

The outmost layer of skin is the epidermis (Figure 13.1). This layer grants a waterproof barrier and tone of our skin (Jackson et al., 2013). It works as a protective barrier against rain, sun rays, and other fundamentals and also protects against infectious bacteria and germs in our organ and blood vessel. The epidermis continually makes new skin cells by replacing the old skin cells that your body blows every day. You have new skin every 30 days.

- **Properties:**
  - **Protects Your Body:** The epidermis layer consists of Langerhans cells. It helps to fight again germs and infection. This layer is part of our immune system.
  - **Provides Skin Color:** Its layer contains melanin pigment which gives the color of our skin. The color of skin, hair, and eyes determines the amount of melanin pigment. Darker skin and more quickly sun tanning people make more melanin.

13.1.1.2 DERMIS (MIDDLE LAYER OF SKIN)

Around 90% of the thickness of the skin is mainly composed of the dermis. This middle layer of skin. Under the epidermis, in the dermis, are sweat glands, hair follicles, and rough connective tissue. Contains elastin and collagen: Protein collagen gives skin cells their strength and resiliency. Elastin, another protein that is present in the dermis, makes skin flexible. It also aids in the form recovery of stretched skin.

- **Properties:**
  - **Grows Hair:** The dermis and hair follicle roots are connected.

- **Keeps You in Touch:** You can also detect pain thanks to these nerve receptors. Dermal nerves alert you when something is very hot, irritating, or extremely soft.
- **Makes Oil:** Oil glands in the dermis help the skin stay supple and smooth. Furthermore, oil keeps moist skin from clenching when you swim or are otherwise immersed in a heavy downpour.
- **Produces Sweat:** With the aid of skin pores, perspiration is secreted by sweat glands, helping to regulate body temperature.
- **Supplies Blood:** Skin layers maintain their health due to the nutrients that blood veins in the dermis provide to the epidermis.

13.1.1.3 HYPODERMIS (BOTTOM LAYER OF SKIN)

A deeper subcutaneous tissue comprised of connective tissue and fat, the hypodermis. The pigments that give skin its color, melanin, are produced by melanocyte cells. The epidermis is where melanocytes are found (Stefanov et al., 2002). The fatty layer is located in the hypodermis, the skin's lowermost layer.

➢ **Properties:**

- Muscles and bones are cushioned by the hypodermis, which contains fat, when you fall or are involved in an accident.
- Contains connective tissue, which joins the skin's layers to the muscles and bones.
- Aids the nerves and blood vessels: In the hypodermis, the middle layer of the dermis, the nerves and blood vessels grow larger. These blood vessels and nerves form the link between the hypodermis and the rest of the body.
- Controls body temperature: The hypodermis's fat prevents you from becoming too hot or cold (Singh et al., 2021).

13.2 NANOTECHNOLOGY

Father of nanotechnology and physicist Richard Feynman Chemistry, biology, physics, materials science, engineering, and other science subjects can all employ nanoscience and nanotechnology to investigate and create incredibly small objects (Panchal et al., 2021). The study of atomic or molecular particles, whose dimensions are measured in nanometers, is known as nanoscience. Around 1 billionth of a meter is known as a nanometer.

Therefore, nanotechnology may be characterized as a collection of procedures and strategies for dispersing materials at the atomic and molecular size to produce goods with unique physicochemical properties in comparison to conventional goods. In contrast, nanobiotechnology deals with the alteration of parts on the biomolecular nanoscale and with tools for investigating it both at the molecular and cellular levels (DeLouise et al., 2012).

Defining Nanotechnology (nanotechnology) The lack of agreement on what constitutes nanotechnology is one of the issues this technology faces. Most focus on understanding and manipulating phenomena and materials with length scales less than 100 nm, and frequently draw comparisons to human hair, which is between 50,000 and 1,00,000 nm in width (Uchechi et al., 2014).

13.2.1 NANOSCIENCE

Nanoscience is the study of materials with typical sizes between 1 and 100 nm. A nanoscience inquiry focuses on the fundamental relationships between physical properties and material dimensions. Nanoscience does not include parts of physics, chemistry, engineering, or biology. Nanoscience is the study of phenomena in systems with nanometer-scale dimensions. Year 2020 will see Mingyue et al. Nanoparticles are defined as particles with a size between 1 and 100 nm (Poole et al., 2003).

13.2.2 NANOWIRES

A nanoscale rod of semiconducting material used in miniature transistors and some laser applications (Madkour et al., 2019).

- **Characteristics of Nanoparticles:**
  - High fraction of atoms/molecules on the surface;
  - Large surface-to-volume ratio;
  - High fraction of atoms/molecules on the surface; large surface-to-volume ratio; (Esposito et al., 2019);
  - Light scattering and plasmon resonance characteristics of metal nanoparticles are distinctive;
  - The electronic band structure of semiconductor nanoparticles may show restricted energy states (e.g., quantum dotes);
  - Can have distinctive physical and chemical characteristics;
  - Shares the same size scale as numerous biological structures (Yetisgin et al., 2020).

13.3 CLASSIFICATION OF NANOTECHNOLOGY-BASED ON SIGNIFICANT USAGES (FIGURE 13.1)

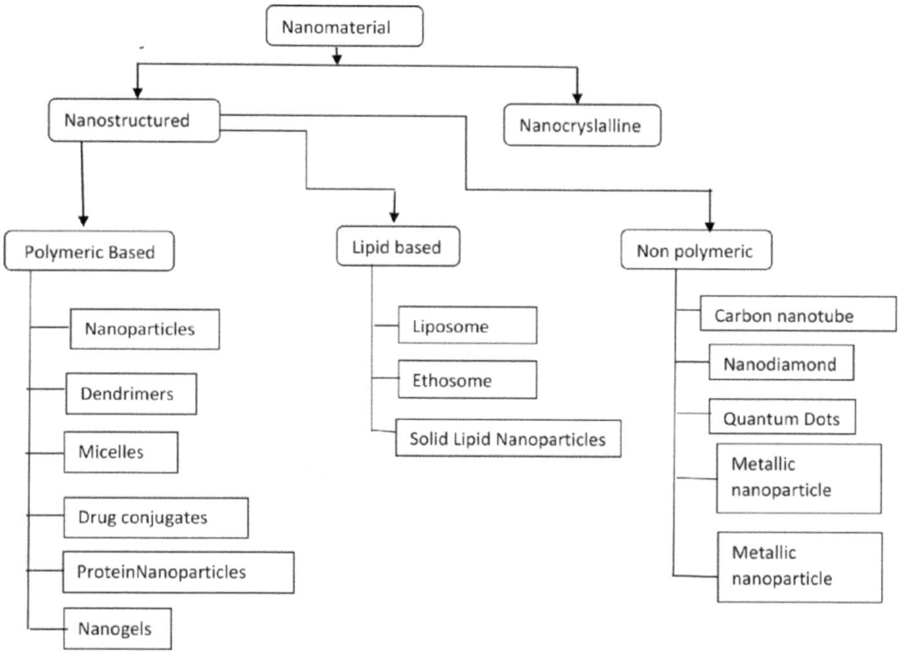

FIGURE 13.1 Elements of nanotechnology, which are utilized in therapeutic applications.
Source: Adapted from Khan et al., 2019

13.4 SKIN BARRIER AND PERMEABILITY

The stratum corneum (SC), the skin's outermost layer, contains the primary barrier. Corneocytes and lipid areas enclose the SC. The structure and makeup of the lipid component are thought to be crucial for the function of the skin barrier since the majority of medications applied to the skin infuse along the lipid domains. Cholesterol, free fatty acids, and long chain ceramides are typically found in this layer (Paiva-Santos et al., 2021). The low pH, the presence of enzymes on the skin, and the transdermal concentration gradient are additional defensive characteristics of the SC that have a detrimental effect on skin penetration. Size, shape, superficial charges, lipophilicity, the presence of penetration enhancers, formulation type, and SC physical state all influence how well topically applied substances penetrate the skin (Lohani, Alka et al., 2014).

13.5 PARTICULATE INTRA- AND TRANSDERMAL DELIVERY SYSTEMS

It has proven successful to target medications or vaccines to specific areas of skin, improve the penetration of those substances into the skin, and control the *in-situ* release of those substances using nano- and micron-sized carriers. Drug absorption into the skin in particle formulations is controlled by physical-chemical characteristics of the carrier, including size, surface area, charge pH, and solubility, and is also influenced by the solvent's properties and chemical makeup. The effects of size and charge are two of these parameters that have been extensively researched. The deepest penetration of particles into hair follicles occurs at the 300–600 nm size range, and they can be stored there for a lot longer than in the SC. Additionally, the biological activity and skin penetration of nanoparticles depend on their form and biological adhesiveness (Castro et al., 2020).

13.5.1 LIPID NANOPARTICLES

Solid lipid nanoparticles (SLNs), nanostructured lipid carriers (NLCs), nano-emulsions (NEs), vesicular nano-systems, and cubosomes (CUBs) are examples of lipid nanoparticles that exhibit sustained active ingredient release over an extended period of time, protection from active ingredient degradation, good admissibility, and physicochemical stability. The ability of lipid nanoparticles to form a thin film on the skin's surface, which encourages greater water retention in the skin layers and keeps the skin more hydrous, distinguishes them from other particles. This hydration process, in turn, permits a better penetration of the formulations through the skin (Hua, Susan et al., 2015).

13.5.2 SOLID LIPID NANOPARTICLES (SLNS)

Solid nanoparticles of lipid SLNs are sub-micron colloidal carriers with sizes ranging from 50 to 1,000 nm. They are made of an amphiphilic surfactant with surfactants between 0.5% and 5% (w/w) in the outer core and a biocompatible lipid core with lipids between 0.1% and 30% (w/w) in the inner core that is solid at body and room temperatures. Since lipids are the primary constituent of SLNs, they define the colloidal properties and are responsible for the SLNs' tiny size, controlled active ingredient release, good skin permeability, and high active ingredient loading. Wax, glycerol esters, and free fatty acids are the most often utilized solid lipids (Singh et al., 2015).

13.5.3 NANOSTRUCTURED LIPID CARRIERS (NLCS)

Nanostructured lipid carriers (NLCs) are very similar to SLNs. However, NLCs have a liquid lipid content entrenched within the solid lipid matrix, allowing superior active ingredient loading and better stability. This can be explained since NLCs do not allow recrystallization of solid lipids, and consequently, the size during the storage time remains almost unaffected. The carriers are mostly composed of nontoxic and biodegradable blends of solid and liquid lipids and nanoparticles (NPs) with a dimension ranging from 50 nm to 1,000 nm. The active ingredient release mainly depends on NLCs composition, which has a lipid matrix that is less organized than SLNs and is composed of medium chain triglycerides, triglycerides of caprylic and capric acid, and/or oleic acid used as the liquid state lipid (Singh, Navdeep et al., 2021).

13.5.4 NANOEMULSIONS (NES)

Nano-emulsions (NEs) are composed of an oil phase, an aqueous phase, and an active ingredient. The hydrophilic active ingredient is retained in the aqueous phase while oily active ingredients are kept in the oil phase. There are available both water in oil and oil in water formulations, but most of them are oil in water. NEs have the advantage of an increased effect on the solubility of the water-soluble active ingredients, by dispersing them on the oily phase (Seeni, Razina et al., 2016).

13.5.5 VESICULAR NANOSYSTEMS

Among the nanocarriers studied, vesicular systems stand out for their versatility (potential to carry a wide range of active substances), good ability to trap the drug and prolongation of the therapeutic effect. They are defined as lamellar structures, where each lamella corresponds to a bilayer formed by amphiphilic molecules immersed in an aqueous medium. The vesicles can encapsulate both hydrophilic molecules, in the aqueous medium present between the bilayers or outside the vesicle, and lipophilic molecules inside the bilayer(s), allowing them to carry different types of active substances. These structures are classified in different ways, depending on their composition, which has a strong influence on their properties, such as size, charge, lamellarity, elasticity, and thermodynamic phase (Jaiswal, Manjit et al., 2015).

13.5.6 LIPOSOMES

Known as nano-sized lipid vesicles, liposomes have potential use in topical medication delivery. One or more lipid bilayers that encapsulate a distinct aqueous phase from them (Figure 13.2). As drug delivery vehicles, liposomes have a number of benefits, including the ability to encapsulate both water-soluble and lipophilic compounds, biodegradability, and non-toxicity. They can permeate the epidermal barrier to a larger extent than other traditional dose forms because they have a lipid content that is similar to that of the epidermis. Most topically applied liposomes to the skin will build up in the SC's upper layers and operate more as a "reservoir," resulting in a more focused activity (Beloqui, Ana et al., 2016).

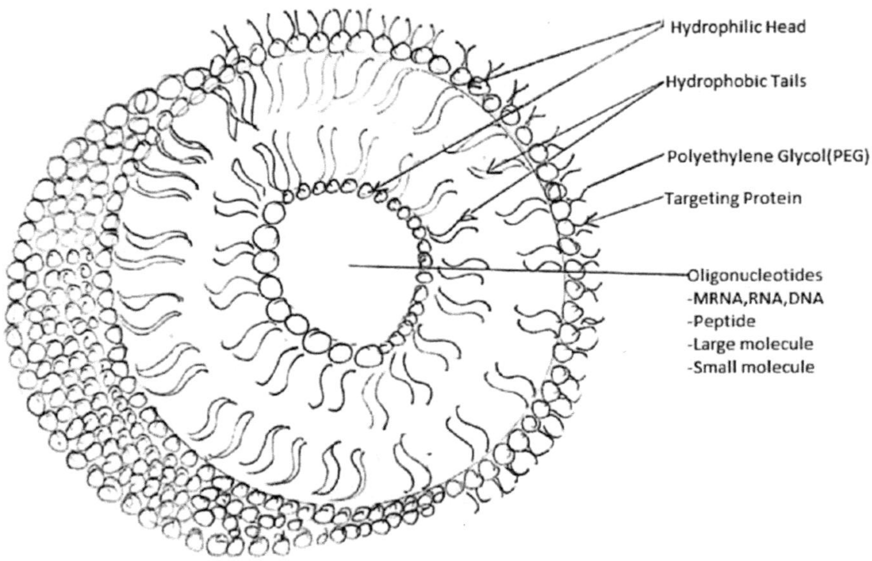

FIGURE 13.2 Structure of liposomes.

13.5.7 NANOCAPSULES

Nanocapsules have an aqueous or oily core that is encased in a thin polymer membrane. Such nano-capsules (Figure 13.3) were produced using two different technologies: interfacial nano-deposition for premade polymer and interfacial nano-polymerization for monomer. The construction of nano-scale vectors that can deliver radionuclides and target tumors has benefited greatly from technological advancements in the pharmaceutical research industry. Lipid nano-capsules (LNCs), a nano-vector-based formulation with biomimetic features, are one of them (Shao, Li et al., 2020).

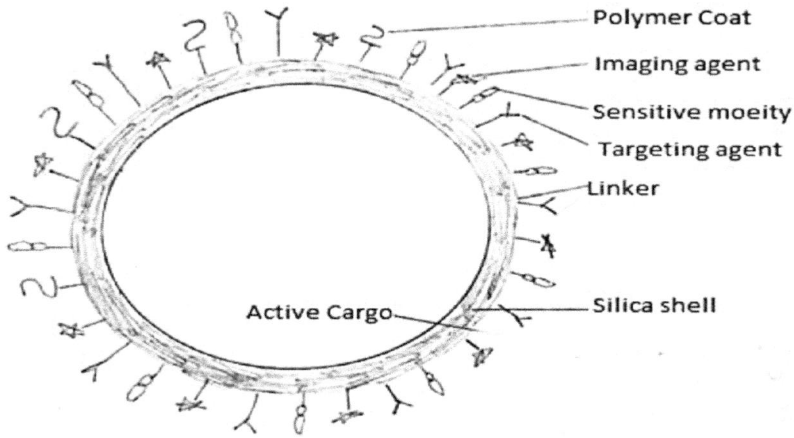

FIGURE 13.3 Structure of nanocapsules.

13.5.8 DENDRIMERS

Highly organized, branching polymeric molecules make up dendrimers (Figure 13.4). Dendrimers can also be referred to as arborols or cascade molecules. Typically, dendrimers acquire a spherical three-dimensional morphology and are symmetric about the center. Dendron is another commonly used word (Abbasi, Elham et al., 2014).

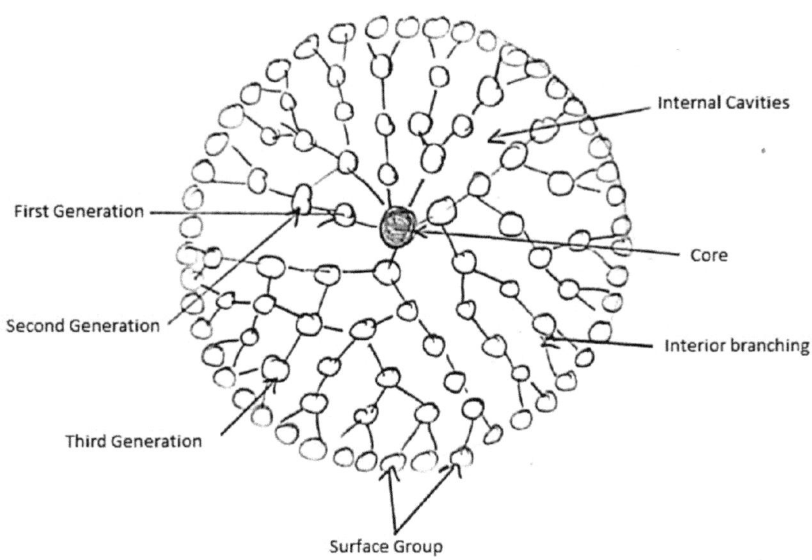

FIGURE 13.4 Structure of dendrimers.

13.5.9 ETHOSOMES (ETOS)

Ethosomes (ETOs) are phospholipidic vesicles composed of phosphatidylcholine, cholesterol, ethanol, and water (Figure 13.5). The profuse amount of ethanol, 20–50%, improves skin permeation, and both ethanol and cholesterol contribute to their elastic properties. ETOs are advantageous by having the faculty of carrying both lipophilic and/or hydrophilic active ingredients, and by so long as an efficient active ingredient delivery in both occlusive and non-occlusive conditions.

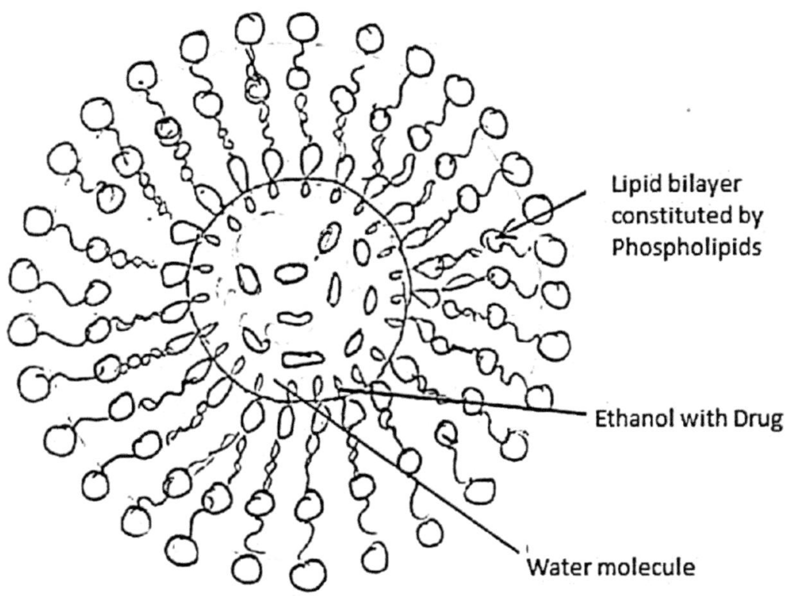

FIGURE 13.5 Structure of ethosomes.

13.5.10 TRANSFERSOMES (TRAS)

Transfersomes (TRAs) are highly deformable vesicles made up of an edge activator and a complex phospholipidic bilayer (Figure 13.6). Because they can alter the interfacial tension, edge activators like sodium deoxycholate, sodium cholate, Span® 60, Span® 65, and Span® 80 provide the bilayer the capacity to deform. TRAs have a number of benefits, including the capacity to flow through tiny holes, the potential to encapsulate a range of active chemicals, and increased deformability (Touitou, 2000).

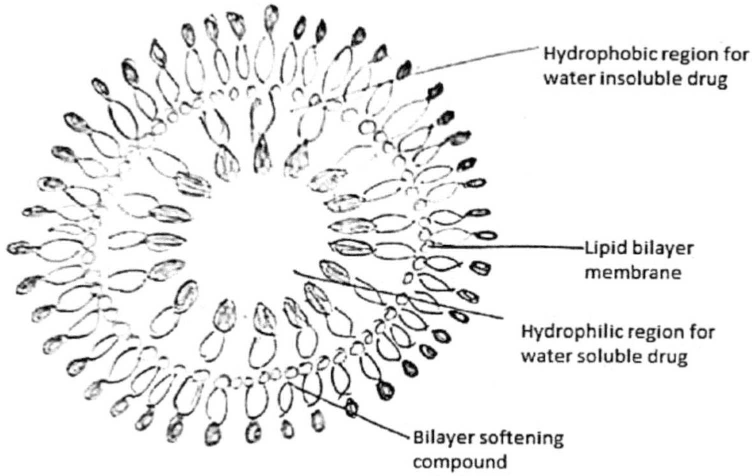

FIGURE 13.6 Structure of transfersome.

13.5.11 CUBOSOMES (CUBS)

Cubosomes round bicontinuous lipid bilayers are arranged in a three-dimensional structure called a CUB, which has a size of 10–500 nm. They are liquid crystalline particles that have self-assembled (Figure 13.7). Skin care, hair care, and antiperspirants are just a few of the personal care product categories that have been the subject of a recent cubosome study. Numerous studies working with cosmetic businesses like L'Oréal and Nivea are attempting to utilize cubosome particles as pollution absorbents and stabilizers for oil-in-water emulsions in cosmeceuticals (Abourehab, Mohammed et al., 2022).

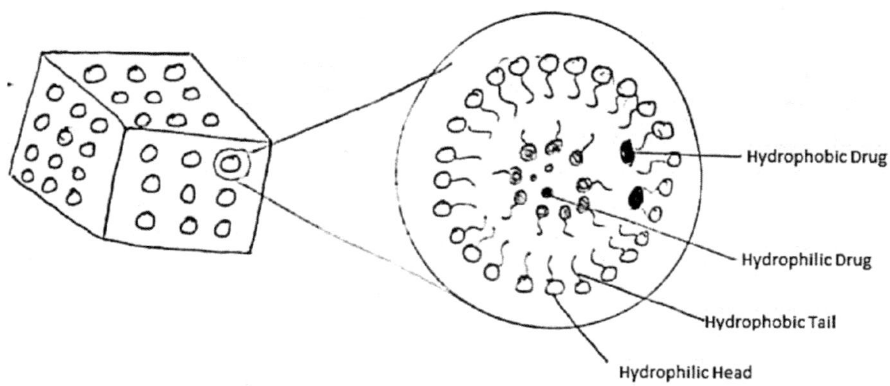

FIGURE 13.7 Structure of cubosomes.

13.5.12 NIOSOME

A niosome is a non-ionic surfactant-based vesicle. Cholesterol is included as an excipient and non-ionic surfactant forms the majority of niosomes. They both feature a bilayer, making them structurally comparable to liposomes. Niosomes are more stable thanks to the ingredients used in their preparation, though. Both lipophilic and hydrophilic medications can be trapped by them (Figure 13.8), either in a vesicular membrane consisting of lipid material (for lipophilic drugs) or in an aqueous layer (for hydrophilic drugs).

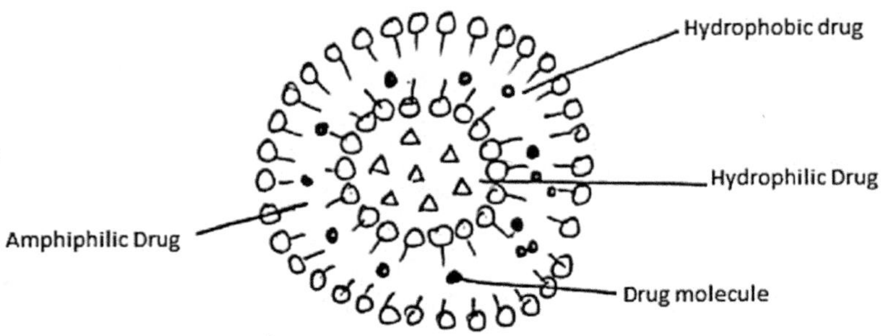

FIGURE 13.8 Structure of niosomes.

13.6 CONCLUSION

Topical treatment is beneficial compared to systemic treatments, however, conventional administration systems to skin present unresolved limitations, such as low bio-distribution, poor effectivity, active ingredient dose dumping, low targeting ability, skin irritability, and communicator toxicity. Nanotechnology-based formulations have been developed to overcome these known limitations, demonstrating remarkable potential as technological approaches for skin treatment and care after skin application.

KEYWORDS

- **dendrimers**
- **micron-sized carriers**
- **nanobiotechnology**
- **nanoparticles**
- **nanotechnology**
- **niosome**
- **topical treatment**

REFERENCES

Abbasi, E., Sedigheh, F. A., Abolfazl, A., Morteza, M., Hamid, T. N., Sang, W. J., Younes, H., et al., (2014). Dendrimers: Synthesis, applications, and properties. *Nanoscale Research Letters 9*(1), 1–10.

Abourehab, M. A. S., Mohammad, J. A., Anshul, S., Ahmed, H., Mohamed, A. A., Prachi, S., Bassam, M. A., et al., (2022). Cubosomes as an emerging platform for drug delivery: A state-of-the-art review. *Journal of Materials Chemistry B.*

Antonio, J. R., Carlos, R. A., Izabela, L. S. C., Julia, M. A. B., & João, R. O., (2014). Nanotechnology in dermatology. *Anais Brasileiros de Dermatologia, 89*, 126–136.

Beloqui, A., María, Á. S., Rodríguez-Gascón, A., António, J. A., & Véronique, P., (2016). Nanostructured lipid carriers: Promising drug delivery systems for future clinics. *Nanomedicine: Nanotechnology, Biology and Medicine, 12*(1), 143–161.

Castro, N. R., Cristal, S. C. P., Elisabete, P. S., & Claudia, R. E. M., (2020). Hybrid vesicular nanosystems based on lipids and polymers applied in therapy, theranostics, and cosmetics. *Critical Reviews™ in Therapeutic Drug Carrier Systems, 37*(3).

Cui, M., Christian, W., Sharon, W. T. C., & Chenjie, X., (2020). Nanodelivery systems for topical management of skin disorders. *Molecular Pharmaceutics, 18*(2), 491–505.

DeLouise, L. A., (2012). Applications of nanotechnology in dermatology. *Journal of Investigative Dermatology, 132*(3), 964–975.

Esposito, E., Claudio, N., Maddalena, S., & Rita, C., (2019). Nanomedicines to treat skin pathologies with natural molecules. *Current Pharmaceutical Design, 25*(21), 2323–2337.

Gharbavi, M., Jafar, A., Kheiri-Manjili, H., Hossein, D., & Ali, S., (2018). Niosome: A promising nanocarrier for natural drug delivery through blood-brain barrier. *Advances in Pharmacological Sciences, 2018.*

Hua, S., (2015). Lipid-based nano-delivery systems for skin delivery of drugs and bioactives. *Frontiers in Pharmacology, 6*, 219.

Jackson, J. E., Zlatko, K., & Allison, J. C., (2013). Nanotechnological advances in cutaneous medicine. *Journal of Nanomaterials, 2013.*

Jaiswal, M., Rupesh, D., & Sharma, P. K., (2015). Nanoemulsion: An advanced mode of drug delivery system. *3 Biotech, 5*(2), 123–127.

Khan, I., Khalid, S., & Idrees, K., (2019). Nanoparticles: Properties, applications, and toxicities. *Arabian Journal of Chemistry, 12*(7), 908–931.

Lohani, A., Anurag, V., Himanshi, J., Niti, Y., & Neha, K., (2014). Nanotechnology-based cosmeceuticals. *International Scholarly Research Notices, 2014.*

Lucia, M., Evelyn, O., Massimo, L., Luisa, F., Luca, P., Davide, P., & Miriam, C., (2021). The emerging role of nanotechnology in skincare. *Advances in Colloid and Interface Science, 293*, 102437.

Madkour, L. H., (2019). Introduction to nanotechnology (NT) and nanomaterials (NMs). In: *Nanoelectronic Materials* (pp. 1–47). Springer, Cham.

Nikalje, A. P., (2015). Nanotechnology and its applications in medicine. *Med. Chem., 5*(2), 081–089.

Opatha, S. A. T., Varin, T., & Romchat, C., (2020). Transfersomes: A promising nanoencapsulation technique for transdermal drug delivery. *Pharmaceutics, 12*(9), 855.

Paiva-Santos, A. C., Mascarenhas-Melo, F., Sara, C. C., Kiran, D. P., Diana, P., Chá-Chá, R., Andre, R. A., et al., (2021). Nanotechnology-based formulations toward the improved topical delivery of anti-acne active ingredients. *Expert Opinion on Drug Delivery, 18*(10), 1435–1454.

Paiva-Santos, A. C., Mascarenhas-Melo, F., Sara, C. C., Kiran, D. P., Diana, P., Chá-Chá, R., Andre, R. A., et al., (2021). Nanotechnology-based formulations toward the improved topical delivery of anti-acne active ingredients. *Expert Opinion on Drug Delivery, 18*(10), 1435–1454.

Panchal, M. (2022). Anti-skin cancer properties of plant & marine organism. *European Journal of Pharmaceutical and Medical Research, 9*(6), 197—201.

Poole, Jr., Charles, P., & Frank, J. O., (2003). Introduction to nanotechnology. John Wiley & Sons, 2003.

Seeni, R. Z., Sangeetha, K., & Juliana, M. C., (2016). Nanoparticles for improved topical drug delivery for skin diseases. In: *Perspectives in Micro-and Nanotechnology for Biomedical Applications* (pp. 275–294).

Shao, L., Bin, H., Xiangquan, H., David, S., Steven, P. K., & Jerry, L. A., (2020). Construction of polymeric metal–organic nanocapsule networks via supramolecular coordination-driven self-assembly. *Journal of the American Chemical Society, 142*(16), 7270–7275.

Singh, H., (2021). Nanotechnology: A novel approach for treatment of skin disorder. *Journal of Drug Delivery and Therapeutics, 11*(4-S), 271–277.

Singh, N., Shivi, S., Sanyam, S., Dheeraj, S., Vishal, K., Kamya, G., & Shammy, J., (2021). Treatment of skin cancer by topical drug delivery of nanoparticles: A review. *Research Journal of Pharmacy and Technology, 14*(10), 5589–5598.

Stefanov, S. R., & Velichka, Y. A., (2021). Lipid nanoparticulate drug delivery systems: Recent advances in the treatment of skin disorders. *Pharmaceuticals, 14*(11), 1083.

Thomas, L. M., & Abeer, H. K., (2020). Nanotechnology-based topical drug delivery systems for management of dandruff and seborrheic dermatitis: An overview. *Iraqi Journal of Pharmaceutical Sciences* (Vol. 29, No. 1, pp. 12–32). P-ISSN: 1683-3597, E-ISSN: 2521-3512.

Touitou, E., Dayan, N., Bergelson, L., Biana, G., & Eliaz, M., (2000). Ethosomes—Novel vesicular carriers for enhanced delivery: Characterization and skin penetration properties. *Journal of Controlled Release, 65*(3), 403–418.

Uchechi, O., John, D. N. O., & Anthony, A. A., (2014). Nanoparticles for dermal and transdermal drug delivery. *Application of Nanotechnology in Drug Delivery, 4*, 193–227.

Yetisgin, A. A., Sibel, C., Merve, Z., Ali, K., & Ozlem, K., (2020). *Therapeutic Nanoparticles and Their Targeted Delivery Applications, 25*(9), 2193.

Index

D

E

F

G

H

I

O

P

Q

R

T